CARDIOLOGY SECRETS

CARDIOLOGY SECRETS

OLIVIA VYNN ADAIR, M.D.

Assistant Professor
Department of Medicine
University of Colorado School of Medicine
Director, Coronary Care Unit and
    Pacemaker Service
Director, Non-invasive Cardiology
Denver General Hospital
Denver, Colorado

EDWARD P. HAVRANEK, M.D.

Assistant Professor
Department of Medicine
University of Colorado School of Medicine
Director, Cardiac Catheterization Laboratory
Denver General Hospital
Denver, Colorado

HANLEY & BELFUS, INC./ Philadelphia

Publisher: HANLEY & BELFUS, INC.
                    210 S. 13th Street
                    Philadelphia, PA 19107
                    (215) 546-7293
                    FAX (215) 790-9330

Library of Congress Cataloging-in-Publication Data

Cardiology secrets / [edited by] Olivia Adair, Edward P. Havranek.
        p.   cm.
    Includes bibliographical references and index.
    ISBN 1-56053-104-5
    1. Cardiology—Miscellanea.   I. Adair, Olivia, 1956-   .
II. Havranek, Edward P., 1955-   .
    [DNLM: 1. Heart Diseases—examination questions.   WG 18 1994]
RC682.C397   1994
616.1'2'0076—dc20
DNLM/DLC
for Library of Congress   94-39122
                                                                        CIP

CARDIOLOGY SECRETS   ISBN 1-56053-104-5

Library of Congress catalog card number   94-39122

Last digit is the print number: 9 8 7 6 5 4 3 2 1

DEDICATION

In loving memory of my mother, Eunice Tanner Adair, and for the support and encouragement of Mark, Lisa, and Matthew

OVA

To Janis, Katie, and Rachel, for their patience and understanding

EPH

CONTENTS

V. VALVULAR HEART DISEASE

VI. CARDIOVASCULAR PHARMACOLOGY

VII. OTHER MEDICAL CONDITIONS WITH ASSOCIATED CARDIAC INVOLVEMENT

CONTRIBUTORS

Olivia V. Adair, M.D.
Assistant Professor of Medicine, Division of Cardiology, University of Colorado School of Medicine; Director, Coronary Care Unit and Pacemaker Service, and Director, Noninvasive Cardiology, Denver General Hospital, Denver, Colorado

Stuart W. Adler, M.D.
Assistant Professor of Medicine, University of Minnesota Medical School, Minneapolis, Minnesota

Bruce E. Andrea, M.D.
Four Corners Heart Clinic, Mercy Medical Center, Durango, Colorado

David B. Badesch, M.D.
Assistant Professor of Medicine, Division of Pulmonary Sciences and Critical Care Medicine, University of Colorado School of Medicine, Denver, Colorado

William M. Bailey, M.D.
Assistant Professor of Medicine, and Director of Cardiac Electrophysiology, University of Colorado School of Medicine, Denver, Colorado

Jennifer L. Calagan, M.D.
Fellow in Cardiovascular Disease, Fitzsimons Army Medical Center, Aurora, Colorado

Robert W. Cameron, M.D.
Chief, Echocardiography and Noninvasive Laboratories, Fitzsimons Army Medical Center, Aurora, Colorado

Arlene Chapman, M.D.
Assistant Professor of Medicine, University of Colorado School of Medicine, Denver, Colorado

Mohamad Chebaclo, M.D., FACC
Assistant Professor of Medicine, State University of New York Health Sciences Center at Brooklyn; Associate Director, Catheterization Laboratory, Brooklyn VA Medical Center, Brooklyn, New York

Luther T. Clark, M.D.
Associate Professor of Clinical Medicine, State University of New York Health Science Center at Brooklyn, Brooklyn, New York

Karen Cooper, M.D.
Private Practice, Hematology/Oncology, Kingston, Pennsylvania

Stephen T. Crowley, M.D., FACC
Assistant Professor of Medicine, Division of Cardiology, University of Colorado School of Medicine, Denver, Colorado

Talley F. Culclasure, M.D.
Fellow in Cardiovascular Disease, Fitzsimons Army Medical Center, Aurora, Colorado

Ira M. Dauber, M.D.
Clinical Assistant Professor of Medicine, University of Colorado School of Medicine, Denver, Colorado

Richard C. Davis, Jr., M.D., Ph.D.
Chief, Cardiology Service, Department of Medicine, Fitzsimons Army Medical Center, Aurora, Colorado

Mark E. Dorogy, M.D.
Cardiology Service, Department of Medicine, and Chief, Cardiovascular Research, Fitzsimons Army Medical Center, Aurora, Colorado

Arnold Einhorn, M.D., FACC
Clinical Instructor, Department of Medicine, Division of Cardiology, University of Florida, Gainesville, Florida

Ashraf S. ElSakr, M.D.
Clinical Assistant Instructor, Division of Cardiology, State University of New York Health Science Center at Brooklyn, Brooklyn, New York

Richard W. Erickson, MD
Senior Fellow in Rheumatology, Department of Medicine, Division of Rheumatology, University of Colorado School of Medicine, Denver, Colorado

Edward A. Gill, M.D.
Assistant Professor of Medicine, and Director, Echocardiography, University of Colorado School of Medicine, Denver, Colorado

Michael E. Hanley, M.D.
Assistant Professor of Medicine, University of Colorado School of Medicine; Staff Physician and Director, Pulmonary Function Laboratory, Denver General Hospital, Denver, Colorado

Edward P. Havranek, M.D.
Assistant Professor of Medicine, University of Colorado School of Medicine, Denver; Director, Cardiac Catheterization Laboratory, Denver General Hospital, Denver, Colorado

Marsha J. Heinig, M.D., Ph.D.
Assistant Professor of Radiology, University of Colorado School of Medicine; Chief of Diagnostic Radiology, Denver General Hospital, Denver, Colorado

William T. Highfill, M.D.
Director, Cardiac Catheterization Laboratory, Cardiology Service, Department of Medicine, Fitzsimons Army Medical Center, Aurora, Colorado

Fred D. Hofeldt, M.D.
Professor of Medicine, University of Colorado School of Medicine, Denver, Colorado

Ali R. Homayuni, M.D., FACC, FCCP
Clinical Assistant Professor of Medicine, Division of Cardiology, Mt. Sinai School of Medicine of the City University of New York, New York, New York

Evelyn Hutt, M.D.
Assistant Professor of Medicine, University of Colorado School of Medicine, Denver, Colorado

David A. Kaminsky, M.D.
Fellow, Pulmonary and Critical Care Medicine, Department of Medicine, University of Colorado School of Medicine, Denver, Colorado

Mark Keller, M.D.
Assistant Professor of Medicine, University of Colorado School of Medicine; Director, Noninvasive Cardiology, VA Medical Center, Denver, Colorado

Christopher M. Kozlowski, M.D., MAJ, MC
Cardiology Fellow, Fitzsimons Army Medical Center, Aurora, Colorado

Norman Krasnow, M.D.
Professor of Medicine, State University of New York Health Science Center at Brooklyn, Brooklyn, New York

Mitchel Kruger, M.D.
Staff Cardiologist, Fitzsimons Army Medical Center, Aurora, Colorado

James C. Lafferty, M.D., FACC
Assistant Clinical Professor of Medicine, Downstate Medical Center, Brooklyn, and Staten Island University Hospital, Staten Island, New York

JoAnn Lindenfeld, M.D.
Professor of Medicine, University of Colorado School of Medicine, Denver, Colorado

Brian D. Lowes, M.D.
Cardiology Fellow, Department of Medicine, University of Colorado School of Medicine, Denver, Colorado

John T. Madonna, Jr., M.D.
Staff Cardiologist, Cardiology Service, Department of Medicine, Fitzsimons Army Medical Center, Aurora, Colorado

Mark Malyak, M.D.
Assistant Professor of Medicine, Department of Medicine, Division of Rheumatology, University of Colorado School of Medicine, Denver, Colorado

Donald A. McCord, M.D., FACC
Assistant Clinical Professor of Medicine, Downstate Medical Center, Brooklyn, and Staten Island University Hospital, Staten Island, New York

Querubin P. Mendoza, M.D.
Chief, Coronary Care Unit, William Beaumont Army Medical Center, El Paso, Texas

Raul Mendoza, M.D., FACC
Private Practice, Lawrence, New York

William P. Miller, M.D.
Associate Professor of Medicine, University of Wisconsin Medical School, Madison, Wisconsin

Thomas A. Neff, M.D.
Professor of Medicine, University of Colorado School of Medicine, Denver; Chief, Division of Pulmonary Medicine, Denver General Hospital, Denver, Colorado

Arvo J. Oopik, M.D. (Deceased)
Assistant Clinical Professor of Medicine, University of Colorado School of Medicine, Denver; Staff Cardiologist, Fitzsimons Army Medical Center, Aurora, Colorado; Public Health Service and U.S. Army Liaison Officer for the Strong Heart Study of Native Americans

Jeffrey Pickard, M.D.
Associate Professor of Medicine, University of Colorado School of Medicine, Denver, Colorado

Robert A. Quaife, M.D.
Assistant Professor, Departments of Medicine and Radiology, and Director, Cardiovascular Imaging Services, University of Colorado School of Medicine, Denver, Colorado

Jane E. B. Reusch, M.D.
Assistant Professor, Department of Medicine, Division of Endocrinology, Metabolism and Diabetes, University of Colorado School of Medicine, Denver, Colorado

John J. Reusch, M.D.
Fellow, Division of Cardiology, University of Colorado School of Medicine, Denver, Colorado

Roy W. Robertson, M.D.
Fellow in Cardiovascular Medicine, Department of Cardiology, University of Wisconsin Medical School, Madison, Wisconsin

David T. Schachter, M.D.
Fellow in Cardiovascular Medicine, Fitzsimons Army Medical Center, Aurora, Colorado

Paul D. Sherry, M.D.
Staff Cardiologist, Fitzsimons Army Medical Center, Aurora, Colorado

Harmeet Singh, M.D.
Clinical Instructor, Department of Medicine, Division of Renal Disease and Hypertension, University of Colorado School of Medicine, Denver, Colorado

Richard A. Stein, M.D.
Professor of Medicine and Chief of Cardiology, State University of New York Health Science Center at Brooklyn, Brooklyn, New York

David J. Tanaka, M.D.
Assistant Professor of Medicine, University of Colorado School of Medicine, Denver, Colorado

Nelson P. Trujillo, M.D.
Cardiology Fellow, Department of Medicine, Division of Cardiology, University of Colorado School of Medicine, Denver, Colorado

Robert A. Vaccarino, M.D.
Clinical Instructor of Medicine, Columbia-Presbyterian Medical Center, New York, New York

Gumpanart Veerakul, M.D.
Director, Cardiology Catheterization Laboratory, Cardiology Department, Bhumibol Adulyades Hospital, Bangkok, Thailand

Douglas P. Voorhees, R.R.T.
Special Imaging Technologist, Cardiology Department, Denver General Hospital, Denver, Colorado

Madeline Jean White, M.D.
Clinical Associate Professor of Community Medicine, University of Colorado School of Medicine, Denver, Colorado

Donald L. Warkentin, M.D.
Clinical Associate Professor of Medicine, University of Colorado School of Medicine, Denver, Colorado

Howard D. Weinberger, M.D.
Cardiology Fellow, Department of Medicine, Division of Cardiology, University of Colorado School of Medicine, Denver, Colorado

Phillip S. Wolf, M.D.
Professor of Medicine and Chief of Clinical Cardiology, University of Colorado School of Medicine, Denver, Colorado

Richard E. Wolfe, M.D.
Staff, Emergency Medicine Services, Denver General Hospital; Assistant Professor, Division of Emergency Medicine, University of Colorado School of Medicine, Denver, Colorado

Kenneth Matthew Wong, M.D.
Cardiovascular Clinic, Baptist Medical Plaza, Oklahoma City, Oklahoma

Marie E. Wood, M.D.
Assistant Professor of Medicine, University of Colorado School of Medicine; Staff, Denver General Hospital, Division of Hematology and Oncology, Denver, Colorado

Robert A. Zaloom, M.D., FACC
Department of Cardiology, Lutheran Medical Center and St. Vincent's Hospital Medical Center, New York, New York

PREFACE

There is no faster growing subspecialty than cardiology. All aspects of medicine require basic knowledge in cardiology no matter if you're in the emergency department, on the medical wards, or conducting your daily office patient visits. We hope this volume of *Cardiology Secrets* will make the acquisition of knowledge exciting, fun, and easy. It should serve as a basic review for the cardiologist and a primary fund of knowledge and references for other health professionals as well as medical students. We hope the reader will be stimulated to learn more and pass on the knowledge to the novice, as the question/answer format is ideal for teaching.

Special acknowledgment to Patricia Ross for her exceptional organizational and secretarial skills, making this book possible. Also special thanks to all the authors who took the time from their busy lives and professional schedules to prepare their chapters.

Olivia V. Adair, M.D.
Edward P. Havranek, M.D.

I. General Examination

1. CARDIOVASCULAR PHYSICAL DIAGNOSIS

Phillip S. Wolf, M.D.

1. What is the proper position for examining the patient? How should auscultation be performed?

The examiner should be on the patient's right side. Both patient and examiner should be comfortable, and the examiner's hands should be warm. *The surroundings must be quiet* and all conversation should cease. Before using the stethoscope, the examiner should inspect the precordium and palpate for abnormal impulses. Auscultation ideally should be performed in the same manner each time—e.g., the stethoscope bell placed at the cardiac apex, then "inched" along to the lower left sternal border, then up to the left and right base. Because the bell records the difficult-to-hear, low-pitched sounds best, it is used first. The diaphragm is useful for registering high-pitched breath sounds, murmurs of aortic and pulmonic valve insufficiency, and splitting of the heart sounds.

2. What is meant by "grading" of heart murmurs?

The grading classification system was developed 60 years ago by Dr. Samuel Levine and is useful for following the course of a murmur in an individual. Murmurs are graded on a scale of 1 to 6:

GRADE	PHYSICAL FINDINGS
1	Barely audible
2	Soft but readily heard
3	Prominent but not loud
4	Loud
5	Audible with stethoscope partially off chest
6	Extremely loud; audible with stethoscope removed from chest

Grades 5 and 6 are uncommon. Using this system, an examiner would list a soft murmur as grade 2 over 6 (2/6).

3. What are the characteristics of an innocent (functional) murmur?

Innocent murmurs are commonly of two types. One, heard in children and young adults, is best heard at the second left intercostal space and is thought to originate from vibrations within the main pulmonary artery. The other, audible between the apex and lower sternal edge, is apt to have a buzzing or vibrating quality and is thought to originate from vibrations of normal pulmonary leaflets. Both murmurs are midsystolic, usually no louder than grade 2/6 or 3/6, and common in young healthy people.

Associated findings help in distinguishing an innocent from a pathologic murmur. For example, wide splitting of the second heart sound in conjunction with a basal systolic murmur favors the diagnosis of atrial septal defect or congenital pulmonary valve stenosis. A sharp, early systolic clicking sound (ejection sound) at the left second interspace suggests pulmonic stenosis. A similar click at the cardiac apex indicates congenital aortic stenosis. Single or multiple clicks that occur in mid or late systole are common with mitral valve prolapse and are best heard at the cardiac apex.

4. Are diastolic murmurs ever "innocent"?
In contrast to systolic murmurs, diastolic murmurs are seldom innocent. The most common diastolic murmurs are due to very mild degrees of regurgitation across the aortic or pulmonic valves, when they are high-pitched and decrescendo in shape. Mitral stenosis, heard precisely over the cardiac apex, has a low-frequency, rumbling characteristic. It is best heard using the stethoscope bell applied with very light pressure, with the patient reclining to the left. On rare occasions, an atrial tumor or clot will produce a noise in diastole. Extracardiac diastolic bruits, on the other hand, may represent normal events. Examples include a venous hum, almost universally present in young people, and best heard over the anterior cervical fossa with the patient sitting and taking a deep breath. A mammary souffle audible over the breast of a nursing mother may occur as a continuous murmur (systole through diastole).

5. What are the cardivascular findings in normal pregnancy?
Plasma volume increases by 40–50% as pregnancy progresses. The elevated diaphragm and increased blood volume displace the apical impulse upward and laterally. Innocent midsystolic murmurs are common, best heard at the upper left sternal border. Splitting of the second heart sound is normal. Occasionally, a systolic–diastolic bruit is audible over the breast or over the gravid uterus, signifying flow through a functional arteriovenous shunt. Blood pressure (especially diastolic) tends to fall in early pregnancy and rise to prepregnancy levels toward term.

6. How can pulmonary hypertension be detected on examination?
The palm of your hand is placed just left of the sternal margin. A diffuse heaving impulse in this region indicates right ventricular enlargement. Prior to listening to the heart, check for an elevation in jugular venous pressure. Typically, the "a-wave" is prominent and the overall level of pressure increased. With right ventricular failure, tricuspid regurgitation develops and the "v-wave" becomes predominant (*see* jugular venous pressure below). Auscultation provides some valuable clues. The second sound tends to be narrowly split, and with concentration, the second (pulmonic) component will be noted to be increased. Finally, an audible S_3 or S_4 at the lower left sternal margin that increases on inspiration provides additional support for the diagnosis.

7. What is a paradoxical pulse?
Pulsus paradoxus is a misnomer, hallowed by decades of misuse. There is neither a pulse nor paradox involved. The term refers to an exaggeration of the normal slight decrease in blood pressure associated with inspiration. With paradoxical pulse, quiet inspiration produces a drop in systolic and diastolic pressure of at least 10 mm Hg. To elicit this finding, the examiner should sit comfortably in order to observe for both the Korotkoff sounds and the patient's respiratory excursions. The pneumatic cuff is slowly deflated, approximately 2 to 3 mm with each quiet breath. With paradox, the initial systolic beats become audible with expiration and disappear on inspiration. The cuff is further deflated until sounds are audible through all phases of respiration. The difference between these two pressures, measured in mm Hg, is recorded as the level of "paradox."

8. What causes a paradoxical pulse?
The abnormality in pericardial tamponade is thought to occur when, with inspiration, intrathoracic pressure becomes increasingly negative and venous return to the right heart increases. The heart distends, but the abrupt rise in volume meets an elevated pressure in the taut pericardial sac, and the right ventricle quickly reaches its limit of expansion. The increased volume in the right ventricle displaces the ventricular septum to the left. This decreases left ventricular volume and,

therefore, left ventricular stroke output over the next few beats. This reduction in cardiac output accounts for a reduction in systolic pressure with inspiration.

Expiration reverses this process. The pulmonary blood volume enters the left heart chambers, restoring the septum to its usual position and raising left ventricular volume. Systolic pressure rises.

Other conditions that abruptly raise right heart volume, such as acute pulmonary embolism, may share this same pathophysiologic process, since the acutely dilated right ventricle may distend against a relatively unyielding pericardial sac and produce septal displacement to the left.

9. How is coarctation of the aorta detected?

This important, reversible cause of hypertension is simple to diagnose, and every new case of hypertension should be screened for it. The most reliable diagnostic technique is to place the thumb of one hand on the brachial pulse and the other on the femoral pulse, and assess them simultaneously. Normally, these pulses are equal in volume and timing. A delay in the femoral impulse, or a reduction or absence of this pulse in a young person, strongly supports the diagnosis of coarctation. Other suggestive features include a vigorous pulsation in the suprasternal notch and a systolic murmur under the left clavicle. Occasionally, a continuous murmur can be heard between the scapulae, signifying collateral circulation via intercostal arteries.

10. I am having difficulty measuring blood pressure in the arm. How can I improve the technique?

Blood pressure (Korotkoff) sounds may be difficult to hear in some patients. An obese or muscular arm, arterial obstruction from previous surgical cutdown or atherosclerosis, or simply repeating blood pressure measurements too quickly in succession may make the readings difficult. Emptying the venous circulation in the arm helps. Have the patient elevate his or her arm above the head, and then open and close the fist several times in succession. The pressure readings will appear much more distinct on subsequent measurement.

11. Which bedside maneuvers are useful in diagnosing murmurs?

The simplest and most readily available maneuver is **exercise,** which increases blood flow and may bring out indistinct murmurs, such as the low-frequency rumble of mitral stenosis. Have the patient perform situps or straight leg raising while recumbent, and listen immediately afterward to the area of interest.

Respiratory maneuvers also are useful. **Inspiration** accentuates all murmurs as well as heart sounds that are of right-sided origin; thus, murmurs of tricuspid or pulmonic disease are brought out by deep inhalation. The obverse holds true: **expiration** magnifies murmurs and heart sounds of left-sided origin.

Another helpful maneuver is the **Valsalva.** Instruct the patient to exhale and strain, while you listen during and immediately after release of the straining maneuver. Demonstrate this by placing the palm of your hand against the patient's abdomen and having the patient strain against it. This technique reduces left ventricular volume; those murmurs that increase due to a relatively empty left ventricle (e.g., murmurs of mitral valve prolapse and hypertrophic cardiomyopathy).

Likewise, **changing body position** accentuates or diminishes some murmurs. Having the patient squat (while you listen to the precordium) increases left ventricular volume by raising systemic vascular resistance and increasing venous return. Murmurs of mitral prolapse and hypertrophic cardiomyopathy will lessen. Standing from the squatting position reverses the volume shift and accentuates these murmurs.

Another useful technique that augments the murmur of mitral stenosis is to listen at the cardiac apex when the patient turns from the recumbent to the left lateral position. This position is also useful for detecting faint left-sided "gallops" (S_3 and S_4). Having the patient cough vigorously three or four times further accentuates these findings.

12. What is the significance of an S₄?

This heart sound represents atrial contraction (the late filling phase of diastole). It becomes more forceful and therefore more easily audible when left ventricular filling is impaired. Causes of impairment include aortic stenosis, hypertension, myocardial ischemia, and almost all instances of acute myocardial infarction. The S_4 is common, especially in people over the age of 60.

The S_4 is often confused with a split S_1. The following points favor an S_4:

1. The S_4 tends to be softer and of lower frequency than a split S_1.
2. The S_4 of left-sided origin is best heard at the cardiac apex and is accentuated by expiration.
3. When the S_4 derives from increased right ventricular "stiffness," it is accentuated on inspiration.
4. Obvious splitting at the apex suggests an S_4, whereas splitting of S_1 is best heard at the lower sternal border.

The S_4 is best heard, as are all low-frequency sounds, with the stethoscope bell applied with very light pressure to the chest wall.

13. What is the significance of an S₃?

The S_3 is a relatively rare heart sound. It is heard in early diastole as blood rushes to the left ventricular apex from the base of the heart. Except for young, healthy adults, in whom an S_3 often normally occurs, its presence denotes more advanced heart disease with cardiac dilatation and congestive failure. It is best heard at the apex and is more easily appreciated with the stethoscope bell and with the patient rolled onto the left side.

14. What are the common abnormalities to consider in evaluating a systolic murmur? How are they differentiated?

Statistically, most murmurs are innocent, especially in young healthy people. The most common murmurs of pathologic origin include mitral and tricuspid regurgitation, aortic stenosis, and hypertrophic cardiomyopathy with outflow tract obstruction. Less common but important considerations in younger people include atrial or ventricular septal defects.

Systolic Murmurs

LESION	QUALITY OF MURMUR	SITE BEST HEARD	COMMENTS
Aortic stenosis (AS)	Harsh, often noisy murmur, especially when severe	Right upper sternal border	Increases in loudness as systole progresses
			Late peaking and duration of murmur correlate with severity of stenosis
			In severe AS, murmur may carry through S_2, which may be muffled or absent
			In LV failure, murmur may be soft or inaudible, but associated with late-rising and feeble arterial pulse
Mitral regurgitation	Evenly pitched sound, "blowing"	Cardiac apex; may radiate to left axilla and sometimes, when very loud, back	Continues through all or part of systole
Tricuspid regurgitation	Evenly pitched sound, "blowing"	Lower left sternal border	Continues through all or part of systole
			Increases with inspiration
			Signs of elevated venous pressure present

Systolic Murmurs (Continued)

LESION	QUALITY OF MURMUR	SITE BEST HEARD	COMMENTS
Hypertrophic cardiomyopathy	Similar to AS	Mid-left sternal border or in path between sternum and cardiac apex	Increases with Valsalva or standing Increases in beat following premature ventricular contraction Vigorous peripheral pulse
Atrial septal defect	Widely split and fixed S_2 that does not vary with respiration; not very loud or harsh	Upper 2nd left interspace	Right ventricular enlargement always present
Ventricular septal defect (VSD)	Loud, harsh murmur, especially when defect is small	Left sternal border at 3rd or 4th interspace	Holosystolic Cardiac exam otherwise normal if VSD is small

15. What is the significance of jugular venous waves?

Two positive waves are seen (*see* figure below). The "**a-wave**" originates from right atrial contraction. It *precedes* the carotid pulse; i.e., it occurs in late diastole. It increases in amplitude as the vigor of atrial contraction increases. Increased right ventricular end-diastolic pressure from pulmonary hypertension is the commonest cause. Occasionally, a giant a-wave, termed "**cannon wave**," will be seen when atrial and ventricular contraction are out of phase and the atrium contracts against a closed tricuspid valve. This occurs in cardiac rhythm disorders such as complete heart block.

The "**v-wave**" begins during ventricular systole just after the carotid pulse. When increased, it signifies tricuspid regurgitation. In this circumstance, the right ventricle ejects some of its volume retrogradely into the atrium. The resultant v wave has a slow and undulatory form and is accentuated with deep inspiration.

The "**x**" descent follows the a wave. When prominent, it suggests pericardial constriction. The "**y**" descent follows the v wave. Abnormalities include a rapid descent as seen in constrictive pericarditis and a slow decline with tricuspid stenosis.

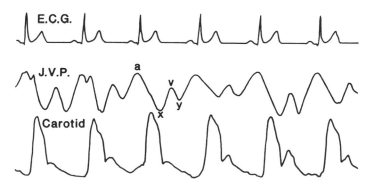

16. How do I measure venous pressure at the bedside?

This technique, with a little practice, is one of the most valuable features of the cardiac examination. It is preferable to examine the internal jugular vein, which lies in the carotid sheath just anterior to the sternocleidomastoid muscle. The patient should be placed in a semi-sitting position with the trunk elevated between 30° and 45°. (The exact position is unimportant—what matters is that the position allows you to observe the top of the oscillating venous column.) The neck should be relaxed so that the sternocleidomastoid muscle is not tensed. With a tongue blade

and centimeter ruler, measure the distance between the top of the venous column and the sternal
angle (the manubriosternal joint) (*see* figure). The sternal angle rests approximately 5 cm above the
center of the right atrium. In the illustration, the venous pressure measurement is 2 cm above the
sternal angle, so that the total venous pressure is 2 + 5 cm, or 7 cm. With the patient's trunk
positioned at 30°–45°, the venous pulse is ordinarily not visible more than 2 cm above the clavicle.

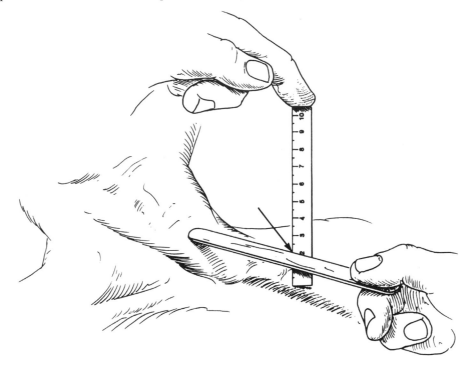

17. How is the venous jugular pulse differentiated from the carotid arterial pulse?

The most common error in assessing the jugular venous pressure, even for experienced observers,
is to mistake the venous for the carotid arterial pulse. The following hints help identify the *venous*
pulse:

    1. It varies with respiration, normally falling with inspiration and rising with expiration.

    2. It is easily obliterated by gentle finger pressure at the base of the neck.

    3. It is amplified, especially when pressure is elevated, by gentle pressure over the abdomen
(hepatojugular reflux).

    4. Multiple waveforms are seen in contrast to the single carotid beat.

BIBLIOGRAPHY

1. Bruns DL: A general theory of the causes of murmurs in the cardiovascular system. Am J Med 27:360–374,
   1959.
2. Craige E: Gallop rhythm. Prog Cardiovasc Dis 10:246, 1967.
3. Leatham A: Auscultation of the heart. Lancet 2:703, 757, 1958.
4. Leathan A: The second heart sound: Key to auscultation of the heart. Acta Cardiol 19:395, 1964.
5. Lembo NJ, Dell'Italia LJ, Crawford MH, O'Rourke RA: Bedside diagnosis of systolic murmurs. N Engl J
   Med 318:1572, 1988.
6. Patel R, Bushnell DL, Sobotka PA: Implications of an audible third heart sound in evaluating cardiac
   function. West J Med 158:606–609, 1993.
7. Perloff JK: Physical Examination of the Heart and Circulation. Philadelphia, W.B. Saunders, 1990.
8. Ravin A, Craddock LD, Wolf PS, Shander D: Auscultation of the Heart. Chicago, Year Book, 1977.

2. MURMURS AND HEART SOUNDS

Kenneth Matthew Wong, M.D.

1. What maneuvers and positions are best for accentuating pericardial rubs?
With the patient lying supine, visceral and parietal pericardial contact can be reinforced by applying the diaphragm with firm pressure while the patient holds expiration. Apposition of visceral and parietal pericardium can be further accentuated while the patient rests on elbows and knees or leans forward.

2. What does handgrip isometric exercise accomplish physiologically? How does it affect murmurs?
- Increases systolic blood pressure, left ventricular systolic pressure, and left ventricular diastolic pressure.
- Mitral and aortic regurgitation murmurs get louder.
- The late systolic murmur of mitral valve prolapse shortens but increases in intensity.
- The click of mitral valve prolapse occurs later in systole.
- The systolic murmur of hypertrophic obstructive cardiomyopathy decreases (due to increased left ventricular volume).

3. What is Kussmaul's sign?
Kussmaul's sign is an increase in the jugular venous pressure with inspiration. Normally during inspiration, the negative intrathoracic pressure causes a fall in systemic venous pressure and therefore a drop in the jugular venous pressure. However, in patients with constrictive pericarditis, the thickened pericardium causes the transmission of intrathoracic pressure to the chambers of the heart to fail; thus the venous pressure does not decrease.

4. What is a continuous murmur? With which cardiac abnormalities is it associated?
A continuous murmur is one that begins in systole and continues without interruption through the timing of the second heart sound into all or part of diastole. It is generated by flow from a zone of high resistance to one of low resistance. Continuous murmurs are associated with aortopulmonary connections, such as patent ductus arteriosus; arteriovenous connections, such as anomalous origin of the left coronary artery from the pulmonary trunk; coronary artery fistulas; and sinus of Valsalva to right heart connections.

5. How do you discern the difference between murmurs of valvular aortic stenosis and hypertrophic obstructive cardiomyopathy?
The systolic murmur of hypertrophic obstructive cardiomyopathy is increased with the Valsalva maneuver, whereas the murmur of aortic stenosis decreases with this maneuver.

6. What are the physical findings in aortic stenosis?
Aortic stenosis produces a diamond-shaped systolic murmur best heard at the aortic area. The murmur is usually transmitted to one or both carotid arteries. It decreases in intensity with the Valsalva maneuver, handgrip, and sudden squatting, and increases with passive leg raising. In moderate or severe stenosis, A_2 is diminished or absent due to slow filling. The carotid pulses may be diminished and delayed (*pulsus parvus et tardus*).

7. What is Hamman's sign?
Hamman's sign is described as a mediastinal crunch. This sound occurs from subcutaneous air, usually due to a pneumothorax. It is frequently loud with a "crunchy" character and may be palpable.

8. What is a pericardial knock?
A pericardial knock is a high- or low-pitched sound that occurs during diastole in constrictive pericarditis. It is caused by the abrupt cessation of ventricular filling during early diastole due to the thickened and stiff pericardium.

9. Describe the auscultative findings in mitral valve prolapse.
In mild mitral valve prolapse, a mid-systolic click may be noted without a murmur. The click is caused by the sudden tensing of the redundant chordae or valve leaflets. In more severe cases, the presence of mitral regurgitation produces a mid-systolic murmur that commences just after the mid-systolic click. The murmur is best heard at the apex and may radiate posteriorly to the mid-axillary line. The murmur may become holosystolic in the most severe cases. Because of the decrease in left ventricular volume, the murmur becomes more intense and commences earlier with the administration of amyl nitrite, upon standing, or with the Valsalva maneuver.

10. Describe the murmur of mitral stenosis.
The murmur of mitral stenosis depends on the turbulence created by the flow across a narrowed mitral valve orifice. The murmur is usually low pitched in frequency, due to the relative low prescribed gradient across the mitral valve, and is best heard at the apex with the bell. The murmur is usually preceded by an opening snap in early diastole and can be accentuated by having the patient lie in the left lateral decubitus position.

11. What are the effects of the Valsalva maneuver, standing, squatting, handgrip, and amyl nitrate on murmurs?
    1. **Valsalva maneuver** (decreases venous return): Most murmurs decrease in intensity, except for those of hypertrophic obstructive cardiomyopathy and mitral valve prolapse, which increase.
    2. **Standing** (decreases venous return): Most murmurs decrease in intensity, except those of hypertrophic obstructive cardiomyopathy and mitral valve prolapse, which increase.
    3. **Squatting** (increases venous return, stroke volume, and systemic resistance): Most murmurs increase in intensity, except those of hypertrophic obstructive cardiomyopathy and mitral valve prolapse, which decrease.
    4. **Handgrip** (increases systemic vascular resistance and cardiac output): Most murmurs across normal or obstructed valves increase; mitral regurgitation, ventricular septal defect, and aortic regurgitation murmurs also intensify. The murmur of hypertrophic obstructive cardiomyopathy decreases, and the murmur of mitral valve prolapse occurs later.
    5. **Amyl nitrate** (potent vasodilator): The murmurs of hypertrophic obstructive cardiomyopathy and aortic stenosis increase, whereas the murmurs of mitral regurgitation, ventricular septal defect, and aortic regurgitation decrease.

BIBLIOGRAPHY

1. Bates B, Hoekelman RA, Thompson JEB: A Guide to Physical Examination and History Taking, 5th ed. Philadelphia, J. B. Lippincott, 1991.
2. Braunwald E (ed): Heart Disease, 4th ed. Philadelphia, W.B. Saunders, 1992.
3. DeGowin EL, Richard L: Bedside Diagnostic Examination, 4th ed. New York, Macmillan, 1981.
4. Leonard JJ, et al: Examination of the Heart: Part IV. Auscultation. Dallas, TX, American Heart Association, 1974.
5. Wilson JD, et al (eds): Harrison's Principles of Internal Medicine, 12th ed. New York, McGraw-Hill, 1991.

3. CHEST X-RAY

Marsha Heinig, M.D., Ph.D.

1. Why order a chest x-ray?

Following history and physical examination, the chest x-ray is one of the least expensive and most noninvasive ways to confirm or exclude suspected diagnoses. Among common cardiovascular problems that may be diagnosed are:

- Congestive heart failure
- Valvular disease
- Congenital malformations of the heart and great vessels
- Left to right shunts
- Pulmonary hypertension (when relatively severe)

The chest x-ray can also diagnose conditions which may mimic cardiac problems, such as a pneumothorax or pneumonia causing chest pain.

2. What cardiovascular disease processes may not be readily apparent on the chest x-ray?

1. Acute myocardial infarction without congestive heart failure
2. Coronary artery disease
3. Systemic hypertension (radiographic signs appear late)
4. Pulmonary hypertension (until advanced)
5. Intracardiac shunts with shunt ratio <1.5–2 to 1
6. Mild valvular disease
7. Pericardial effusion (unless large)
8. Aortic dissection
9. Remember that a normal (or "normal for age") x-ray does not mean that the patient is normal!

3. What do you look for on the chest x-ray?

Start with an overview—do not forget the forest for the trees! What does the patient look like: male or female, fat or thin, young or old, straight up or bent over? Then, work from outside in: soft tissues, bones, pleura (not normally visible), lungs, mediastinal contour, heart size and configuration, great vessels, hila. Remember to check technical factors such as patient ID and side marker (right vs. left).

4. What are the major cardiovascular "bumps" that form the silhouette of the mediastinum on the frontal chest x-ray working from top to bottom?

Right side:
1. Ascending aorta (should not be prominent in patients under 50 years of age)
2. Right atrium

Left side:
1. Aortic knob (should be thumb-sized in patients under 50)
2. Left pulmonary artery
3. Left atrial appendage (should be nearly concave)
4. Left ventricle

5. How do you know if the heart is big on the chest x-ray?

Look at both the frontal and lateral views. If the heart looks too big on both views, it probably is. How do you know your Aunt Minnie is short? She's smaller than everyone around her. Remember to take into account the many uncontrolled variables among patients and techniques. Does the heart look as if it fits the patient?

6. What patient factors can affect heart size on the chest x-ray?

- Size of the patient (obese or thin)
- Degree of inspiration

- Presence of emphysema (long skinny heart)
- Systole or diastole (up to 1.5 cm difference in size on frontal view)
- Heart rate and cardiac output (low heart rate and large stroke volume lead to increased ventricular filling)
- Configuration of the chest (very thin chest or pectus excavatum can "squish" the heart and make it look big on the frontal view)

7. What technical factors can affect the heart size on the chest x-ray?

1. **Direction of the x-ray beam:** posterior to anterior with film in front (PA) or anterior to posterior with film in back (AP). The heart is farther away from the film on the AP view and thus looks larger because the x-ray beam is diverging.

2. **Distance of x-ray tube from the patient and film:** Portable examinations are often done at a 40-inch source-to-image distance, whereas PA examinations in the x-ray department are done at 72 inches. The heart looks bigger on a 40-inch film because of greater beam divergence.

3. **Patient position:** supine or standing. The heart looks bigger if the patient is supine.

4. **Degree of inspiration:** Shallow inspiration makes the heart look bigger.

8. When cardiac enlargement is suspected, how do you know which chambers are enlarged?

Ventricular enlargement usually displaces the lower heart border to the left and posteriorly. This is true whether it is right ventricle (RV) or left ventricle (LV), as the RV, when enlarged, tends to push the LV to the left and back. The best way to tell RV from LV enlargement is to look at their outflow tracts. If the pulmonary arteries are enlarged and the aorta is diminutive, the RV is probably enlarged. If the aorta (ascending, knob, or overall) looks enlarged, it is probably the LV. Remember, both may be enlarged at the same time!

Left atrial enlargement makes a convexity between the left pulmonary artery and LV on the frontal view and may make a round "double density" just inferior to the carina and seen through the right atrial contour on the frontal view. It also displaces the descending left lower lobe bronchus backward on the lateral view. **Right atrial enlargement** (rare as an isolated finding in adults) causes the lower right heart border to bulge rightward.

9. What are the most common cardiovascular findings on adult chest radiographs? What is the differential diagnosis?

Mild enlargement of left ventricle (lower left heart border) with leftward bulging apex, enlarged aortic knob, and calcification in the aortic wall. These findings represent atherosclerotic disease and/or hypertension.

10. What are the cardinal signs of congestive heart failure on the chest x-ray?

- Cardiac enlargement
- Pulmonary arterial enlargement
- Peribronchovascular haziness and thickened septal lines representing interstitial edema
- Fuzzy air-space-filling disease representing alveolar edema
- Pleural effusion, especially on the right.

With early congestive failure, one may merely see mild cardiac and pulmonary arterial prominence and a "perihilar haze" of early transudative pulmonary edema. The transudative edema of congestive failure tends to be quite mobile and accumulate in dependent portions of the chest; thus, it may appear to be entirely in the lower chest in the upright patient.

11. Which sided heart failure—right or left—causes pleural effusions?

Both. The pleural space is in direct anatomic contiguity with the lung interstitium. Thus, the interstitial edema of left-sided heart failure, as it is mobile, easily enters the pleural space. However, pleural fluid is absorbed into the parietal pleural lymphatics and thus into the **systemic** venous system. Therefore, right-sided heart failure with systemic venous hypertension may also lead to pleural effusions.

12. What disease processes mimic congestive heart failure on the chest x-ray?

Multiple disease processes of the lungs may occupy the same spaces—peribronchovascular interstitium, interlobular septa, air space, and pleura—as the edema of congestive heart failure. These disease processes, when accompanied by a prominent-looking heart, may mimic congestive failure. Examples are airways disease with thick bronchi which may be mistaken for edema, early acute respiratory distress syndrome (ARDS, injury edema), diffuse pneumonias, and occasionally, lymphangitic spread of carcinoma. It is impossible to distinguish renal failure and consequent fluid overload from congestive heart failure.

13. What is the differential diagnosis of a big, baggy-looking heart on the chest x-ray (e.g., cardiomegaly without specific chamber enlargement)?

1. Cardiomyopathy (of multiple causes)
2. Pericardial effusion
3. Polyvalvular disease (becoming rarer with decrease in rheumatic fever).

This appearance is sometimes called a "water bottle" heart, because the normal chamber outlines cannot be seen. I personally have not seen many "water bottles" of that shape, but perhaps your grandmother had a hot water bottle that looked like that.

14. Can you differentiate a pericardial effusion on the chest x-ray?

Often, you cannot. Occasionally, the lateral view will show the outline of the effusion anterior to the heart shadow. There will be a thin lucent (relatively black) line adjacent to the heart representing "epicardial fat" (actually associated with the visceral pericardium), then a fatter soft-tissue stripe representing the effusion, and then most anteriorly, a thin lucent fat stripe representing the "pericardial fat" (mediastinal fat).

15. Is the chest x-ray sensitive for diagnosing a pericardial effusion?

The chest radiograph is not at all sensitive to even moderate amounts of pericardial fluid. Echocardiography is the most sensitive method for distinguishing pericardial fluid from myocardial dilatation.

16. What is the *sine qua non* of significant pulmonary arterial hypertension on the chest x-ray?

Calcification in the pulmonary arteries (a very rare finding). A more common sign is big distorted globs where the pulmonary arteries should be, although this appearance is sometimes difficult to differentiate from hilar adenopathy. On the frontal view, the left pulmonary artery always looks bigger because its profile in the left mediastinum and hilum is closer to its origin. The lateral view is quite helpful in distinguishing pulmonary hypertension from adenopathy. An enlarged left pulmonary artery looks like an aorta curving over the left upper lobe bronchus, and an enlarged right pulmonary artery makes a large circle anteroinferior to the carina. If these shadows are distinguishable, pulmonary hypertension can be differentiated from adenopathy.

17. What are the causes of pulmonary arterial hypertension?

The most common cause is lung disease—chronic obstructive pulmonary disease—or hypoxia of multiple causes. Lung disease usually causes enlarged pulmonary arteries that seem to taper quickly but do not appear anatomically distorted centrally. Three diseases cause marked pulmonary hypertension with distorted-looking arteries and normal-looking lungs: idiopathic pulmonary hypertension (in young females), chronic pulmonary emboli, and Eisenmenger reaction (from chronic shunt).

18. What congenital cardiovascular malformations may be seen on an adult chest x-ray?

Congenital Cardiovascular Malformations Seen on Adult X-rays

1. Anomalies of the aortic arch and great vessels
   Right aortic arch
   Aberrant subclavian arteries
   Coarctation of the aorta
   Aortic stenosis
2. Mild shunts
   Atrial septal defect
3. Mild right-sided outflow obstructions
   Pulmonic stenosis
   Ebstein's anomaly
4. Partial anomalous pulmonary venous return
5. Corrected transposition of the great vessels

19. An adult patient shows a right-sided aortic arch on his chest x-ray and no other signs of cardiovascular disease. What other abnormality does this patient almost certainly have?
Aberrant left subclavian artery. Patients with "mirror-image" branching of a right-sided aortic arch have a 95% chance of having congenital heart disease.

20. What acquired valvular diseases are most commonly demonstrated on the chest x-ray? What are their radiographic signs?
  Mitral stenosis: Enlarged left atrium and enlarged upper-lobe pulmonary vessels.
  Mitral regurgitation: Enlarged left atrium and left ventricle (may look like a big baggy heart) and enlarged pulmonary arteries.
  Aortic stenosis: Bulging left ventricular apex and enlarged ascending aorta (upper right mediastinal border).

21. How is magnetic resonance imaging (MRI) useful in diagnosing cardiovascular diseases?
MRI is a noninvasive test for distinguishing vascular abnormalities from mediastinal or hilar masses. It is useful in evaluating several types of congenital cardiovascular diseases: aortic arch anomalies, aberrant subclavian arteries, coarctation of the aorta, and aberrant pulmonary arteries and veins. It may also be useful in evaluating complex congenital lesions such as transposition of the great vessels. Multiplanar imaging is particularly helpful. MRI also can be used to evaluate rare intracardiac tumors.

CONTROVERSIES

22. What is "vascular redistribution"?
Vascular redistribution occurs when the upper-lobe pulmonary arteries and veins, which are usually smaller than those of the lower lobe because of less blood flow, actually become **larger** than the vessels in the lower lobes. This finding is detected by comparing the size of the vessels coming from the upper hilum on the chest x-ray to those coming from the lower hilum. If the upper ones do not look clearly larger and the lower ones look clearly too skinny, then there is probably *not* "redistribution" present.

23. When does "vascular redistribution" occur in congestive heart failure?
Many sources describe "vascular redistribution" as a cardinal feature of congestive heart failure. However, this may be a particularly unhelpful sign. It is probably **chronic** pulmonary venous hypertension (e.g., mitral valve disease, chronic left ventricular failure) that causes vascular redistribution. The theory is that chronic venous hypertension may affect the lower-lobe arteries to a greater extent because of the greater blood flow to lower lungs and greater venous return

pressure due to gravity. Thus, in the body's attempt to maintain more normal blood flow and oxygenation, blood flow is diverted to the upper lungs.

Thus, redistribution is usually not helpful in the ICU patient with acute congestive failure. All of the pulmonary arteries probably look big, and upper-lobe vessels probably look about the same size as or a little smaller than the lower-lobe vessels. The upper-lobe vessels are larger than normal because of stasis of blood flow and because the patient is often supine, but there is not a true "redistribution."

24. What is the best test for evaluating aortic dissection? Why may dissection be missed by aortography?

Three techniques have been touted recently for evaluation of aortic dissection: contrast-enhanced computed tomography (CT), MRI, and transesophageal echocardiography. Aortography, though, probably remains the "gold standard." All of these imaging methods have advantages and disadvantages, and all have claimed superiority.

CT scan is probably the easiest test to do in the acute situation and is readily available and reliable (90% accuracy). True and false lumens can usually be readily demonstrated, as can the intimal flap in the ascending aorta if it is involved. Imaging before, during, and after contrast administration increases sensitivity.

The multiplanar imaging capability of **MRI** makes it an ideal method to image the aorta. Dissections are especially well demonstrated if the false lumen is partially clotted or if there is a dramatic difference in rate of blood flow between true and false lumens. However, because of pulsatile motion in the aorta, a thin intimal flap may be missed. MRI is also nearly impossible to perform in the critically ill patient.

Transesophageal echocardiography has been claimed to be quite sensitive for type B (descending) aortic dissection, but it is operator-dependent. A multiplane, or omniplate, scope is now available which visualizes the ascending aorta with accuracy.

Aortography images only contrast flowing in a lumen. If the false lumen is clotted, dissection may be only indirectly diagnosed by aortography as narrowing of the lumen of the aorta or thickening of the wall. Aortography is useful, however, in evaluating the origins of the great vessels in type A aortic dissection, as well as in evaluating associated aortic regurgitation.

BIBLIOGRAPHY

1. Chen JT: The plain radiograph in the diagnosis of cardiovascular disease. Radiol Clin North Am 21:609–621, 1983.
2. Daves ML. Cardiac Roentgenology. Chicago, Year Book, 1981.
3. Gedgaudas E, Moller JH, Castaneda-Zuniga WR, Amplatz K: Cardiovascular Radiology. Philadelphia, W.B. Saunders, 1985.
4. Gomes A: MR imaging of congenital anomalies of the thoracic aorta and pulmonary arteries. Radiol Clin North Am 27:1171–1181, 1989.
5. Gross GW, Steiner RM: Radiographic manifestations of congenital heart disease in the adult patient. Radiol Clin North Am 29:293–317, 1991.
6. Matthay RA, Shub C: Imaging techniques for assessing pulmonary artery hypertension and right ventricular performance with special reference to COPD. J Thorac Imag 5:47–67, 1990.
7. Milne ENC, Pistolesi M, Miniati M, Guintini C: The radiologic distinction of cardiogenic and noncardiogenic edema. AJR 144:879–894, 1988.
8. Newell J (ed): Diseases of the thoracic aorta: A symposium. J Thorac Imag 5:1–48, 1990.
9. Swischuk LE, Sapire DW: Basic Imaging in Congenital Heart Disease. Baltimore, Williams & Wilkins, 1986.
10. Win EK, Reeves JT (eds): Pulmonary Hypertension. Mount Kisco, NY, Futura, 1984.

4. BEDSIDE HEMODYNAMIC MONITORING

Edward P. Havranek, M.D.

1. What is a Swan-Ganz catheter?

A Swan-Ganz catheter is a relatively soft, flexible right heart catheter with an inflatable balloon at its tip. This balloon allows the catheter to "float" with the flow of blood from the great veins, through the right heart chambers, and into the pulmonary artery.

2. How is a Swan-Ganz catheter constructed?

Most catheters in clinical use in intensive care units have four lumens. One is connected to the end hole of the catheter, allowing for measurement of pressure in the pulmonary artery. The second lumen is attached to a temperature-sensing thermocouple 5 cm from the catheter's tip, allowing for measurement of cardiac output. A third lumen is connected to a port 15 cm back from the tip of the catheter, allowing for measurement of pressure in the right atrium or for infusion of drugs or fluid into the central circulation. The last lumen is used to fill the balloon with air and to deflate it after insertion is completed. In addition, some catheters contain an additional port for infusion of drugs or fluid, fiberoptics for continuous monitoring of pulmonary oxygen saturation, or a lumen through which a temporary pacing electrode can be passed into the apex of the right ventricle.

3. How is the Swan-Ganz catheter inserted?

Most commonly, a catheter known as a sheath is inserted into the subclavian or internal jugular vein. The Swan-Ganz catheter is passed through this sheath into the central vein. The balloon is inflated, and the catheter advanced. It follows blood flow through the right atrium and ventricle, and into the pulmonary artery. Its position is monitored by watching the pressure recorded from the distal port. The catheter is advanced until a wedge tracing is obtained; the balloon is then deflated. This generally occurs when the catheter has been advanced a total of about 55 cm. In some circumstances, it may be preferable to insert the catheter via the femoral vein or a peripheral vein in the antecubital fossa.

4. What information can be gained from the Swan-Ganz catheter?

Basically two main types of data are obtained from the catheter: cardiac output and left ventricular preload.

Cardiac output is measured by injecting saline colder than the blood through the "proximal port" of the lumen into the right atrium, and the temperature of the blood in the pulmonary artery is measured continuously by a temperature sensor (actually, a thermocouple) positioned 5 cm back from the tip of the catheter. The brief dip in the blood's temperature with time is related to cardiac output by a somewhat complicated formula, which, luckily, is calculated by computer.

Left ventricular preload is estimated by measuring the pulmonary capillary wedge pressure (PCW), also known as the pulmonary artery wedge pressure (PAW). The wedge pressure is obtained by inflating the balloon while the catheter is positioned in the left or right main pulmonary artery. Blood flow carries the catheter distally, until the diameter of the branch of the pulmonary artery is smaller than the diameter of the balloon. The catheter tip becomes stuck or "wedged." The tip of the catheter is now shielded from the pressure in the pulmonary artery, and records pressure in the pulmonary arterioles. It turns out that this pressure closely approximates left atrial pressure, which in turn is a good measure of left ventricular preload.

5. Why are cardiac output and left ventricular preload important?

Cardiac output and left ventricular preload are important physiologic parameters because knowing them allows one, in actual clinical situations, to apply Starling's law: an increase in preload produces an increase in cardiac output at any given level of myocardial contractility. For instance, in a patient with a low cardiac output and a wedge pressure below normal, intravenous fluid would be expected to improve cardiac output.

6. Does the "wedge" really mean anything?
As improbable as it seems, the wedge pressure correlates nicely with left atrial pressure.

7. In what situations is a Swan-Ganz catheter useful for managing patients?
Whenever knowledge of cardiac output or pulmonary artery pressure would change management, a Swan-Ganz catheter is useful, because clinical data are unreliable for predicting these parameters. It is most often used in the following situations:
    1. To differentiate cardiogenic from noncardiogenic pulmonary edema
    2. In the management of congestive heart failure refractory to conventional treatment, especially in the setting of acute myocardial infarction
    3. Following cardiac surgery
    4. In the management of patients in shock
    5. In the management of patients with large shifts in intravascular fluid volume, such as following extensive burns or trauma or after major surgery

8. What diagnoses can the catheter help make?
In addition to its use in the management of patients, the catheter can be useful in making some difficult diagnoses at the bedside. Constrictive pericarditis and pericardial tamponade have distinctive pressure waveforms detectable with the catheter. An acute ventricular septal defect resulting from myocardial infarction can be diagnosed by finding an increase in oxygen saturation between samples drawn from the proximal and distal ports. Another complication of acute myocardial infarction, right ventricular infarction, shows a typical "dip-and-plateau" pattern in the right ventricular pressure tracing. Atrial flutter may be diagnosed from a right atrial pressure tracing showing a waves occurring at a rate of 300/minute. Ventricular tachycardia may be diagnosed by dissociation of the a and v waves in a patient with wide complex tachycardia.

9. What complications are associated with use of a Swan-Ganz catheter?
    1. All the complications of central venous cannulation
    2. Risk of infection (increases the longer the catheter remains in place)
    3. Right bundle branch block (especially in patients with preexisting left bundle branch block)
    4. Ventricular tachyarrhythmias
    5. Pulmonary infarction (if the tip migrates into a permanently wedged position)
    6. Pulmonary rupture (if the balloon is overinflated)
    7. Catheter knotting (from careless insertion)

10. How can complications be minimized?
Think twice about the need to insert a pulmonary artery catheter in the first place. Consider removing the catheter after the first set of data have been obtained. Try to leave it in place for no more than 48 hours. Use fluoroscopy.

11. I cannot get a good wedge tracing. What do I do?
    1. Check the chest x-ray for proper catheter position.
    2. Aspirate and flush the catheter to remove clots and bubbles.
    3. Check all connecting lines and stopcocks.
    4. Check to see that the pressure transducers are at right atrial level.
    5. The balloon might be over inflated; try letting the air out and refilling it slowly.
    6. Consider the possibility that the tracing really is a wedge tracing with a giant v wave, such as is seen in acute severe mitral regurgitation and several other conditions.

12. The cardiac output does not make any sense. What's wrong?
Check to see that at least three values were averaged and that the range of these values is no greater than 20% of the mean. Check the chest x-ray; is the distal tip of the catheter in the pulmonary artery and the proximal port in the right atrium? Check to see if the computer is calibrated to the proper temperatures. Finally, if the computer can display the time versus temperature curve, check to see that the curve is shaped properly (see figure below).

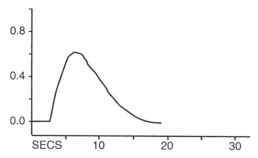

Typical time versus fall-in-temperature curve obtained from a thermodilution cardiac output computer. The curve rises steeply, then falls slowly. The downsloping limb of the curve is not perfectly concave, indicating some early recirculation of the indicator (cold saline). This tracing was obtained from a patient with heart failure; the recirculation is probably the result of tricuspid regurgitation, and does not affect the accuracy of the cardiac output determination.

CONTROVERSY

13. Does pulmonary artery catheterization really help?
Despite widespread use of these devices in intensive care units, some physicians point out that few if any studies have shown that their use decreases mortality and that randomized studies have not been widely performed. Proponents point out that many studies have shown that clinical data predict wedge pressure poorly and that insertion of the catheter changes management plans frequently. In at least one study of critically ill postoperative patients, management based on cardiac output data improved survival. The truth lies somewhere between. Pulmonary artery catheterization at the bedside is not without risk. It should be used only after careful consideration of its possible benefits and with thorough knowledge of its capabilities.

BIBLIOGRAPHY

1. Gore JM, Goldberg RJ, Spodick DH, et al: A community-wide assessment of the use of pulmonary artery catheters in patients with acute myocardial infarction. Chest 92:721–731, 1987.
2. Hillis DL, Firth BG, Winniford MD: Analysis of factors affecting the variability of Fick versus indicator dilution methods of cardiac output. Am J Cardiol 56:764–768, 1985.
3. Robin ED: The cult of the Swan-Ganz catheter. Ann Intern Med 103:445–449, 1985.
4. Sharkey SW: Beyond the wedge: Clinical physiology and the Swan Ganz catheter. Am J Med 83:111–122, 1987.
5. Sise MJ, Hollingsworth P, Brimm JE, et al: Complications of the flow-directed pulmonary-artery catheter: A prospective analysis in 219 patients. Crit Care Med 9:315–318, 1981.
6. Walston A, Kendall ME: Comparison of pulmonary wedge and left atrial pressure in man. Am Heart J 86:159–164, 1973.

II. Diagnostic Procedures

5. ELECTROCARDIOGRAM

Donald L. Warkentin, M.D.

1. Can the ECG offer useful information about supraventricular tachycardia (SVT)?
Ordinarily, identifying the various types of SVT from the standard ECG is difficult. In many cases, electrophysiologic intracardiac testing is required. Of the major types of SVT—sinus node reentry, intra-atrial reentry, accelerated conduction syndromes with narrow QRS complex, and AV nodal reentry—the latter condition makes up about 60% of the total. If the P waves are inverted in the inferior leads, and when they are present before or immediately after the QRS complex, they allow accurate diagnosis. Unfortunately, many times, the P waves are superimposed in the QRS complex and prevent easy diagnosis. Thus, the standard ECG is only occasionally helpful. Sinus node reentry and AV nodal reentry usually can be terminated by carotid sinus massage.

2. How does the signal-averaged electrocardiogram aid clinical decision-making?
The signal-averaged ECG (SAECG) amplifies exceedingly weak electrical signals generated by the heart and passes them through an electronic filter. The remaining signals from many cardiac cycles are averaged by a computer and printed out as a single QRS complex. Of particular importance are low-amplitude potentials (usually <40 μV) occurring late in the QRS complex. To a lesser extent, the magnitude of the QRS vector and the total duration of the QRS complex are also important.

Abnormal SAECG findings have been recorded in many patients with episodes of sustained ventricular tachycardia and may indicate which of those patients, as well as those with unexplained syncope, might benefit from electrophysiologic testing. A potential application of SAECG is in risk stratification of patients after myocardial infarction; there is a high correlation between late potentials and inducible ventricular tachycardia, and the test may pinpoint individuals at high risk of sudden death.

3. What are the criteria for ventricular hypertrophy?
In **left ventricular hypertrophy** (LVH), the increased muscle mass generates increased QRS voltage, often with secondary changes in ST and T waves. Because some of these changes are subtle, numerous (at least 25) specific ECG criteria have been proposed to aid the diagnosis of LVH. Voltage criteria appear to be the most helpful:
  Limb lead: R amplitude in aVL > 11 mm
      R wave in aVF > 14 mm
      R wave in lead I plus S wave in lead III > 25 mm
  Precordial lead: R wave in V_5 or V_6 > 26 mm
      R wave in V_{5-6} plus S wave in V_1 > 35 mm
Most cases of LVH can be diagnosed by these criteria. If some of the more arcane criteria from textbooks of electrocardiology are used, the accuracy of diagnosis is generally improved.

In **right ventricular hypertrophy** (RVH), diagnosis also depends on voltage amplitude. In RVH, however, frontal plane axis deviation is also helpful. Among the important criteria of RVH are:

Right axis deviation of ≥ 110°
R wave in V_1 ≥ 7 mm
R/S ratio in V_1 > 1
qR patterns in V_1 and rSR′ in V_1 with R′ ≥ 10 mm
When both RVH and LVH occur in the same patient, most bets are off because the forces counterbalance each other.

4. Is non-Q-wave infarction an ECG diagnosis?

The short answer is no! For positive diagnosis of non-Q-wave infarction, confirmatory evidence (such as elevated cardiac muscle enzyme levels) must accompany these highly suspicious ECG findings. Q waves have long been recognized as a hallmark in transmural infarct, but experience shows that using that criterion alone will result in missing a large number of acute infarctions. It is also true that occasionally Q waves will be recorded in nontransmural infarcts. The ECG changes that occur with non-Q-wave infarctions are those involving the ST segment and T waves. Both ST-segment elevation and depression may be recorded, although depression numerically outnumbers elevation. A particularly striking ECG finding, and one that should raise a high level of suspicion for infarction, is the exceedingly deep symmetric inversion of the precordial T waves. Indeed, the presence of ST segment depression and the above T-wave changes is almost always a result of nontransmural infarction. It is clinically important to diagnose non-Q-wave infarction accurately since this subset of patients has a high risk of further ischemic events.

5. What is torsade de pointes?

By definition, torsade de pointes is an intermediate arrhythmia between ventricular tachycardia and ventricular fibrillation. The term was coined by Dessertenne to describe cycles of tachyar-rhythmia with alternating peaks of QRS amplitude appearing to twist around the isoelectric line. That said, torsade de pointes is a strident alarm to alert clinicians to underlying pathophysiology and the possibility of sudden death.

The basic prerequisite for this condition is thought to be a prolonged QT interval but any condition or drug affecting the QT interval may spark the arrhythmia. Quinidine is the most common cause, but other class I antiarrhythmics also have been implicated. Of paramount importance is to discontinue any possible offending drugs. Electrolyte imbalance, intrinsic heart disease, marked bradycardia, and the prolonged QT syndrome also can stimulate the disorder. When the ECG finding occurs, immediate efforts must be made to determine the underlying cause of QT lengthening, lest the arrhythmia become irreversible.

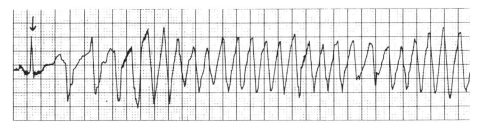

Torsade de pointes. A single sinus beat (arrow) is followed by ventricular tachycardia with an oscillating or swinging pattern of the QRS complexes. (From Seelig CB: Simplified EKG Analysis. Philadelphia, Hanley & Belfus, 1992, p 75, with permission.)

6. What are the ECG features of bradycardia-tachycardia syndrome?

Bradycardia-tachycardia syndrome is a particular manifestation of the sick sinus syndrome in which the sinus node is faulty either in its impulse formation or the transmittal of the impulse to the atrium. In such cases, it is often associated with episodes of supraventricular tachycardia. Detection of the bradycardia-tachycardia syndrome usually requires ambulatory monitoring. Sinus pauses of > 2 seconds are generally considered abnormal, particularly if symptoms accompany the rhythm disturbances. Between one-half and three-quarters of patients with the sick sinus node syndrome have episodes of tachycardia and may develop syncope when there is prolonged asystole following a run of supraventricular tachycardia. Many patients with this syndrome also have additional conduction defects, such as atrioventricular block, intraventricular condition defect, and/or bundle branch block. One confounding feature of the syndrome is its intermittent nature. Repeat episodes of ambulatory monitoring may be required to document the diagnosis.

7. Why three degrees of heart block?

Heart block, or atrioventricular (AV) block, is either complete or incomplete. The term **third-degree AV block**, or complete heart block, is applied when there is no relationship between the atrial and ventricular beats and the atrial rate is faster than the ventricular. Incomplete AV block is divided into first-degree, second-degree, and advanced AV block. By definition, **first-degree AV block** occurs when the PR interval is > 0.20 seconds and each atrial beat is followed by a ventricular complex. **Second-degree AV block** results in intermittent failure of atrial impulses to be conducted to the ventricles and is divided into two basic types: **Type I** or Wenckebach (also called Mobitz I) shows progressive lengthening of the PR interval from beat to beat until an atrial complex is blocked. Because of these periodic pauses, "grouped beating" occurs and, when present, aids in the diagnosis of Mobitz I block. It may be seen transiently in acute inferior wall myocardial infarction. **Type II** AV block (advanced or Mobitz II) shows intermittent blocked P waves where the PR intervals of the conducted beats are constant. In these situations, the block is usually below the His bundle and may be accompanied by an associated bundle branch block.

Mobitz II is usually considered more serious than Mobitz I and may require artificial pacemaker treatment. In third-degree block, pacemaker cells in the AV node or in the His Purkinje system may initiate ventricular contraction. Except for some cases of congenital third-degree AV block, this condition usually requires an artificial pacemaker.

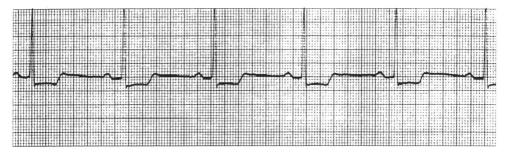

First-degree block (PR interval = 0.26 seconds).

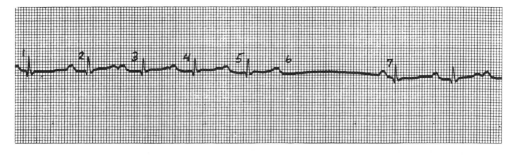

Mobitz type I second-degree AV block (Wenckebach). Note the gradual prolongation of the PR interval (1–5), the missing QRS complex after the sixth P wave, and the return of the PR interval to its shortest duration (7).

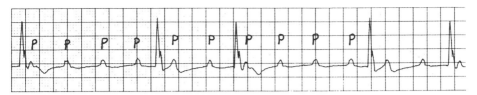

Mobitz type II second-degree AV block. Note that when beats are conducted, the PR interval is unvarying.

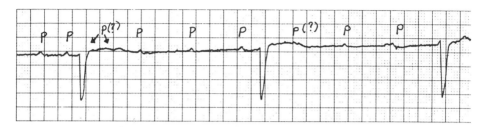

Third-degree AV block with a ventricular escape rhythm at 32 bpm. P-wave activity is somewhat irregular.

Figures from Seelig CB: Simplified EKG Analysis. Philadelphia, Hanley & Belfus, 1992, pp 77–80, with permission.

8. What is the power spectrum of the ECG?

Recent interest in autonomic nervous system dysfunction and its effect on mortality from cardiac events has led to power spectrum ECG measurements. There seems to be a significant relationship between decreased heart rate variability and mortality in ECGs recorded from patients following myocardial infarction. Further autonomic nervous system activity in patients can be evaluated by spectral frequency analysis of the ECG. This analysis is divided into ultra low, very low, low, and high frequencies. Such analysis demonstrates a marked decrease in variability in all four frequency categories in postmyocardial infarct patients. It is postulated that high-frequency power and heart rate variability are modulated by the parasympathetic nervous system, whereas low-frequency power is modulated by both the sympathetic and parasympathetic systems. This effect appears to last for at least 12 months following infarction. The recovery of normal heart rate variability and the declining rate of mortality following infarction appear to occur nearly simultaneously, although further analysis is needed to rule out a coincidental finding.

9. How important are the signs of atrial abnormality?

Because atrial hypertrophy is usually of minor degree, the ECG findings of atrial abnormality are more dependent on the duration of atrial contraction than on its amplitude. Likewise, the common increase in P-wave amplitude suggestive of right atrial hypertrophy or dilation (P pulmonade) often correlates poorly with clinical and anatomic findings—hence, the descriptive term, *atrial abnormality*. Prolongation and notching of P waves often indicate enlargement or delayed conduction within the atria, and these signs are helpful, but not diagnostic, in those conditions. Therefore, most electrocardiographers use the finding of atrial abnormality as an adjunct to the diagnosis of other conditions, such as rheumatic heart disease and left or right ventricular hypertrophy. Atrial enlargement may result in numerous arrhythmias, the most common being atrial fibrillation. There is some correlation between the amplitude of the fibrillatory waves and atrial size. Overall, the signs of atrial abnormality seem less important than other ECG criteria of abnormal size or function.

10. Can right ventricular infarction be determined on the ECG?

Myocardial infarction involving the right ventricular wall is rarely isolated. It has been found with equal frequency in both anterior and inferior infarction. Because the right ventricular muscle mass is small in comparison to the left ventricle, the ECG diagnosis depends on the finding of acute inferior or inferoposterior myocardial infarction plus ST-segment elevation of 1 mm or more of the right precordial leads. Of significant help is the finding of ST-segment elevation in leads V_3R and V_4R. Thus, in patients with inferior infarcts, these leads should be included with the standard 12-lead ECG. When anterior infarction is present, the diagnosis of right ventricular infarction is difficult. Right ventricular infarction can clinically mimic severe left heart failure, and because present treatment for the two conditions is quite different, the importance of proper diagnosis is evident.

11. What are the common causes of ST-segment elevation?

The most dramatic and worrisome ST segment elevations occur as a result of severe coronary ischemia. The elevation occurring with transmural myocardial infarction is the best known and may be the earliest ECG finding during the acute process. Less frequent, but still a result of coronary ischemia, is the elevation seen in a small percentage of treadmill exercise tests and in patients with Prinzmetal's variant angina. Usually, the ST segment must be > 1 mm above baseline to merit attention. Adding spice to the evaluation is the fact that a goodly proportion of normal ECGs will have significant ST elevation. This is attributed to the early repolarization phenomenon and can be seen in healthy individuals. Of help in differentiating normal from abnormal elevations is the shape of the initial portion of the segment. In normals, it has an upward concavity, whereas in severe ischemia it usually has an upward convexity. The normal is often accompanied by a notched J point and prominent T wave.

12. How helpful is the ECG in "wide complex" tachycardia?

With the advent of surgical and ablation therapy for tachycardias, it becomes imperative to discern the correct type and site of origin of the arrhythmia. A regular tachycardia of 120–200 beats/min and a QRS duration of ≥ 0.12 seconds may be either ventricular or supraventricular. Unfortunately, definitive diagnosis may require invasive electrophysiologic studies. Wide complexes appear with supraventricular tachycardia if there is preexisting bundle branch block, anterograde conduction through bypass tracts, or aberrant ventricular conduction. Ventricular tachycardia is more likely if there is AV dissociation, right bundle branch block with QRS duration > 0.14 seconds or left bundle branch block with QRS duration > 0.16 seconds, QRS axis in right upper quadrant ($-90°$ to $+180°$), positive QRS deflections in all precordial leads (V_1–V_6), captive or fusion beats, or a QRS pattern identical to that of premature ventricular beats during sinus rhythm.

13. Can the ECG diagnose electrolyte abnormalities?

ECG abnormalities due to electrolyte imbalance, particularly potassium and calcium, have been evident for years. However, because multiple electrolyte may be involved and because of the patient's underlying disease or even drug effects, the ECG should not be used in lieu of direct laboratory electrolyte determination. When an abnormality has been identified, the ECG may be used as a guide to the effectiveness of therapy.

The classic ECG changes of hyperkalemia are tall, narrow, peaked T waves, intraventricular conduction defect, decreased amplitude or absence of P waves, bradyarrhythmias, and AV blocks (see figure on p. 22). Hypokalemia causes ST-segment depression, decreased T amplitude, prominent U waves, cardiac arrhythmias, and rarely QRS prolongation. Serum calcium primarily alters the QT interval, with calcium excess causing shortening and deficiency causing prolongation. Currently, serum magnesium levels are assuming importance, but unfortunately are unlikely to be detected by the ECG.

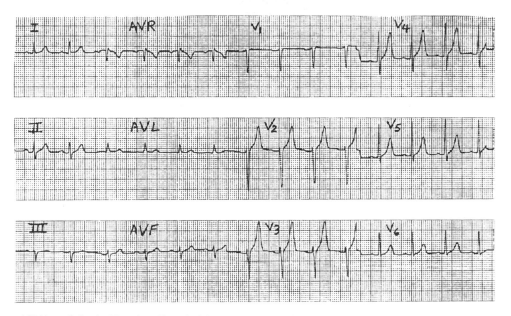

Mild hyperkalemia. Note the tall, peaked T waves, most prominent in V_2-V_5. (From Seelig CB: Simplified EKG Analysis, Philadelphis, Hanley & Belfus, 1992, pp 107–110, with permission.)

14. What are the ECG signs of "drug effect"?

Although many drugs and substances can affect the ECG, most do so subtly. Certain compounds, however, leave a characteristic mark. Digitalis causes classic depression and coving of the ST segment. Toxic doses primarily affect AV conduction, resulting in various degrees of heart block. Many class I antiarrhythmics cause classic QT-interval prolongation. Toxic quantities of these and other antiarrhythmics can cause intraventricular conduction abnormalities and QRS prolongation. Some substances, such as cocaine, cause shortening of both the PR and QT intervals, and their adrenergic effect results in sinus tachycardia. Toxic doses of cocaine can result in ventricular tachycardia and/or fibrillation. Conversely, beta adrenergic blockers, such as propranolol, cause sinus bradycardia as a most common ECG side effect.

15. When is ambulatory ECG monitoring most useful?

Holter (ambulatory) monitoring initially was used to detect cardiac arrhythmia. With increasing sophistication of recording hardware, it is now possible to detect ST-segment changes indicative of myocardial ischemia. Programs are also available to detect abnormal changes in the circadian variability of cardiac rate. At present, Holter monitoring is used both in detection of arrhythmia and in monitoring efficacy of treatment. Overt and silent myocardial ischemic episodes in patients can be detected and are powerful predictors of future serious illness. The predictive value of heart rate variability is less certain. The highest return of information comes from monitoring patients at highest risk of disease—i.e., those with coronary artery disease, unexplained syncope, or known cardiac arrhythmias. It should be noted that 24-hour monitoring may not be sufficient to truly detect disease and that ambulatory recordings should always be correlated with the standard ECG.

BIBLIOGRAPHY

1. Abildskov JA: The atrial complex of the electrocardiogram. Am Heart J 57:930–941, 1959.
2. Bigger JT Jr, Fleiss JL, Rolinski LM, et al: Time course of recovery of heart period variability after myocardial infarction. J Am Coll Cardiol 18:1643–1649, 1991.

3. Braat S, Brugada P, DeZwaan C, et al: Value of electrocardiogram in diagnosing right ventricular involvement in patients with an acute inferior wall myocardial infarction. Br Heart J 49:368–372, 1983.
4. Chou T: Electrocardiography in Clinical Practice, 3rd ed. Philadelphia, W.B. Saunders, 1991.
5. Damato AN, Law SH, Helfant Retal: A study of heart block in man using His bundle recordings. Circulation 39:297–305, 1969.
6. Goldberg RJ, Gore JM, Alpert JS, Dalen JE: Non-Q wave myocardial infarction: Recent changes in occurrence and prognosis: A community-wide perspective. Am Heart J 113:273–279, 1987.
7. Josephson ME, Koster JA: Supraventricular tachycardia: Mechanisms and management. Ann Intern Med 87:346–358, 1977.
8. Kennedy HL, Wiens RD: Ambulatory (Holter) electrocardiography and myocardial ischemia. Am Heart J 117:164–167, 1989.
9. Lansdown LM: Signal-averaged electrocardiograms. Heart Lung 19:329–336, 1990.
10. Rubenstein JJ, Schulman CL, Yurchak PM, et al: Clinical spectrum of the sick sinus syndrome. Circulation 46:5–13, 1972.
11. Scott RC: Ventricular hypertrophy. Cardiovasc Clin 5:220–253, 1973.
12. Surawicz B: Electrophysiologic substrate of torsade de pointes: Depression of repolarization or early afterdepolarization? J Am Coll Cardiol 14:172–184, 1989.

6. HOLTER MONITORING AND SIGNAL-AVERAGED ELECTROCARDIOGRAPHY

Olivia V. Adair, M.D.

1. What symptoms lead to suspicion of arrhythmia?
Symptoms that commonly lead to suspicion of arrhythmia are palpitations, syncope, presyncope, or congestive heart failure. The physician must evaluate the patient's overall status rather than the rhythm disturbance in isolation.

2. What are the major indications for Holter monitors?
- Detection of a suspected rhythm disturbance
- Syncope work-up
- Evaluation after myocardial infarction
- Evaluation of high-risk cardiac patient
- Risk stratification
- Evaluation after cardiac surgery
- Diagnosis of silent ischemia
- Diagnosis of suspected myocardial ischemia
- Evaluation of therapy, i.e., antiarrhythmic drugs, pacemaker function, cardiac ablation
- Evaluation of heart-rate variability

3. Should tests for patients with established or suspected arrhythmia be done in a particular order?
The clinical setting has as great a significance as the arrhythmia on choice of work-up and possible risk to the patient. Some arrhythmias are potentially fatal *regardless of* the clinical setting, whereas others are potentially dangerous *because of* the clinical setting. The usual progression is from the less expensive, simpler noninvasive test to tests that are more complex and invasive. Certain clinical circumstances, however, necessitate a more complex initial study (e.g., electrophysiology study) before a Holter monitor or signal-averaged electrocardiogram (SAECG). The Holter monitor and SAECG are usually the initial tests. SAECG is especially appropriate if ventricular arrhythmias are expected. The type of Holter monitor should be individualized to the patient, depending on associated symptoms as well as frequency and awareness of arrhythmia. An important consideration in the work-up of rhythm disturbance is underlying heart disease (e.g., valve disease, cardiomyopathy, myocardial infarction). A resting ECG and echocardiogram may answer several of these questions and help to categorize the patient as high risk (e.g., low ejection fraction) or low risk (a normal ejection fraction and normal ECG). If the rhythm disturbance is associated with ischemia, an exercise stress test may be appropriate. If the data are positive or if a diagnosis is not established but symptoms or potentially fatal arrhythmias recur, an electrophysiology test should be performed.

4. Is there a particular subset of patients post myocardial infarction (MI) who should have a Holter monitor evaluation before discharge?
The whole patient needs to be considered for risk stratification, but certain patients are likely candidates for Holter monitoring after MI. Patients with an anterior infarction and bundle-branch block are at high risk for arrhythmia. Up to 35% have late ventricular fibrillation (VF) in the hospital, and the risk persists for 6 weeks after infarction. In addition, atrioventricular (AV) block and intraventricular conduction abnormalities were found in 90% of patients who had recurrent VF during hospitalization and prehospital resuscitation for cardiac arrest. Patients with frequent ventricular ectopy after approximately 48 hours post MI or high-grade heart block after 48–72 hours following an acute MI should be evaluated with Holter monitoring before discharge,

along with patients in whom marked bradycardia persists for 48–72 hours after MI. Finally, patients at risk for sudden death (e.g., low ejection fraction) may be considered for predischarge Holter monitoring.

5. Should patients with suspected arrhythmias have a Holter monitor and an exercise tolerance test (ETT)?

During ETT about one-third of patients with normal hearts may develop ventricular ectopy, usually occasional monomorphic pairs or even 3–6-beat nonsustained runs. Ectopy may occur in older patients with no coronary artery or other heart disease and is not a predictor of increased mortality or morbidity. Although ETT is more sensitive than a resting, standard 12-lead ECG in detecting ventricular arrhythmias, a Holter monitor is more sensitive than ETT. However, because each may uncover serious arrhythmias that the other does not detect, both tests may be indicated in selected patients, such as those with known or suspected coronary artery disease.

6. What types of monitoring devices are available for long-term recording of the ECG?

Traditional Holter monitors record on 2 or 3 ECG channels for 24 hours. Recorders are currently available in four types:

1. Continuous recorders, with every beat recorded and available for analysis

2. Patient-activated recorders, which are especially useful when a patient can predict symptoms of the arrhythmias and activate the recorder

3. Arrhythmia-activated recorders, in which the monitor turns on when a rhythm disturbance begins and off when it terminates (accuracy depends on the arrhythmia-detection algorithm)

4. Transmitters for on-line or stored transtelephonic sending of ECG signals during a detected arrhythmia or during symptoms (especially helpful with infrequent but predicted symptoms; not indicated for arrhythmias associated with syncope)

Event monitors, continuous or transmitted, have the disadvantage of requiring patient perception of the arrhythmias. Many patients may be unaware of significant or serious bradyarrhythmias or tachyarrhythmias but able to detect others. Therefore, significant arrhythmias may be missed and incorrect treatment strategies employed. Each system has advantages and disadvantages; selection must be tailored to the individual. With any system, however, patients must record in some fashion (e.g., diary) symptoms and activities during the monitored period.

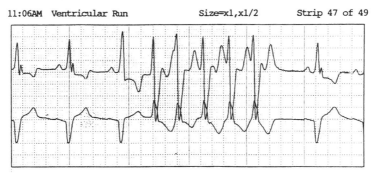

11:06AM Ventricular Run   Size=x1,x1/2   Strip 47 of 49

Holter monitor strip with two-channel recording shows 5-beat run of ventricular tachycardia.

7. What percentage of patients have symptoms during the monitoring? What percentage of such symptoms occur with a rhythm disturbance?

Approximately 25–50% of patients experience a complaint or symptom during a 24-hour recording. Of such symptoms, only 2–15% correlate with or are believed to be caused by arrhythmia.

8. In general, when is a Holter monitor considered positive?
It is rather uncommon for healthy, young persons to have significant rhythm disturbances; in fact, several arrhythmias are not necessarily abnormal, including sinus bradycardias (35–40 beats/ minute), sinus arrhythmias (with pauses up to 3 seconds), sinoatrial exit block, Wenckebach block (second-degree AV block type I), wandering atrial pacemaker, junctional escape complexes, and premature atrial or ventricular contractions.

Of concern are frequent and complex atrial and ventricular rhythm disturbances that are less commonly observed in normal subjects, including second-degree AV block type II, sinus pauses > 3 seconds, and brady- or tachyarrhythmias associated with symptoms. Results of the Holter monitor need to be analyzed with the diary to correlate specific symptoms to the rhythm and rate recorded.

9. What is the role of the Holter monitor in patients with known ischemic heart disease?
Patients post MI and those with other forms of ischemic heart disease frequently have premature ventricular contractions (PVCs). After MI the frequency of PVCs increases for several weeks and then declines after 6 months. The frequency and complexity of PVCs are independent markers for sudden death or acute cardiac event; risk may be increased 2–5 times. Patients with symptoms and known ischemic heart disease are in a higher risk group and should be evaluated with both a Holter monitor and SAECG.

10. Can Holter monitors assist in the diagnosis of suspected ischemic heart disease?
Yes. Transient ST-segment depressions ≥ 0.1 mV for less than 30 seconds are rare in normal subjects and correlate strongly with myocardial perfusion scans that show regional ischemia.

11. What have Holter monitors demonstrated about angina and its pattern of occurrence?
Holter monitoring has shown that the majority of ischemic episodes that occur during normal daily activities are silent (asymptomatic) and that symptomatic and silent episodes of ST-segment depression exhibit a circadian rhythm, with ischemic ST-changes more common in the morning. Studies also have shown that nocturnal ST-segment changes are almost always an indicator of two- or three-vessel coronary artery disease or left mainstem stenosis.

12. Do certain groups of patients benefit from Holter monitoring for detection of silent ischemia?
The answer depends on the clinical picture, but patients with an "anginal equivalent" and risk factors for coronary artery disease (e.g., exerctional shortness of breath) are also at high risk for ischemia. Patients with type II diabetes mellitus also have a greater incidence of asymptomatic ischemia as well as silent myocardial infarctions and may benefit from Holter evaluation for silent ischemia.

13. What is heart-rate variability?
Holter monitor recordings can be used to assess heart-rate variability as a measurement of the standard deviation of the sinus rhythm cycle length (or fluctuation around the mean RR interval). Heart-rate variability reflects the parasympathetic and sympathetic balance of the autonomic nervous system and therefore offers insight into the risk for sudden cardiac death.

14. What is the clinical significance of heart-rate variability?
Recent studies show that analysis of heart-rate variability is important in evaluation of postinfarction and diabetic patients. In both groups decreased heart-rate variability is associated with an increased risk of sudden cardiac death. Lower heart-rate variability is also recorded with acute MI. Here a predominance of sympathetic activity and reduction in parasympathetic cardiac control result in increased sympathetic activity, which decreases the fibrillation threshold and predisposes to ventricular fibrillation. In addition, anterior-wall MI results in a more profound reduction in heart-rate variability than inferior-wall infarction.

15. What is signal-averaged electrocardiography (SAECG)?

SAECG is a method of recording the ECG in which amplifiers and filters record cardiac signals with amplitudes of only a few microvolts. Electrical potentials corresponding to delayed and fragmental conduction in the ventricle are recorded in microvolts and waveforms continuous with the QRS complex. Three criteria are of importance: (1) QRS duration, (2) low-voltage signals in the last 40 msec of the QRS, and (3) low-frequency waveforms lasting > 30 msec after terminal QRS complex.

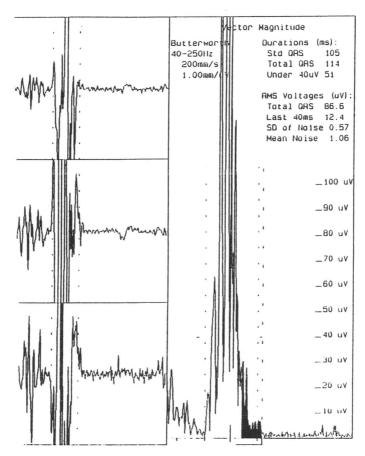

Positive SAECG with late potentials highlighted are the end of the QRS complex between 150 and 190 ms. The low-amplitude signals (< 25 mV) exceed the voltage for noise at the terminal 40 ms. The QRS duration is normal (114 ms). QRS 114 ms (normal < 120 ms) LA S - 51 ms (normal < 40 ms). RMS 40 12.5 mV (normal > 25 mV).

16. How is the SAECG used clinically?

Late potentials have been detected in 73–92% of patients with sustained and inducible ventricular tachycardia after MI. Late potentials also have been identified in patients with nonischemic heart disease and ventricular tachycardia, such as those with dilated cardiomyopathy. Early use of thrombolytic agents reduces the prevalence of late potentials after coronary occlusion and therefore the risk of sudden death, ventricular fibrillation, and tachycardia.

Late potentials after MI are an independent marker of patients at high risk for ventricular tachycardia. SAECG results combined with other noninvasive data (e.g., Holter, ETT, ejection fraction) provide a highly sensitive and highly specific method of identifying patients at risk for ventricular tachycardia or sudden death.

BIBLIOGRAPHY

1. DiMarco JP, Philbrick JT: Use of ambulatory electrocardiographic (Holter) monitoring. Ann Intern Med 113:53–68, 1990.
2. El-Sherrif N, Ursell SN, Bekheit S, et al: Prognostic significance of the signal-average ECG depends on the time of recording in the post-infarction period. Am Heart J 118:256, 1989.
3. Gomes JA, Winters SL, Martinson M, et al: The prognostic significance of quantitative signal-averaged variables relative to clinical variables, site of myocardial infarction, ejection fraction and ventricular premature beats: A prospective study. J Am Coll Cardiol 13:377, 1989.
4. Hauer RN, Lie KI, Liem KL, Dureer D: Long-term prognosis in patients with bundle branch block complicating acute anteroseptal infarction. Am J Cardiol 49:1581, 1982.
5. Kennedy HL: Long-term (Holter) electrocardiogram recordings. In Zipes DP, Jalife J (eds): Cardiac Electrophysiology: From Cell to Bedside. Philadelphia, W.B. Saunders, 1990, p 791.
6. Kuchar DL, Thorburn CW, Sammel NL: Prediction of serious arrhythmic events after myocardial infraction: Signal-averaged electrocardiogram, Holter monitoring and radionuclide ventriculography. J Am Coll Cardiol 9:531, 1987.
7. Langer A, Freeman MR, Josse RG, et al: Detection of silent myocardial ischemia in diabetes mellitus. Am J Cardiol 67:1073, 1991.
8. Turitto G, Fontaine JM, Ursell SN, et al: Value of the signal-averaged electrocardiogram as a predictor of the results of programmed stimulation in nonsustained ventricular tachycardia. Am J Cardiol 61:1272, 1988.
9. Van Ravenswaaij-Arts MA, Kollee AA, Hopman JC, et al: Heart rate variability. Ann Intern Med 118:436–47, 1993.
10. Yeung AC, Barry J, Orav J, et al: Effects of asymptomatic ischemia on long-term prognosis in chronic stable coronary disease. Circulation 83:1598, 1991.

7. ECHOCARDIOGRAPHY AND DOPPLER/ COLOR-FLOW IMAGING

Olivia V. Adair, M.D.

1. Why has echocardiography become so popular in assessment of cardiovascular diagnosis?

Echocardiography has become the most common imaging and hemodynamic modality for the following reasons.

    1. It allows high-quality imaging.

    2. As a biologically safe modality, with no cumulative effects, it lends itself to serial studies as well as use in children and pregnant women.

    3. It is painless.

    4. No preparation is required (except for transesophageal echocardiography).

    5. It is mobile and quick and allows on-line interpretation.

    6. Doppler imaging provides anatomic as well as hemodynamic data.

    7. It can be used as an early screening test.

2. What are the major anatomic data obtained with echocardiography?

Although the number of possible cross-sectional planes through which the heart can be viewed is almost infinite, standard sections are based on the transducer position—parasternal, apical, subcostal, and suprasternal—whereas the planes are long-axis, short-axis, four-chamber, and

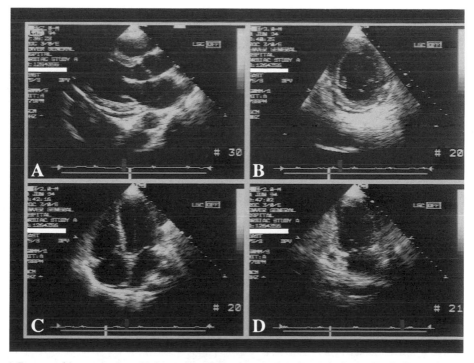

A, Parasternal long-axis view of left ventricles, left atrium, aortic valve, and mitral valve. **B,** Short-axis view of left ventricle. *C,* Four-chamber view. *D,* Two-chamber view of left ventricle, mitral valves, and left atrium.

two-chamber. Chamber size and function are well imaged, as are the mitral, aortic, tricuspid and pulmonic valves. The thickness of the walls is easily evaluated as well as the septum; wall motion is evaluated by segments in each view (inferior, posterior, anterior, and lateral walls). The aorta and sometimes even coronary arteries are visualized. The pericardium can be evaluated as well as the pulmonary artery and right ventricular outflow tract. The left atrial appendage is occasionally seen on transthoracic echocardiography.

3. Is Doppler/color-flow imaging a separate imaging technique from echocardiography?
Doppler imaging uses the direction and velocity of blood flow to evaluate cardiovascular hemodynamics, and color-flow imaging (CFI) provides real-time, two-dimensional imaging of blood flow. Echocardiography, Doppler imaging, and CFI are complementary rather than competitive; the best studies integrate the three techniques.

4. What are the major hemodynamic measurements and clinical applications of Doppler echocardiography?
Multiple hemodynamic measurements and analyses are possible with Doppler acquisition, but the major categories of application are ventricular performance, valvular function, and shunt lesions. **Stroke volume** can be obtained with measurements of the left ventricular outflow tract, blood flow into the ascending aorta, and flow velocities. Doppler evaluation of pulmonary artery flow allows measurement of **right ventricular output.** Measurement of time intervals aids in the evaluation of **systolic and diastolic ventricular function.** The differences in flow volumes can be used to calculate **intracardiac shunts** and **regurgitant flows.** One of the most valuable uses of Doppler is to evaluate **valve function,** especially pressure gradients, which can be used to calculate the area of the stenotic valve and maximal velocity across the valve. Flow disturbances (turbulence) are used to diagnose **valvular regurgitation** and to evaluate its severity.

5. What are the limitations to echocardiography and Doppler imaging?
The major limitation is the lack of anatomic quantitative measurements in echocardiography, which necessitates technical skill in performance and interpretation. Another limitation is the acquisition of total cardiac anatomic information, which is achieved in 80–90% of studies. Moreover the complexity of anatomic and hemodynamic information often leads to incorrect or incomplete interpretations by examiners who are not well versed or adequately experienced. In transesophageal echocardiography the images are frequently clear but should be interpreted only by an experienced cardiologist. Misinterpretation also may be due to technical limitations, misreading of artifacts, or extraneous echoes.

6. What are the clinically useful recommendations for echocardiography and Doppler imaging?
- Evaluating ventricular systolic and diastolic performance
- Estimating right-sided heart hemodynamics
- Measuring pressure gradients and valvular orifice areas in stenotic valves or other discrete narrowings
- Detecting valvular regurgitation and estimating its hemodynamic significance
- Evaluating function of valvular prostheses
- Establishing the presence and determining the significance of intracardiac shunts

7. What is contrast echocardiography? How is it applied clinically?
Contrast echocardiography is used to delineate structures not readily seen (superior and inferior vena cava, descending aorta, right ventricular outflow tract, pulmonary arteries) as well as to evaluate intracardiac shunts, regurgitant lesions, and complex congenital heart problems. Contrast echocardiography uses microbubbles by agitating approximately 8 cc of saline between two 10-ml syringes connected to a three-way stopcock and an intravenous line. The agitated saline is injected with extreme force into the intravenous line while recording in the four-chamber view or focusing on the suspected site. Apical or subcostal four-chamber views allow visualiza-

tion of a small number of microbubbles crossing a right-to-left shunt as well as a negative jet of left-to-right flow that causes a defect in the otherwise bubble-filled right chamber. If a large shunt is suspected, the number of injections and amount of contrast should be limited. An appropriate routine is first to inject 3 cc, record and evaluate; if a large shunt is not present, 8–10 cc are then injected. If the study is negative at this point, reinjection, with the patient coughing when the right atrium is filled, increases right-sided pressure and allows even the smallest shunt to be identified. This technique is extremely sensitive and specific for shunt diagnosis, which can be confirmed with only a few microbubbles; it is even more sensitive than oximetry and dye dilation and can detect shunts as small as 3%. It is also sensitive enough to evaluate patency of the foramen ovale or surgical repairs of shunts. The noninvasive laboratory at our institution uses contrast in the echocardiographic evaluation of all patients with stroke or transient ischemic attacks (TIAs).

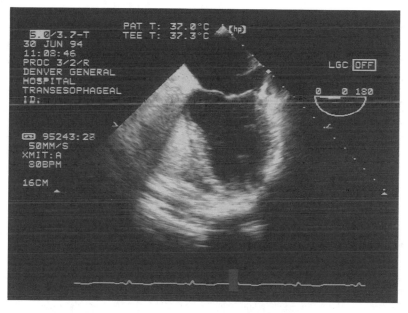

Normal contrast echocardiography. Four-chamber view shows complete filling of right atrium and ventricle (to left) with microbubbles and no bubbles in left atrium or ventricle (to right).

8. How do echocardiography and Doppler imaging help in the evaluation of the patient with suspected ischemic heart disease?

Echocardiography is useful in evaluating possible ischemic heart disease, chest pain syndromes, and left ventricular function and in establishing risk stratification and complications of acute myocardial infarction. Assessment of regional wall motion and absence of systolic thickening of the myocardium may implicate coronary artery disease. Serial studies can be evaluated in side-by-side formats to compare wall motion abnormalities or to evaluate myocardial remodeling. Also, exercise echocardiography adds sensitivity and specificity to routine stress electrocardiography and has been advocated as especially useful in diagnosing coronary artery disease in women, with a sensitivity and specificity comparable to radionuclear stress studies. Whereas only 50% of ECGs are diagnostic for acute myocardial infarction, the detection of regional wall motion abnormalities is much more sensitive (though less specific). A negative echocardiogram during chest pain predicts a very low risk of ischemia. Another advantage of using echocardiography with chest pain syndromes is the additional diagnostic information about other causes of chest pain, such as aortic stenosis, aortic dissection, mitral valve prolapse, pericardial effusions, or hypertrophic cardiomyopathy.

9. Why is echocardiography the imaging technique of choice for valvular disease?

Echocardiology is the imaging technique of choice for evaluation of valvular disease, because it provides hemodynamic, structural, and functional data as well as assesses the severity of valvular disease, its possible etiology, and prognosis. Evaluation of the valve may include information about leaflet calcification, pliability, and mobility; any coexisting pathology also can be assessed along with left ventricular function and thrombi. Because echocardiography and Doppler imaging are safe for serial studies, they can be used to follow the patient or to evaluate interventions and management. Doppler imaging and CFI enable more accurate location of the lesion as well as better assessment of pressure gradient, valve areas, and regurgitant flows.

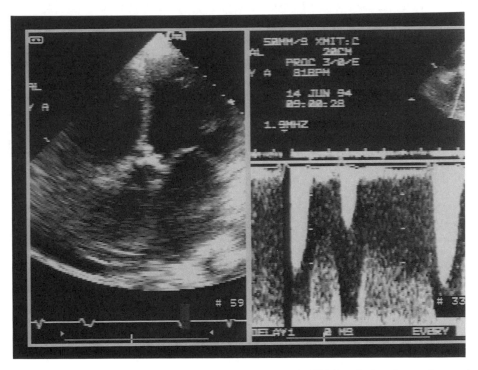

Left, Aortic stenosis with thickened and calcified aortic valve. *Right,* With Doppler imaging, aortic stenosis velocity is demonstrated by the white envelope, flow direction away from transducer (downward), maximal velocity of 3.5 m/s, and peak gradient of 49 mmHg.

10. What are the applications for stress echocardiography? How is it performed?

Stress echocardiography is an important imaging technique for evaluating ventricular function, global ejection fraction, regional wall motion, and myocardial thickening and for assessing hemodynamic or cardiac function at baseline as well as at maximal stress or point of symptoms. Among the most common clinical applications is hemodynamic assessment of mitral stenosis in symptomatic patients in whom resting hemodynamic status is insufficient for a clinical decision. In addition, other dynamic lesions are better assessed with stress, including hypertrophic cardiomyopathy, recoarctation of the aorta, and dysfunction of prosthetic valves. The most common use is diagnosis of ischemic heart disease with a pre- and intermediate post-exercise echocardiography to evaluate wall motion. The test is relatively inexpensive and is as sensitive and specific as single-photon emission computed tomography (SPECT) with thallium during exercise for assessment of ischemic heart disease. For patients who cannot do conventional treadmill stress tests, dobutamine or dipyridamole can be used.

11. What is the role of echocardiography in patients with acute myocardial infarction?
Because electrocardiography is not always diagnostic for acute infarction, echocardiography is easily used to detect wall motion abnormalities. Immediate evaluation of ischemia and the amount of myocardium at risk is especially important for decisions about early intervention, such as use of thrombolytic agents or angioplasty. Echocardiography also assesses patients with infarction for complications such as severity of ischemic mitral regurgitation, postinfarction ventricular septal defect, aneurysm (true vs. false), and right-sided pressures. Serial studies can evaluate reperfusion. Because the most powerful prognostic indicator after infarction is left ventricular function, the larger the infarct, the higher the risk for subsequent cardiac events; echocardiography and Doppler imaging are essential in risk stratification and prognostic evaluation, both of which help to determine the management plan.

12. What are the indications for transesophageal echocardiography (TEE)?
TEE has increased imaging abilities tremendously through multiplane windows from the stomach and esophagus that provide high-resolution tomographic imaging views. TEE is used both in the awake patient and intraoperatively. A study of TEEs done at the Mayo Clinic over 5 years shows three major indications: (1) source of emboli, (2) native and prosthetic valve disease, and (3) endocarditis. For the intraoperative patient the most frequent applications are monitoring of cardiac function, intraoperative diagnosis, and assessment of postoperative results. Victims of trauma often are best evaluated with TEE because of its mobility, speed, and capacity for on-line interpretation.

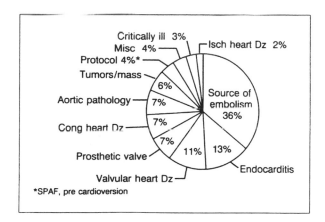

Indications for TEE examination at the Mayo Clinic from November 1987 to November 1992 (5,441 procedures). Three major indications are source of embolism, native and prosthetic valve disease, and endocarditis. (*SPAF* = Stroke Prevention in Atrial Fibrillation trial). Isch = ischemic Cong = congestive, Dz = disease. (From Freeman WK, et al (eds): Transesophageal Echocardiography. Boston, Little, Brown. © 1994 by Mayo Foundation, Rochester, Minnesota. Used with permission.)

13. What are the risks in TEE? How invasive is TEE?
TEE is a low-risk procedure that provides a tremendous amount of clinically important data. TEE should be performed only by trained echocardiographers fully aware not only of the diagnostic interpretation but also of technique, potential complications, and contraindications. Two large

studies reported only 1 death each (0.02%). In one study the cause of death was unclear; in the other study, a malignant lung tumor infiltrating the esophagus was lacerated during probe introduction and caused massive hemorrhage and subsequent death. The Mayo Clinic reports a complication rate of 0.18–0.5% among over 5,000 procedures. Most complications are minor and easily treatable.

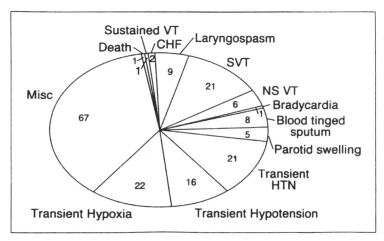

Classification of 180 complications (3.3%) of TEE examinations encountered in the Mayo Clinic experience with 5,441 procedures between November 1987 and November 1992. Major complications included laryngospasm, sustained ventricular tachycardia (VT), acute congestive heart failurre (CHF), and one death. SVT = supraventricular tachycardia, NS = nonsustained, HTN = hypertension. (From Freeman WK, et al (eds): Transesophageal Echocardiography. Boston, Little, Brown. © 1994 by Mayo Foundation, Rochester, Minnesota. Used with permission.)

Overall TEE is a safe procedure and is used to complement transthoracic echocardiography in approximately 10% of patients. The physician should be aware of contraindications to avoid complications.

Contraindications to TEE

ABSOLUTE CONTRAINDICATIONS	RELATIVE CONTRAINDICATIONS
Esophageal obstruction (stricture, neoplasm)	Recent gastroesophageal operation
Esophageal fistula, laceration, or perforation	Esophageal varices
Esophageal diverticulum	Upper gastrointestinal bleeding
Cervical spine instability	Atlantoaxial arthritis
	Unexplained symptoms of dysphasia or odynophagia

14. How should a patient with a prosthetic valve be evaluated and followed?
Patients with a prosthetic valve are best managed by using the patient as his or her own control and obtaining early postoperative echocardiography and Doppler evaluations, which can be compared with follow-up evaluations. This approach is helpful because the gradients of prosthetic valves are inherently higher than the gradients of native valves and may vary with positioning. The transthoracic (TTE) approach in echocardiography, and less so in Doppler imaging, is limited by acoustic shadowing, whereas TEE circumvents many of these imaging problems. Assessment of mitral valve prostheses is especially difficult with TTE, but TEE sensitively detects and quantitates regurgitation, valvular or perivalvular leaks, abnormal morphology, vegetation, thrombi, abscess, and leaflet tear. Although aortic valve prostheses are easier to view via TTE, TEE is much superior in evaluating vegetation or abscess cavities, especially when a mitral prosthesis is also present. Certainly TEE should be considered strongly for any patient with

suspected or proven prosthetic valve endocarditis because of its high sensitivity and ability to detect complications. Serial echocardiography and Doppler imaging have replaced cardiac catheterization as the procedure of choice for hemodynamic and morphologic evaluation.

15. How useful is TEE in the diagnosis of infectious endocarditis? How does it help in the management of patients?

TEE has been shown in several large studies to have higher sensitivity than TTE for native valves (94–100% vs. 44–63%) and prosthetic valves (75% vs. 25%); both have high specificity (98%). TTE detection of vegetation depends largely on the extent of the vegetation, whereas TEE can detect much smaller vegetations. TEE also has an effect on patient management, because it detects complications such as abscesses, chordal rupture, and secondary valve involvement. Because mortality is higher and prognosis is worse with such complications, identification of affected patients should prompt consideration of early interventions.

16. What are the echocardiographic findings in patients with hypertrophic obstructive cardiomyopathy (HOCM)?

Echocardiography is the best method of diagnosing HOCM and is extremely sensitive. The classic finding is asymmetric septal hypertrophy, but symmetric hypertrophy may be seen, as well as other varieties (e.g., apical or midventricular hypertrophy). Echocardiography also assesses systolic anterior motion of the mitral valve and contact of the anterior leaflet and the septum. The aortic valve closes early in mid-systole, either partially (notch) or completely. The left ventricle cavity is usually decreased, whereas the left atrium is dilated.

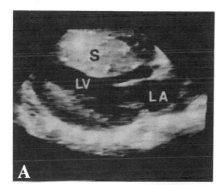
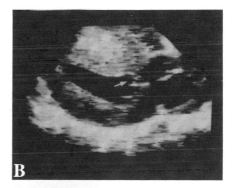
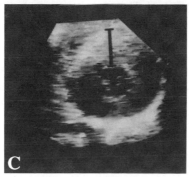

Two-dimensional echocardiographic images show asymmetric septal hypertrophy and systolic anterior motion of the mitral valve, two classic signs of hypertrophic cardiomyopathy. *A,* Long-axis view, diastole. *B,* Long-axis view, systole. *C,* Short-axis view. S = septum; LA = left atrium; LV = left ventricle. (From Pandian NG, Simonetti J: Echocardiography in hypertrophic cardiomyopathy. Cardiovasc Rev Rep Oct 1988, p 60, with permission.)

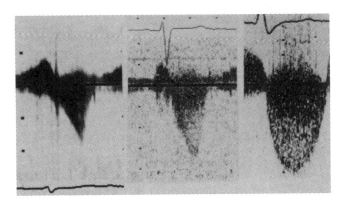

Continuous wave Doppler recordings along the LV outflow tract from two patients with hypertrophic obstructive cardiomyopathy (*Left* and *middle*) and from a patient with valvular aortic stenosis (*right*). In HOCM, the rise in velocity during early systole is gradual, but then the dynamic obstruction causes a steep rise, to a maximum in late systole, giving a characteristic dagger-shaped flow velocity profile different from that seen in valvular aortic stenosis. (From Pandian NG, Simonetti J: Echocardiography in hypertrophic cardiomyopathy. Cardiovasc Rev Rep Oct 1988, p 60, with permission.)

17. What is the imaging technique of choice to evaluate the aorta?
TEE has become the modality of choice in patients with suspected aortic dissection, especially with the involvement of the descending aorta, which is poorly visualized by TTE. TEE also can be used for evaluations of other aortic abnormalities, such as plague, aneurysm, or thrombus. The reported sensitivity for aortic dissection is 97–100%; the reported specificity, 98–100%.

BIBLIOGRAPHY

1. Crouse LJ, Harbrecht JJ, Vacek JL: Exercise echocardiography as a screening test for coronary artery disease and correlation with coronary angiography. Am J Cardiol 67:1213–1218, 1991.
2. Daniel WG, Mugge A, Martin RP, et al: Improvement in the diagnosis of abscesses associated with endocarditis by transesophageal echocardiography. N Engl J Med 324:795–800, 1991.
3. Felner JM, Martin RP: The echocardiogram. In Schlant R, Alexander R (eds): The Heart Arteries and Veins, 8th ed. New York, McGraw-Hill, 1994.
4. Freeman WK, Seward JB, Khandheria BK, Tajik AJ: Transesophageal Echocardiography. Boston, Little, Brown, 1994.
5. Khandheria BK, Seward JB, Tajik AJ: Transesophageal echocardiography. In Braunwald E (ed): Heart Disease: A Textbook of Cardiovascular Medicine, 3rd ed. Philadelphia, W.B. Saunders, 1992, p 290.
6. Pearlman AS: Technique of Doppler and color flow Doppler in the evaluation of cardiac disorders and function. In Schlant R, Alexander R (eds): The Heart Arteries and Veins, 8th ed. New York, McGraw-Hill, 1994.
7. Pearson AC: Transthoracic echocardiography versus transesophageal echocardiography in detecting cardiac source of embolism. Echocardiography 10:397–403, 1993.
8. Shivey BK, Gurule FT, Roldan CA, et al: Diagnostic value of transesophageal compared with transthoracic echocardiography in infective endocarditis. J Am Coll Cardiol 18:391–397, 1991.

8. ECHOCARDIOGRAPHY IN THE CRITICALLY ILL PATIENT

Olivia V. Adair, M.D., and Douglas Paul Voorhees, R.R.T.

1. Why has echocardiography emerged as such an important diagnostic tool in critically ill patients?

Critically ill patients need urgent diagnostic evaluation and expedient, appropriate intervention to improve the course of disease and chance of survival. Often their clinical condition and medical environment (e.g., respirator, multiple intravenous lines, cardiac monitoring) limit diagnostic options, because transport involves major effort and risk. Therefore, echocardiography has become extremely popular because of (1) bedside mobility, (2) high-quality imaging, (3) noninvasive nature, (4) immediate on-line image analysis, and (5) extensive yield of data, including structural, functional, and hemodynamic information. In addition, transesophageal echocardiography (TEE) has increased the quality of studies in patients on respirators, with chest injuries requiring chest tubes, or surgical wounds of the chest, all of which limit the transthoracic windows.

2. How important is an echocardiography study in a critically ill patient?

The bedside echocardiography study gives immediate data to direct management strategies. The extensive differential diagnosis of hemodynamic instability includes critical valve disease, intracardiac shunt, cardiomyopathy, and tamponade, all of which are easily diagnosed with echocardiography and require different management despite similar clinical presentations. Therefore, emergent echocardiography is important to help to eliminate several of the possible etiologies and either to make the diagnosis or to establish a foundation for initial management.

3. Are different risks or procedural problems involved in the use of TEE in critically ill patients?

TEE is semiinvasive. Passing the probe into the stomach of critically ill patients requires more experience and manual guidance. The patient may be agitated, unable to cooperate and confined to the supine position. Adequate sedation and prophylaxis for endocarditis in patients with prosthetic valves are necessary before passage of the probe. Problems with hemodynamically unstable and critically ill patients are uncommon, except in the presence of extensive neck and facial trauma. A laryngoscope is often helpful if the procedure proves difficult. Although patients are often hemodynamically unstable, clinically significant complications are rare. TEE should be performed by a cardiologist ready to manage hemodynamic deterioration, fully trained in endoscopic intubation procedures, and experienced in TEE interpretation.

4. What are the common indications for TEE in the intensive care unit?

The primary reason for TEE in critically ill patients in our institution is hemodynamic instability, which may result from hypotension, pulmonary edema, acute myocardial infarction, endocarditis, tamponade, trauma, or cardiogenic shock. Patients frequently present with shock syndrome that requires prompt intervention. Several reports show favorable results from the use of TEE in such patients. For example, of 44 patients with shock syndrome, only 48% were partially diagnosed by transthoracic echocardiography (TTE), whereas 100% were diagnosed with TEE. Critical information was obtained in 68%, with 30% undergoing urgent cardiac surgery (including mitral valve replacement, tamponade relief, correction of postinfarction ventricular septal rupture and aortic rupture, and closure of patent foramen ovale). Of the 4 patients with normal TEEs, all had a noncardiovascular cause of hemodynamic compromise, as established by other investigations. Pearson et al.[11] reported similar success with different indications (aortic dissection, 29%; source of emboli, 26%; postinfarction complications, 10%); critically important clinical information, not seen on TTE, was obtained in 44%.

5. What is the best diagnostic procedure when aortic dissection is suspected?

Although magnetic resonance imaging (MRI) permits visualization of the thoracic aorta in multiple planes with high sensitivity, delay and transport of patients often pose problems. Moreover, multiple support systems, such as intravenous pumps, respirators, and monitors, make transport impossible or involve an unacceptably high risk. Newer generation computed tomography also has 95% accuracy but involves similar problems of transport and time for acquisition. TEE, on the other hand, is portable and quick, providing on-line interpretation. Transthoracic echocardiography has a sensitivity of 75–85%; sensitivity is lower for distal dissection. TEE has both a sensitivity and a specifity of 98%. TEE is also useful for detecting extracardiac complications of dissection, such as pericardial effusion (seen in ~25%) and coronary artery dissection, as well as conditions that mimic dissection. Traumatic rupture of the aorta, as well as contained intimal disruption with thrombus, is also diagnosed by TEE, especially with multiplane imaging, with high sensitivity and specificity. Furthermore, TEE has the advantage of providing added diagnostic information, particularly in patients with chest trauma (e.g., from automobile accidents) that may result in pericardial effusions or hematomas, contusion, and infarction. Intravascular ultrasound also has gained popularity in diagnosing aortic dissection, especially in victims of trauma, but requires an invasive test as well as specialized training and equipment; it also lacks the advantage of additional echocardiographic data. More studies are needed to make direct comparisons.

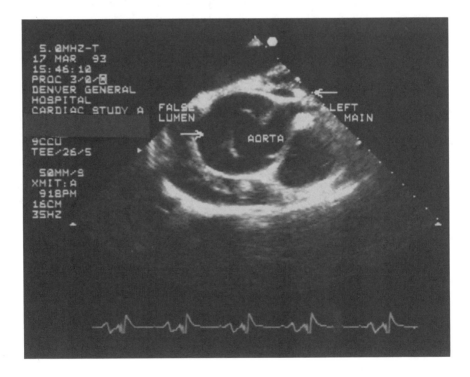

TEE of proximal aortic dissection.

6. How common is trauma to the heart? When should it be suspected and evaluated?

Accidental or intentional trauma is the leading cause of death and hospitalization, especially in young people, among whom violent injuries are increasing. Cardiac and great-vessel injuries are major contributors to mortality and morbidity secondary to penetrating and nonpenetrating trauma.

Any penetrating injuries to the precordium, chest, neck, or upper abdomen should prompt investigation for cardiac trauma; such injuries usually involve knife or gunshot wounds. Of special concern are signs of tamponade or hemothorax. Over 50% of victims with penetrating cardiac trauma die immediately; in the others, who survive for varying lengths of time, immediate evaluation is essential. TEE is an important procedure, because small-caliber bullets and tears can be missed on TTE. The majority of nonpenetrating injuries are due to automobile accidents (50% involve fatal or severe chest injuries); contact sports, falls, and altercations also result in such injuries. TEE is the procedure of choice to evaluate patients for pericardial, myocardial, valvular, coronay artery, and aortic injury.

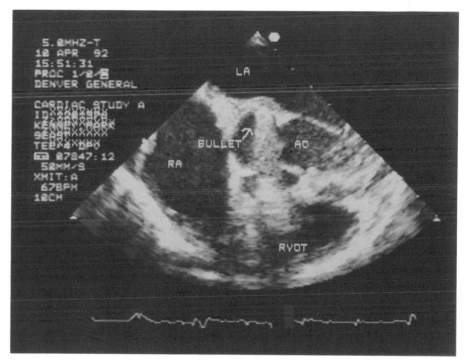

TEE of bullet in proximal aortic root.

7. What role should TEE play in the evaluation of potential cardiac donors?

TEE should be considered an important part of donor evaluation. Many donors are victims of motor vehicle accidents or violent crimes, both of which may result in significant cardiac or chest trauma. Such injuries may cause ventricular contusion (right or left), coronary thrombus, regional wall motion abnormalities, tricuspid valve disruption and regurgitation, or aortic dissection. Affected patients may not be easily imaged by transthoracic echocardiography. As high as one-half of the significant findings in potential donors on TEE are not diagnosed by TTE. Donor candidates, therefore, should undergo TEE before cardiac status is established. Surgical repair of detected lesions should be considered, and more appropriate data for specific recipients' urgency of need should be employed.

BIBLIOGRAPHY

1. Brathwaite CEM, Weiss RL, Baldino WA, et al: Multichamber gunshot wounds of the heart: The utility of transesophageal echocardiography. Chest 101:287–288, 1992.
2. Brooks SW, Young JC, Cmolik B, et al: The use of transesophageal echocardiography in the evaluation of chest trauma. J Trauma. 32:761–766, 1992.
3. Daniel WG, Mügge A, Martin RP, et al: Improvement in the diagnosis of abscesses associated with endocarditis by transesophageal echocardiography. N Engl J Med 324:795–800, 1991.
4. Davis GA, Sauerisen S, Chandrassekaran K, et al: Subclinical traumatic aortic injury diagnosed by transesophageal echocardiography. Am Heart J 123:534–536, 1992.
5. Font VE, Obarski TP, Klein AL, et al: Transesophageal echocardiography in the critical care unit. Cleve Clin J Med 58:315–322, 1991.
6. Foster E, Schiller NB: The role of transesophageal echocardiography in critical care: UCSF experience. J Am Soc Echocardiogr 5:368–374, 1992.
7. Freeman WK, Seward JB, Khandheria BK, Tajik AJ: Transesophageal Echocardiography. Boston, Little, Brown, 1994.
8. Nienaber CA, von Kodolitsch Y, Nicolas V, et al: The diagnosis of thoracic aortic dissection by non-invasive imaging procedures. N Engl J Med 328:1–9, 1993.
9. Oh JK, Seward JB, Khanderia BK, et al: Transesophageal echocardiography in critically ill patients. Am J Cardiol 66:1492–1495, 1990.
10. Oh JK, Sinak LJ, Freeman WK, et al: Transesophageal echocardiography in patients with shock syndrome [abstract]. Circulation 84 (Suppl 2): 127, 1991.
11. Pearson AC, Castello R, Iabovitz AJ: Safety and utility of transesophageal echocardiography in the critically ill patient. Am Heart J 119:1083–1089, 1990.
12. Smyllie JH, Sutherland GR, Geuskens R, et al: Doppler color flow mapping in the diagnosis of ventricular septal rupture and acute mitral regurgitation after myocardial infraction. J Am Coll Cardiol 15:1449–1455, 1990.

9. EXERCISE TESTING

John J. Reusch, M.D.

1. When is an exercise test useful?

Most commonly, exercise testing is used to aid in the diagnosis of coronary artery disease in patients (1) who have chest pain or (2) who are thought to be at risk for coronary disease because of the presence of risk factors, such as family history or hypertension. In patients known to have cardiopulmonary disease, exercise testing is often used to assess therapeutic interventions (e.g., medications, surgery, angioplasty) and in following symptoms related to the disease. In addition, exercise testing can be helpful in determining a prognosis in patients with recent myocardial infarction, valvular heart disease, or known congestive heart failure.

2. How reliable is an exercise test for the diagnosis of coronary artery disease?

The reported sensitivity of exercise electrocardiography (ECG) ranges from 55–85%, and the specificity ranges from 70–90%. An exercise test clearly is an imperfect study, and interpretation of the results is best thought of in terms of the "**predictive value**" of an abnormal test result, which depends heavily on factors related to the patient and to the study itself. The following table illustrates some of these factors and describes how they influence the predictive value of a test result.

Factors Influencing Predictive Value of Exercise ECG Testing

	PREDICTIVE VALUE	
FACTORS	Better	Worse
Patient factors		
Age	Older	Younger
Gender	Male	Female
Cardiac risk factors	Present	Absent
Angina	Typical	Atypical/none
Test factors		
Heart rate	Higher	Lower
ST depression	More	Less
ST morphology	Downsloping	Horizontal
Exercise chest pain	Present	Absent

According to the table, a patient having an abnormal exercise ECG is more likely to have obstructive coronary artery disease if one or more of the "better" factors are present, and less likely if the "worse" factors are present. For example, a 45-year-old man with typical angina and 2 mm of horizontal ST-segment depression on exercise ECG has a >95% chance of having obstructed coronary arteries, whereas a 45-year-old asymptomatic woman with the same exercise ECG has only a 10% likelihood of obstructive coronary disease.

3. What is the Bruce protocol?

The Bruce protocol specifies how the intensity of exercise progresses during the test. Protocols have been developed by many investigators. The one developed by Bruce and coworkers is the most popular, both because it is the most extensively validated and because it can be performed relatively quickly. In the Bruce protocol, each stage lasts 3 minutes. During Stage I, the patient walks at 1.7 mph up a 10% grade. Energy expenditure for the average person is estimated to be 4.8 METS during this stage. Both speed and grade rise with each stage. It is unusual for a patient to complete Stage V (5.0 mph, 18% grade).

4. What is a MET?

MET is an abbreviation for **metabolic equivalent**. It is arrived at by measuring the oxygen consumed by the patient, which reflects the energy the patient is expending. One MET is 3.5 ml O_2/kg/min, the oxygen consumption by an average individual at rest. It is estimated that most people need to be able to perform exercise at an intensity of at least 5 METs in order to carry out adequately activities of daily living.

5. What are the differences between a normal and abnormal exercise ECG?

The single most reliable indicator of exercise-induced ischemia is **ST-segment depression.** One millimeter or more of horizontal or downsloping ST depression is generally considered indicative of an abnormal ischemic change. Greater amounts of ST depression and downsloping morphology increase specificity for ischemia. Upsloping ST depression is a less specific ECG change. Some suggest that 1.5 mm of upsloping ST depression should be considered diagnostic of ischemia, but more rapidly upsloping ST depression is a nondiagnostic finding.

ST elevation with exercise is an infrequent finding that may represent severe ischemia. When it occurs in an area of prior infarction (in leads with pathologic Q waves), it is a nonspecific finding that is thought to be caused by abnormal wall motion. ST elevation in lead aVR is also a nonspecific finding.

T wave changes, such as inversion or "pseudonormalization," in the absence of ST-segment shift are also nonspecific findings. Finally, changes in **R-wave amplitude** and in **U-wave axis** have been associated with ischemia but are not of great clinical utility.

6. Does blood pressure change with exercise?

Yes. Normally during exercise, there is a widening of the pulse pressure caused by a gradual rise in systolic pressure and a slight fall or no change in diastolic pressure. Failure of the systolic pressure to rise at least 30 mmHg is considered abnormal and may be related to heart failure and/or severe ischemia (occasionally, these conditions may even cause a fall in systolic pressure). Antianginal or antihypertensive medications (e.g., beta blockers or calcium channel blockers) usually cause a mild blunting of the rise in systolic blood pressure. A rise in systolic pressure significantly above 200 mmHg is considered a hypertensive response to exercise.

7. How is an individual's expected maximum heart rate determined?

The maximum predicted heart rate (MPHR) varies among individuals but is reasonably well predicted by the formula MPHR = 220 − age.

8. Can anything be learned from the exercise heart rate response?

Mainly, the heart rate is considered an index of the intensity of exercise. In general, the closer a patient gets to his or her predicted maximum heart rate, the more intense the exercise is, the more stress is placed on the cardiopulmonary system, and the more sensitive the test will be for detecting an abnormal condition. By convention, most clinicians accept a heart rate of 85% of predicted maximum as reflective of near-maximal exercise—a level of exercise that yields a sufficiently sensitive test.

A rapidly rising heart rate at low levels of exercise can indicate severe deconditioning and/or severe cardiopulmonary disease. Rarely, severe cardiac disease can cause an inadequate heart response to exercise. This is referred to as *chronotropic incompetence.*

9. List four factors that interfere with the ability to interpret an exercise ECG.

1. Left ventricular hypertrophy
2. Left bundle branch block
3. Baseline ST-T abnormality > 1 mm
4. Digitalis (with or without baseline ECG abnormality)

Even in the absence of an interpretable exercise ECG, the exercise test can still yield useful information about exercise capacity, presence or absence of symptoms or arrhythmias, and the patient's heart rate and blood pressure response to exercise.

10. What does it mean when a patient gets chest pain during an exercise test?

Chest discomfort is fairly common and often nonspecific during exercise testing. However, the symptoms must be assessed in an attempt to decide how closely they match the classic description of angina. Chest discomfort is classified into one of three categories: clearly cardiac, clearly noncardiac, or uncertain. Obviously, chest discomfort in the first two categories helps with interpretation of the test, whereas discomfort in the latter category leaves the clinician uncertain.

Overall, the presence of exercise chest pain makes the likelihood of obstructive coronary disease greater, but absence of chest pain does not rule it out. Asymptomatic ischemia with exercise may be more likely in patients with diabetes.

11. List the absolute contraindications to maximum exercise testing.
1. Myocardial infarction within the prior 3 weeks
2. Uncontrolled heart failure
3. Unstable angina
4. Uncontrolled hypertension (systolic >250 mmHg, diastolic >120 mmHg)
5. Acute myocarditis, pericarditis
6. Acute febrile illness
7. Severe aortic stenosis

12. What is a "submaximal" exercise test?
A submaximal test typically is used for patients undergoing stress testing within 1 week after an acute myocardial infarction. In a submaximal test, the goal is not for the patient to reach his or her maximum tolerated exercise capacity, but to stop at a level lower than that. This goal can be defined as a heart rate of 70% of maximum predicted, a heart rate of 120 bpm, or the completion of a certain stage of a protocol.

13. When should an exercise test be stopped?
- Patient desires to stop
- Severe chest pain, dyspnea, dizziness, or other symptoms
- Increasingly severe ventricular ectopy
- New-onset atrial fibrillation or supraventricular tachycardia
- Second- or third-degree heart block
- New bundle branch block
- Severe ST-segment shifts (e.g., >3 mm ST depression)
- Fall in blood pressure below resting level or a ≥20-mmHg fall in systolic blood pressure
- Systolic blood pressure >300 or diastolic blood pressure >130

14. What are the risks of exercise testing?
Overall, there is minimal risk associated with performing maximal exercise testing when patients are chosen properly. The frequently quoted risk of serious complication, such as death, myocardial infarction, or life-threatening arrhythmia, is approximately 1 in 10,000 (0.01%).

15. When is a test considered to have been "strongly positive"?
A strongly positive test indicates a relatively high likelihood (>70%) of severe coronary artery disease being present. Several definitions have been suggested, but most would agree that a test is strongly positive when there is a progressive fall in systolic blood pressure during exercise or when there is evidence for ischemia (angina or significant ST depression) during the first or second stage of the Bruce protocol, especially if exercise is terminated by the patient during one of those stages.

BIBLIOGRAPHY

1. Ellestad MH: Stress Testing: Principles and Practices. Philadelphia, FA Davis, 1986.
2. Mark DB, Hlatky MA, Harrell FE, et al: Exercise treadmill score for predicting prognosis in coronary artery disease. Ann Intern Med 106:793–800, 1987.
3. Schlant RC, Blomqvist CG, Brandenburg RO, et al: Guidelines for exercise testing: A report of the joint American College of Cardiology/American Heart Association Task Force on Assessment of Cardiovascular Procedures (Subcommittee on Exercise Testing). Circulation 74:653A–667A, 1986.
4. Weiner DA, Ryan TJ, McCabe CH, et al: The role of exercise testing in identifying patients with improved survival after coronary artery bypass surgery. J Am Coll Cardiol 8:741–748, 1986.

10. NUCLEAR CARDIOLOGY, MAGNETIC RESONANCE IMAGING, AND COMPUTED TOMOGRAPHY

Robert A. Quaife, M.D.

1. What is myocardial perfusion imaging?

Myocardial perfusion imaging is a noninvasive method for assessing regional myocardial blood flow and the cellular integrity of myocytes. This technique uses radiotracers or cationic compounds, such as thallium-201, which cross the myocyte cellular membrane and are trapped intacellularly. Such perfusion agents rely on regional coronary blood flow to distribute the tracer and require viability of living tissue for uptake. Tissues supplied by an unobstructed coronary vessel and with adequate diastolic flow within the coronary vascular tree will possess normal regional myocardial perfusion; however, regions supplied by a stenosed coronary vessel have lower coronary blood flow and therefore less relative myocardial perfusion. The relative difference between these two regions allows detection of myocardial perfusion defects.

When cardiac tissues face increased metabolic demand, as with exercise, the relative difference in blood flow between normal and "stenotic" vascular regions is markedly disparate. Despite maximal coronary vasodilatation beyond the point of coronary artery narrowing, the resultant improvement of blood flow during exercise is minimal, producing a perfusion interface between normal and ischemic myocardium. This maximum difference between normal and stenotic vascular territories during stress forms the basis for myocardial perfusion imaging.

2. What diagnostic questions are addressed by myocardial perfusion imaging?

1. Myocardial perfusion imaging's major utility centers around diagnosis of **coronary artery disease.** In this setting, the overall sensitivity of the test ranges from 70–95% and specificity from 70–85% for static (planar) imaging versus three-dimensional single-photon computed tomography imaging techniques (SPECT), respectively.

2. A second diagnostic question concerns **coronary artery stenoses.** Stress perfusion imaging is used to define the severity or physiologic significance of a stenosis already identified by coronary angiography.

3. **Perioperative risk assessment** is another use of myocardial perfusion studies. Dipyridamole myocardial perfusion imaging with thallium-201 is highly predictive of either perioperative or postoperative cardiac-related death and/or myocardial infarction in patients with reversible perfusion defects prior to surgery. These reversible defects are the equivalent of ischemic tissue or myocardium at-risk, of which perfusion imaging assesses the tissue quantity and severity.

4. Myocardial perfusion imaging has been used to evaluate and define **prognosis following acute myocardial infarction,** identifying fixed defects (suggesting myocardial infarction) as well as reversible defects in other vascular distributions are risk factors for subsequent myocardial events. Dipyridamole–thallium-201 stress myocardial perfusion imaging early following a myocardial infarction (within 48–96 hours) may be useful for identifying patients at greatest risk for subsequent myocardial events, especially when reversible defects are identified within the supposed ECG documented territory.

5. Myocardial perfusion imaging with thallium-201 has been used to identify **living tissue** that will recover function following resupply of normal coronary blood flow termed "viability." Subsequent coronary revascularization with angioplasty or coronary artery bypass surgery then achieves reversal of wall motion abnormalities and complete recovery of cardiac systolic function.

44

3. Compare the radionuclide tracers used to assess myocardial perfusion.

Thallium-201, a potassium analog, is the most widely used and standard myocardial perfusion agent. It is primarily distributed within the myocardium via regional myocardial blood flow but requires cell integrity and intact sodium–potassium ATPase pump activity for intracellular uptake. Thallium-201 is less than optimal for imaging large patients or those with prominent soft tissue outside their chest, due to the low inherent γ-energy (80 KeV) of the radionuclide, a major factor determining image resolution.

New **technetium-based agents** have been developed that employ the improved energy and imaging characteristics of technetium-99m. One such agent is technetium-99m-methoxy-isobutyl-isonitrile (Tc-MIBI), a cationic compound which is distributed via myocardial blood flow and traverses the cell membrane to concentrate within the mitochondrial wall. Tc-MIBI is similar to thallium-201 in its myocardial physiologic perfusion properties, although it possesses improved imaging characteristics resulting from the greater γ-photon energy emission (140 KeV).

Both perfusion agents have similar sensitivity for detecting significant coronary artery disease, although Tc-MIBI has a slightly higher specificity due to its improved image quality. Technetium agents lend themselves to techniques which simultaneously assess myocardial perfusion and myocardial systolic performance from the same study.

4. Perfusion agents allow noninvasive study of coronary blood flow. What is the physiologic basis for such imaging techniques?

Myocardial territories supplied by a significantly stenosed coronary artery have reduced perfusion or blood flow, which is accentuated during physiologic stress. For this reason, exercise treadmill testing is added to myocardial perfusion imaging to enhance the difference between normally perfused and underperfused myocardium. Stress-induced perfusion defects are used to define myocardium at risk for an ischemic and/or infarction event. The comparison of a stress-induced perfusion defect with later normal perfusion (redistribution) on delayed imaging, termed "reversibility," defines the imaging equivalent of myocardial ischemia. Pharmacologic agents, either dipyridamole or adenosine, can also be used to induce relative perfusion differences between normal and stenotic vascular distributions.

The comparison between stress-induced defects and resting perfusion defects may be used to define irreversibly damaged or infarcted tissue, termed a "fixed defect," in which no significant change in relative perfusion is noted between stress and rest. However, some of these fixed defects possess viable tissue. In "hibernating" (viable) myocardium, metabolism is altered to conserve cellular energy at the expense of contraction resulting from severe resting ischemia. Identification of severe resting ischemia or myocardial viability may be obtained by allowing longer redistribution times or by increasing the total quantity of the radiotracer available with reinjection of additional tracer when thallium-201 imaging is performed.

5. Can perfusion imaging define the presence, region, and amount of myocardial tissue involved in an acute myocardial infarction?

Gibbons and coworkers demonstrated that patients presenting with an acute myocardial infarction who are undergoing thrombolytic therapy, myocardial perfusion imaging can accurately predict the amount of myocadium salvageable by thrombolytic therapy. These authors injected Tc-MIBI and imaged presumed infarction patients prior to and then following thrombolytic therapy to determine the amount of myocardium salvaged from thrombolytic therapy (difference of the two images).

Recently, myocardial perfusion imaging has shown diagnostic utility in identifying patients who require hospitalization for acute ischemic syndromes. Patients presenting with acute chest pain without classic electrocardiographic (ECG) abnormalities were studied to define the presence of significant perfusion defects. Perfusion defects noted at the initial evaluation were highly correlated with patients documented to have either acute myocardial infarctions and/or significant coronary artery disease.

6. When is pharmacologic stress perfusion imaging of added utility over standard treadmill exercise testing?

Pharmacologic stress, induced by using either dipyridamole or adenosine, is primarily reserved for patients who cannot complete standard exercise treadmill testing, usually due to some physical limitation. Pharmacologic stress methods may also be important in patients who are deconditioned due to prolonged hospital stays or other chronic diseases.

7. Why is it important to characterize which stress-induced perfusion defects are reversible and whether myocardial viability is present?

When territories are supplied by a subtotal or critical coronary stenosis, these severely underperfused but viable tissues switch to primarily glycolytic metabolism from normal fatty acid metabolism. Such altered cellular biochemistry may be imaged using the glucose analogue 2-deoxy-glucose labeled with ^{18}F. Positron emission tomographic (PET) imaging with FDG identified glycolytically active tissue that is viable. This phenomenon, severe resting ischema, occurs in up to 40% of fixed thallium-201 defects classified as dead or scarred myocardium. When normal coronary blood flow is resupplied to these regions, otherwise ischemic myocardium normalizes thallium-201 perfusion and regional wall motion recovers, demonstrating the importance of detecting such severely ischemic tissue.

8. Is it possible to assess both myocardial perfusion and left ventricular (LV) systolic performance from the same myocardium perfusion study?

The new myocardial perfusion agents, such as Tc-MIBI, allow greater doses of the radiotracer to be administered as well as provide improved inherent imaging characteristics. Therefore, a bolus injection of the radiotracer can be used to assess LV performance at peak stress using the ''first-pass'' LV imaging techniques. Second, gated perfusion imaging using single-photon emission computed tomography (SPECT) 3-D analysis may quantify LV end-diastolic and end-systolic relative volumes and LV ejection fraction (LVEF). Gating or triggering of the imaging camera at the onset of the R-wave over multiple cardiac cycles provides a 16-frame average of multiple cardiac beats necessary for assessing cardiac motion and capturing end-systole and end-diastole, both of which are required for EF determinations.

9. Functional assessment of cardiac performance is determined using which nuclear cardiology techniques?

Standard LV performance may be assessed in two ways: A **first-pass bolus technique** may be used that quantitates individual end-systolic and end-diastolic relative volumes as the bolus passes through the right heart into the lungs and through the LV. Regions of interest are manually determined around the LV at end-diastole and end-systole to provide the counts necessary for calculation of LVEF. (end-diastole volume minus end-systolic volume divided by end-diastolic volume).

Alternatively, **gated equilibrium blood pool imaging** (multiple gated acquisition, MUGA) of the left and right ventricles may be performed to assess myocardial performance. An aliquot of the patient's red blood cells is labeled with sodium pertechnetate and reinjected for subsequent imaging in three static-image cardiac positions. The camera is triggered at the onset of each R-wave for each cardiac cycle; the R-R interval is divided into 16 frames and is compiled into summed images. These average data in image format are subsequently processed and displayed as a continuous cinematic loop to stimulate cardiac motion during the cardiac cycle. From this display, a region of interest is identified around LV end-diastolic and end-systolic volumes again to calculate LVEF. Also from the display, regional myocardial wall motion may be determined from each LV segment.

10. How important is assessment of LVEF by radionuclide techniques?

1. Overall, the LVEF is one of the most powerful predictors of future myocardial events and sudden death in patients with coronary artery disease. Its predictive value in coronary artery disease is probably related to global LV dysfunction manifested as the combination of poor

myocardial perfusion and the presence of underlying scar tissue from previous myocardial infarctions, which is the substrate for future ischemic events or life-threatening cardiac arrhythmias.

2. LVEF is important in evaluating valvular heart disease, as baseline reduced LVEF suggests already-compromised LV function and is a poor prognostic sign when considering surgical intervention.

3. Exercise LVEF may be useful in the early detection of compromised LV systolic performance. When semi-erect or supine bicycle testing is used, the lack of increase in LVEF with exercise may predict loss of LV reserve, signaling the need for early intervention.

4. Both hypertrophic and dilated cardiomyopathy patients may benefit from diagnostic and prognostic information gained from determinations of LV systolic and diastolic performance. From idiopathic dilated cardiomyopathy to doxorubicin-induced cardiomyopathy, reduced LVEF is one of the greatest predictors of subsequent severe congestive heart failure and death.

11. When is computed tomography (CT) important for the diagnosis of cardiac or cardiac-related diseases?

Standard state-of-the-art CT imaging systems, although much faster than their earlier counterparts, still have limited temporal resolution for the beating heart. Therefore, investigations of intracardiac structures—except within the atria, pericardial space, or aorta—are limited. CT has been useful for evaluating suspected constrictive pericarditis or other pericardial diseases (determining pericardial thickness) and intracardiac thrombi (usually in the pulmonary arteries or atria, where there are less cardiac motion artifacts). In many centers, CT has become the first-line assessment for abnormalities of the ascending and descending aorta, especially in suspected aortic dissection.

12. What are the limitations of standard CT imaging?

Cardiac evaluation by CT is primarily limited by insufficient temporal resolution to allow stop-frame assessment of cardiac structures, therefore limiting evaluations of LV chamber thickness, contraction, and intracardiac structures. Additionally, this technique requires administration of an iodinated contrast agent to opacify the intravascular regions and to identify abnormalities within these structures. These contrast agents can provoke adverse reactions. Recently, the introduction of Fastrak Rapid CT (Picker International) provides assessment of multiple cardiac slices within 10–20 cardiac beats at a temporal resolution of approximately 50 ms. Unlike standard CT, this modality has high resolution for intracardiac structures and masses. It also allows bolus contrast injections to study intracardiac transit times and coronary artery bypass graft flow. Unfortunately, rapid CT imaging is not widely available and is of limited general use except for thoracic pathology.

13. How does CT compare to other imaging modalities for the diagnosis of aortic dissection?

A recent comparison of aortic dissection detected by multiple imaging modalities found that, overall, CT had a 93% sensitivity and 87% specificity for detecting dissecting aortic aneurysm. The difficulty in defining a second lumen and the potential false-positive of artifacts resulting from the streaming of contrast and other issues reduced the sensitivity of standard CT. Overall, the sensitivity and specificity are acceptable for a screening test for aortic dissection. Additionally, CT allows assessment of the ascending aorta as well as aortic arch and descending aorta; however, this evaluation requires administration of intravenous contrast. This potentially renal toxic contrast, when combined with either total ischemic time or cardiopulmonary bypass pump use at surgical dissection repair, can induce acute and prolonged renal failure postoperatively.

14. What are the advantages of magnetic resonance imaging (MRI) over standard imaging techniques?

MRI employs inherent physiologic properties of tissues to create images of body structures. This technique provides a wide field of view for assessing structures within the thoracic cage, specifically for cardiac imaging. The ability to orient images in multiple planes and off-axis planes is key to the technique's diagnostic utility and allows images to be oriented within specific oblique or perpendicular views for careful inspection of cardiac structures and/or the great vessels. Additionally, gating or triggering of the MRI scanner based on the R wave of the patient's ECG for each cardiac cycle allows stop-frame imaging of the heart and great vessels. The inherent characteristics of flowing blood result in contrast enhancement of vascular structures without the administration of iodinated contrast agents. Major uses include the assessment of congenital heart disease (adult and pediatric), intracardiac structures, and the great vessels.

Unlike other imaging modalities, such as CT or planar blood pool imaging, MRI provides three-dimensional assessment of myocardial structures. Its advantages, including image resolution and field of view, outweigh some of its limitations, such as placing the patient within a closed area, potential difficulties with cardiac gating, and increased cost.

15. What role does MRI play in diagnosing aortic aneurysm and dissection?
MRI provides full field-of-view assessment of the ascending aorta, aortic arch, and descending aorta. With use of spin-echo techniques, static views of the cardiac structures and great vessels are assessed in a multi-slice format. Spin-echo MRI has a reported high sensitivity for detecting false lumens and intramural flaps associated with dissection, identifying areas of intraluminal thrombosis, and assessing potential rupture of dissecting aortic aneurysms into visceral spaces or pericardium. Contrast enhancement using special imaging sequences provides evaluation of the site of aortic tear into the intima and potential flow within the false lumen of the aortic dissection free of iodinated contrast administration.

Aortic insufficiency may also be assessed as one of the associated markers of aortic dissection, and the reported sensitivity and specificity of MRI for detecting aortic dissection were 98% for both type A and B dissection. In a comparison of transthoracic and transesophageal echocardiography, CT, and MRI for the diagnosis of aortic dissection, the primary limitations of MRI involved its inability to image significantly unstable patients, and its limited availability in emergency situations at all centers. Therefore, CT or transesophageal echocardiography may be indicated for evaluating aortic dissection, depending on the availability and expertise within specific hospitals.

16. Is it possible to assess intracardiac masses, both intramural and intracavitary, by MRI?
Tissue characterizations resulting from MRI-induced physical properties allow the assessment of intracardiac masses, with the greatest sensitivity in the atria and great vessels. There is somewhat less sensitivity, although greater specificity, for detecting intramural cardiac masses, due to the similar image intensity between tumors and myocardial tissues. MRI provides assessment of pericardial and pleural spaces and localization of masses extending into or arising from these structures. MRI and echocardiography are probably the two most sensitive techniques for determining the extent of intracardiac masses.

17. What is the diagnostic accuracy of MRI for congenital heart disease?
Congenital heart disease imaging with MRI is significantly enhanced by the simultaneous evaluation of visceral, vascular, and cardiac structures. Complex congenital heart disease often involves not only cardiac abnormalities but also abnormalities of the associated vascular structures or visceral organs. With MRI, the wide field of view provides associated information important for correct diagnosis. For example, transposition of the great vessels is easily evaluated by MRI, since the orientation of the aorta, pulmonary artery, and cardiac chambers is visualized together rather than separately.

Recently, the increased survival of patients with congenital heart disease into adulthood has supported diagnostic-niche MRI. Many of these patients have surgical shunts or vascular procedures that are not well studied or investigated by standard imaging techniques, but flow, size of vessels, and physiologic function of these shunts may be assessed using the multiple orientations of MRI.

In general, prosthetic intracardiac valves are not a contraindication to MRI (except for the early Starr-Edwards 1200 series ball-cage valves); however, assessment of structures in the region of prosthetic heart valves is limited due to absorption of imaging signal by metallic structures within the heart.

BIBLIOGRAPHY

1. Beller GA: Evaluation of myocardial viability using thallium-201 imaging. Cardiol Rev 1(2):78–86, 1993.
2. Bonow RO, et al: Prognostic implications of symptomatic vs asymptomatic (silent) myocardial ischemia induced by exercise in mildly symptomatic and in asymptomatic patients with angiographically-documented coronary artery disease. Am J Cardiol 60:778, 1987.
3. Dilsizian V, Rocco TP, Freedman NMT, et al: Enhanced detection of ischemic but viable myocardium by the reinjection of thallium after stress-redistribution imaging. New Engl J Med 323:141–146, 1990.
4. Fletcher BD, Jacobstein MD, Nelson AD, et al: Gated magnetic resonance imaging of congenital cardiac malformations. Radiology 150:137–40, 1987.
5. Leppo JA, et al: Dipyridamole thallium-201 scintigraphy in the prediction of future cardiac events after acute myocardial infarction. N Engl J Med 310:1014, 1984.
6. Mohiaddin RH, Longmore DB: Functional aspects of cardiovascular nuclear magnetic resonance imaging. Circulation 88:264, 1993.
7. Nienaber CA, Kodolitsch Y, Nicolas V, et al: The diagnosis of thoracic aortic dissection by noninvasive imaging procedures. N Engl J Med 328:1, 1993.
8. Tillisch J, Brunken R, Marshall R, et al. Reversibility of cardiac wall motion abnormalities predicted by positron tomography. N Engl J Med 314:884–1986, 1986.
9. Yamada T, Tada S, Harada J: Aortic dissection without intimal rupture: Diagnosis with MR imaging and CT. Radiology 163:347–352, 1988.

11. CARDIAC CATHETERIZATION AND ANGIOGRAPHY

Roy W. Robertson, M.D., and William P. Miller, M.D.

1. What are the general indications for performing cardiac catheterization?
Assessment of patients with:
1. Known or suspected coronary artery disease
2. Valvular heart disease
3. Congenital heart disease
4. Cardiomyopathy
5. Sudden cardiac death
6. Pericardial constriction or tamponade
7. Following cardiac transplantation

2. What are the indications for coronary angiography in patients with known or suspected coronary artery disease?
In order of most to least agreed-upon indications:
1. Exercise test predictive of left main and/or multivessel coronary artery disease
2. Limiting angina pectoris
   a. In patients who have failed medical therapy
   b. Most patients with unstable angina
3. Following myocardial infarction
   a. Cardiogenic shock
   b. Clinically failed thrombolysis
   c. Postinfarction angina
   d. Assessment of acute mechanical complications (e.g., ventricular septal defect)
   e. Failed low-level predischarge exercise stress test
   f. Following most non-Q-wave myocardial infarctions
4. Positive exercise and/or pharmacologic stress test
5. Diagnostic evaluation and assessment of "atypical" chest pain and/or suspected coronary spasm
6. Evaluation of high-risk patients prior to a major noncardiac surgical procedure
7. Asymptomatic patients at increased risk for coronary artery disease
   a. Occupational status (e.g., pilot)
   b. Significant cardiovascular risk factors (diabetes mellitus, hyperlipidemia, hypertension)
   c. Abnormal resting electrocardiogram

3. What predisposing factors place patients at high risk for complications from cardiac catheterization?
1. Age (<1 year or > 60 years of age)
2. Functional class: Patients classified as New York Heart Association Class IV are at 10 times higher risk than patients in Class I or II.
3. Severity of coronary atherosclerosis: Left main occlusive stenosis poses a 10 times higher risk than single-vessel occlusive coronary disease.
4. Valvular heart disease
5. Left ventricular dysfunction: Mortality rate is 10 times higher for patients with ejection fraction < 30% compared to those with ejection fraction > 50%.
6. Severe noncardiac disease (e.g., diabetes mellitus, renal insufficiency, peripheral vascular disease, chronic lung disease).

4. List some of the potential complications from a diagnostic cardiac catheterization and their frequencies.

Major Complications of Cardiac Catheterization

Death	0.1–0.2%
Myocardial infarction	0.1–0.3%
Cerebrovascular accident	0.1–0.3%

Minor, Transient, or Reversible Complications of Cardiac Catheterization

Vasovagal reactions	1.5–2.5%
Local vascular complications at access site	1–3%
Serious arrhythmias	0.3–0.5%
Allergic reaction to contrast agent	<2%
Infection	<0.5%
Nephropathy	<0.5%

Complication rates depend on operator experience, equipment, and patient characteristics.

5. Describe the two most common sites of vascular access for cardiac catheterization.
Catheterization can be accomplished by introduction of catheters into the brachial or femoral artery and brachiocephalic or femoral vein. Whereas brachial artery cutdown and arteriotomy (Sones) was the original approach, the percutaneous femoral (Judkins) approach is now used most commonly. Choice of access site depends on preference and experience of the operator and the extent of peripheral vascular disease in the patient.

6. What are the major components of routine left and right cardiac catheterization?
Initially, pressures are measured in the aorta, right heart, and left heart. Right heart pressures include pulmonary capillary wedge pressure, pulmonary artery pressures, right ventricular pressures, and right atrial pressure. Left heart pressures are the left ventricular systolic, early diastolic, and end-diastolic pressures. Pressure measurement is followed by determination of cardiac output. Contrast opacification of the left ventricular chamber (left ventricular cineangiography) and other chambers if clinically indicated is also included—e.g., contrast opacification of the left atrium in the assessment of an atrial septal defect. Selective angiography of the coronary arteries follows.

7. How is cardiac output measured?
Cardiac output is commonly measured by dilutional techniques (e.g., thermodilution) or by the Fick method. In the Fick method, cardiac output (CO) = oxygen consumption (VO_2)/ arteriovenous oxygen difference ($AVO_2\Delta$). Oxygen consumption is measured directly by a mask that fits over the patient's mouth or face, and blood is sampled from the pulmonary artery and femoral artery to compute $AVO_2\Delta$.

8. What are the normal values for intracardiac chamber pressures in the human heart?
Recalling this information is made easy by applying the **"rule of fives."** In this rule, all pressures are estimated as multiples of five. The right atrial pressure (central venous pressure) is normally ~5 mmHg. The right ventricular systolic pressure is ~25 mmHg with an end-diastolic pressure of ~5 mmHg. The left atrial pressure (estimated by the pulmonary capillary wedge pressure) is ~10 mmHg. The left ventricular systolic pressure is normally ~125 mmHg with a left ventricular end-diastolic pressure of 10 mmHg.

9. What information is obtained from the left ventricular cineangiogram?
Left ventricular (LV) volumes can be measured using quantitative ventriculography. The LV ejection fraction provides a measure of LV systolic function. Regional systolic wall motion is assessed by grading each segment of the left ventricle as hyperkinetic, normal, hypokinetic,

akinetic, or dyskinetic. Space-occupying lesions might also be identified, if present, within the LV chamber (e.g., thrombus). Stroke volume is determined by subtracting the end-systolic LV chamber volume from the end-diastolic LV chamber volume. Ejection fraction (EF) is the stroke volume divided by the end-diastolic LV volume. Finally, an assessment of mitral valve competence is made. Mitral incompetence (regurgitation) is graded as mild (1+), moderate (2+), moderately severe (3+), or severe (4+).

10. Typically the left ventriculogram is obtained in one (or ideally two) projections to assess ventricular function. What LV wall segments are assessed in each of the views and how are they graded?
    Each segment is graded as hyperkinetic, normal, hypokinetic, akinetic, or dyskinetic.

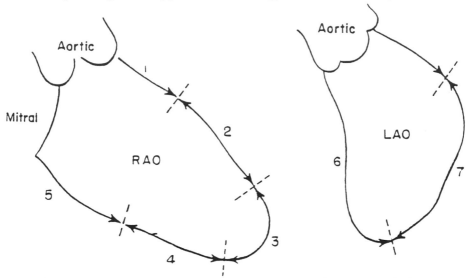

Right anterior oblique (RAO) projection:
1 = Anterobasal
2 = Anterolateral
3 = Apical
4 = Diaphragmatic
5 = Posterobasal

Left anterior oblique projection:
6 = Septal
7 = Posterolateral.

11. Define coronary dominance.
The nomenclature which describes the coronary artery as dominant can be misleading. It is not simply the degree of importance, but instead identifies the coronary artery which crosses the crux of the heart (junction of the posterior atrioventricular groove with the posterior interventricular groove) and therefore generally supplies the basal posterior interventricular septum of the left ventricle. This same artery commonly gives rise to the atrioventricular nodal artery in the region of, or just beyond, the crux. In approximately 85% of humans, the right coronary artery is dominant. In most of the remaining 15%, the left circumflex artery is dominant; however, "codominance" does occur.

12. How is the degree of coronary artery stenosis assessed on a coronary angiogram?
For routine clinical evaluation of coronary angiograms, an experienced angiographer qualitatively estimates the degree of stenosis visually. Multiple views of the regions of interest are obtained over a range of projection angles to best define the three-dimensional geometry of the lesions. The result is generally reported as a percent reduction in lumen diameter (e.g., a 75% stenosis is a lesion that narrows the lumen diameter by approximately 75%). Quantitative

coronary angiography can also be applied using algorithms based on computer image processing, although this method is generally cumbersome and is used almost exclusively as a research tool in clinical trials.

13. Name the coronary arteries and their major branches as they are commonly identified by coronary angiography.

This drawing depicts right-dominant coronary anatomy:

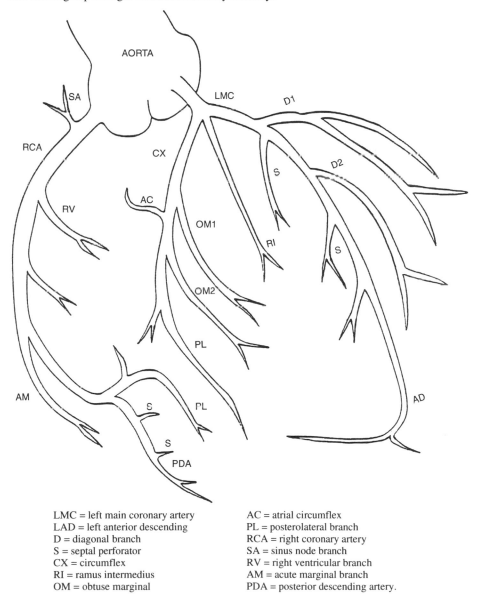

LMC = left main coronary artery	AC = atrial circumflex
LAD = left anterior descending	PL = posterolateral branch
D = diagonal branch	RCA = right coronary artery
S = septal perforator	SA = sinus node branch
CX = circumflex	RV = right ventricular branch
RI = ramus intermedius	AM = acute marginal branch
OM = obtuse marginal	PDA = posterior descending artery.

14. How do angiographers commonly categorize the severity of coronary artery stenoses?

A grading system of reduction in percent lumen diameter has been designed that incorporates the limitations of the qualitative nature of assessing the significance of coronary artery disease.

Coronary atherosclerosis is graded as absent (normal), intimal, 25%, 50%, 75%, 90%, 99% (subtotal occlusion), and 100% (occluded). A ≥75% reduction in luminal diameter is considered to be a "significant" stenosis in that a lesion of this severity will affect that artery's ability to increase coronary blood flow as needed during increased demand. The left main coronary artery is "unique" in that a ≥50% stenosis is prognostically significant. Lesion characteristics such as presence of calcium, length of stenosis, location within the coronary artery tree, concentric vs. eccentric morphology, presence of an ulcerated plaque, and intraluminal thrombus are also important and should be described.

15. How does the degree of coronary artery stenosis affect coronary blood flow both at rest and with maximal vasodilatation?
Under resting conditions, progressive reduction of vessel luminal diameter does not reduce resting coronary blood flow until the vessel luminal diameter is approximately 90% stenosed. A normal distal coronary artery bed is able to dilate and increase coronary blood flow to about four to five times its resting value. This is a normal coronary flow reserve and can be achieved during maximal vasodilation, such as occurs with maximal exercise. A 50% reduction in luminal diameter will prevent a coronary vessel from achieving this normal four to five times increase in coronary blood flow during maximal vasodilation. For this reason, a ≥75% reduction in coronary luminal diameter is considered "significant."

16. Additional procedures in the cardiac catheterization laboratory are applied to special patients. List several procedures and their indications.

1. Procedure: Serial blood sampling to measure percent oxygenation at different points in the circulation.
   Indication: a. Determination of cardiac output (Fick method)
       b. Assessment of intracardiac shunting

2. Procedure: Measurement of oxygen consumption.
   Indication: a. Determination of pulmonary and systemic cardiac output by the Fick method.

3. Procedure: Right ventricular endomyocardial biopsy
   Indication: a. Monitoring of antirejection therapy in patients with heart or heart/lung transplantation
       b. Diagnostic evaluation in cardiomyopathy or myocarditis

4. Procedure: Pericardiocentesis
   Indication: a. Treatment of cardiac tamponade
       b. Diagnostic evaluation of pericardial effusion

5. Procedure: Aortography
   Indication: a. Assessment of aortic valve competence
       b. Assessment of suspected aortic dissection
       c. Evaluation of aortic root dilatation
       d. Localization of reverse saphenous vein bypass grafts

6. Procedure: Coronary artery bypass angiography
   Indication: a. Assessment of coronary artery bypass graft patency

7. Procedure: Hemodynamic assessment during exercise or pharmacologic intervention
   Indication: a. Assessment of valvular heart disease
       b. Determination of "reversibility" of pulmonary hypertension.

BIBLIOGRAPHY

1. Franch RH, King SB III, Douglas JS Jr: Techniques of cardiac catheterization including coronary arteriography. In Schlant RC, Alexander RW (eds): Hurst's The Heart, 8th ed. New York, McGraw-Hill, 1994, pp 2381–2418.
2. Gould KL, Kirkeeide RL, Buchi M: Coronary flow reserve as a physiologic measure of stenosis severity. J Am Coll Cardiol 15:459–474, 1990.
3. Grossman W, Baim DS (eds): Cardiac Catheterization, Angiography, and Intervention, 4th ed. Malvern, PA, Lea & Febiger, 1991.
4. Grossman W, Barry WH: Cardiac catheterization. In Braunwald E (ed): Heart Disease: A Textbook of Cardiovascular Medicine, 4th ed. Philadelphia, W.B. Saunders, 1992, pp 180–203.
5. Hillis DL, Lange RA: Cardiac catherization. In Kloner RA (ed): The guide to cardiology. Cardiovasc Rev Rep 11(1):56–74, 1990.
6. Johnson LW, Lozner EC, Johnson S, et al: Coronary arteriography 1984–1987: A report of the Registry of the Society for Cardiac Angiography and Interventions: I. Results and complications. Cathet Cardiovasc Diagn 17:5–10, 1989.
7. Levin DC, Gardiner GA: Coronary arteriography. In Braunwald E (ed): Heart Disease: A Textbook of Cardiovascular Medicine, 4th ed. Philadelphia, W.B. Saunders, 1992, pp 235–275.
8. Lozner EC, Johnson LW, Johnson S, et al: Coronary arteriography 1984–1987: A report of the Registry of the Society for Cardiac Angiography and Interventions: II. An analysis of 218 deaths related to coronary arteriography. Cathet Cardiovas Diagn 17:11–14, 1989.
9. Ross J Jr, Brandenburg RO, Dinsmore RE, et al: Guidelines for coronary angiography: A report of the American College of Cardiology/American Heart Association Task Force on assessment of diagnostic and therapeutic cardiovascular procedures (Subcommittee on Coronary Angiography). J Am Coll Cardiol 10:935–950, 1987.

12. PERCUTANEOUS TRANSLUMINAL CORONARY ANGIOPLASTY AND OTHER INTERVENTIONS

Robert Zaloom, M.D.

1. What are the current indications for coronary angioplasty in single-vessel disease?
Percutaneous transluminal coronary angioplasty (PTCA) is now well accepted as an effective nonsurgical treatment for coronary artery disease. The American College of Cardiology/ American Heart Association (ACC/AHA) Task Force on Assessment of Diagnostic and Therapeutic Cardiovascular Procedures has provided guidelines for performing PTCA. In **symptomatic patients** with a significant lesion in a major vessel supplying a large area of viable myocardium, PTCA is indicated if any of the following exist:
- Inducible ischemia on stress testing done on medical therapy
- Intolerance to medical therapy
- Continued anginal symptoms despite medical therapy

In the **asymptomatic patient,** PTCA is indicated for single-vessel disease affecting a large area of myocardium if any of the following are present:
- Significant inducible ischemia on stress testing
- Survivor of a "near-death episode" without a myocardial infarction
- History of myocardial infarction with an ischemic stress test
- Planned high-risk noncardiac surgery with objective evidence of ischemia present

2. What are the current indications for coronary angioplasty in multivessel disease?
For **symptomatic patients,** significant lesions should involve each of two major arteries, both supplying moderate areas of viable myocardium, before considering PTCA. Furthermore, there should be objective evidence for ischemia on stress testing, angina unresponsive to maximal medical therapy, and/or intolerance to medications. Lesion characteristics should suggest a moderate to high success rate, and patients should be in a low-risk group for morbidity and mortality from PTCA.

Selection of **asymptomatic patients** with multivessel disease for PTCA generally depends on the presence of the same conditions for PTCA in asymptomatic patients with single-vessel disease (*see* question 1). However, it is with the stipulation that a large area of myocardium must be at risk from the diseased vessel. Additional lesions supply small or nonviable regions.

3. How does the AHA/ACC classify lesion-specific characteristics?
Type A lesions generally have a high success rate (≥85%) and are of low risk. Their characteristics include:

Discrete lesions (< 10 mm length)	Smooth contour and without calcification
Concentric lesions	Not involving major branches
Readily accessible to angioplasty	Not ostial
Nonangulated	No thrombus present

Type B lesions have a moderate success rate (60–85%) and are of moderate risk. Their properties include:

Tubular lesions (10–20 mm in length)	Ostial location
Eccentric lesions	Recent total occlusion (< 3 months)
Moderate angulation	At points of bifurcation (often requiring
Irregular contour	two wires)
Moderate tortuosity of proximal segment to the lesion	Moderately heavy calcification
	Some thrombus present

Type C lesions have a low success rate (<60%) and are of high risk. Their characteristics include:

Diffuse lesions (> 2 cm in length)   Chronic total occlusions (> 3 months)
Excess tortuosity of proximal segment   Extremely angulated
Inability to protect major branches   Vein grafts with friable lesions

4. What is the success rate for elective angioplasty?

The primary success rate for elective PTCA now exceeds 90% for most cases. What previously were considered to be risk factors for adverse outcome (i.e., female gender, distal lesions, or anatomy such as circumflex lesions) may no longer be so. Rather, success is more affected by the presence of significant calcification, severe stenosis, and/or thrombus.

5. What are the major acute complications of PTCA?

Ischemia, acute coronary artery closure, myocardial infarction, and death. The incidence of these complications relates to patient selection, lesion type, operator skill, and technology.

6. What causes these complications? How are they managed?

The more common causes of **ischemia** during PTCA are coronary artery dissection and intracoronary artery thrombus. When dissection occurs and ischemia is present, repeat dilation with longer inflations may result in an adequate result.

Repeated reclosure should be treated with bailout catheters and surgical revascularization. Newer techniques including intracoronary stenting may prove useful in this setting to obviate the need for surgery.

Thrombus is a more difficult complication to deal with. Generally, intracoronary thrombolysis with urokinase may be successful, especially when followed by intravenous heparin. Otherwise, bypass surgery may be the preferred treatment, particularly when infarction is likely to ensue.

The risk of death is greatest in the above settings when acute arterial closure occurs and a significant amount of myocardium is at risk. In various studies, mortality from acute closure is greatest with:

- Multivessel disease
- Female gender
- Elderly patients over 70 years old
- History of congestive heart failure
- Left ventricular dysfunction (ejection fraction < 30%)

7. How often does restenosis occur following angioplasty?

In general, the restenosis rate is approximately 20–30%, and it can be even greater in complex lesions. This process depends on a number of factors which together can cause restenosis. The most important factor is probably elastic recoil of the vessel at the site of the PTCA, which is aided by platelet adhesion and aggregation, as well as thrombus formation. Platelets release factors that aggregate more platelets, activate the clotting system, and cause vasoconstriction. Smooth muscle proliferation at the site of injury also plays a role.

8. List lesion-specific characteristics that promote restenosis after angioplasty.

1. Ostial lesions
2. Left anterior descending artery lesions over circumflex and right coronary artery lesions
3. Saphenous vein graft lesions
4. Multivessel disease
5. Totally occluded vessels
6. Multilesion disease
7. Post-PTCA residual stenosis

   8. Lesions located on bends
   9. Lesions at points of bifurcation
  10. Lengthy lesions

9. What are the proposed pathophysiologic mechanisms of PTCA?
The original explanation given by Andreas Gruentzig for enlargement of a vessel lumen by PTCA was compression of plaque, but we now know that this is a minor effect. Also contributing minimally is extrusion of some liquid components from a soft plaque. More important, however, is that PTCA leads to cracking of the intimal plaque with resultant stretching of media and adventitia and expansion of the outer diameter of the vessel. This is apparent on postmortem histologic examination of these vessels.

10. How is PTCA performed when disease occurs at points of bifurcation?
When both branches of a bifurcation of a coronary artery are diseased, angioplasty of one lesion may cause shifting of plaque to the other lesion, resulting in worsening stenosis or occlusion. Thus, to avoid this problem, the operator uses two steerable guidewires simultaneously. The wires are positioned down each limb of the bifurcation and then dilated one at a time. In some instances, two balloons are used and inflated simultaneously. This prevents shifting of plaque from one branch to the other and is known as the "kissing balloon technique."

11. Describe the patient risk factors for restenosis following angioplasty.
The restenosis rates are fairly similar for men and women, but slightly higher for men. Other traditional risk factors for atherogenesis seem to be operative after angioplasty as well. Diabetes promotes restenosis, as demonstrated in various studies. Hypertension, however, has not been proved sufficiently to cause restenosis. Continued smoking following PTCA is clearly a major risk factor due to its vasoconstricting effects and platelet-stimulating properties. Variable results have been reported regarding hypercholesterolemia and restenosis, but it does not seem to be a major risk factor. Unstable angina at the time of PTCA is an independent risk factor for restenosis when compared to those with stable symptoms.

12. Name some of the minor complications associated with angioplasty.
   1. Embolization of plaque constituents, thrombi, calcium, and others (fortunately rare)
   2. Ventricular fibrillation (usually due to ischemia)
   3. Loss of branch vessels during PTCA of a main vessel
   4. Hypotension from bleeding, tamponade, medications, hypovolemia
   5. Femoral artery complications, including hematoma, pseudoaneurysms, arteriovenous fistulas, etc.
   6. Coronary artery aneurysm at the site of PTCA (rare)

13. Describe the newer interventional devices that can overcome some of the problems of conventional PTCA.
When conventional PTCA results in abrupt closure or restenosis or suboptimal results, newer interventional techniques may be preferred:
   1. **Intravascular stents** are endovascular "splints" used to maintain vascular patency. Different types of stents have been used, but now the balloon expandable ones are preferred. They are useful for reversal of abrupt closure when due to dissection. Its most important complication is thrombosis, which is prevented by a vigorous antithrombotic regimen.
   2. **Directional coronary atherectomy (DCA)** enlarges the coronary lumen by actually removing plaque by high-speed rotation. It is useful in cases of restenosis, vein graft disease, ulcerated plaque, eccentric lesions, or ostial lesions.
   3. **Laser balloon angioplasty** applies both heat and pressure to the arterial wall in an attempt to dilate the lumen. This combination may result in desiccation of thrombus and decreased elastic recoil. Although still in its early stages, there is a high restenosis rate with this technique.

BIBLIOGRAPHY

1. American College of Cardiology/American Heart Association Ad Hoc Task Force on Cardiac Catheterization: ACC/AHA guidelines for cardiac catheterization and cardiac catheterization laboratories. J Am Coll Cardiol 81:1149–1182, 1991.
2. Ellis SG, De Cesare NB, Pinkerton CA, et al: Relation of stenosis morphology and clinical presentation to the procedural results of directional coronary atherectomy.Circulation 84:644–653, 1991.
3. Ellis S, et al: Angiographic and clinical predictors of acute closure after native vessel coronary angioplasty. Circulation 77:372–379, 1988.
4. George B, et al: Multicenter investigation of coronary stenting to treat acute or threatened closure after percutaneous transluminal coronary angioplasty: Clinical and angiographic outcomes. J Am Coll Cardiol 22:135–143, 1993.
5. Gibbons RJ, Holmes DR, Reeder GS, et al: Immediate angioplasty compared with the administration of a thrombolytic agent followed by conservative treatment for myocardial infarction. N Engl J Med. 328:685–691, 1993.
6. Grines CI, Browne KF, Marco J, et al: A comparison of immediate angioplasty what thrombolytic therapy for acute myocardial infarction. N Engl J Med 328:673–679, 1993.
7. Grossman W, Baim DS (eds): Cardiac Catheterization, Angiography, and Intervention. Philadelphia, Lea & Febiger, 1992.
8. Hinohara T, Vetter JW, Rowe MH, et al: The effect of angiographic risk factors on the outcome of directional coronary atherectomy [abstract]. J Am Coll Cardiol 17:23A, 1991.
9. National Heart, Lung, and Blood Institute Balloon Valvuloplasty Registry Participants: Multicenter experience with balloon mitral commissurotomy: NHLBI Balloon Valvuloplasty Registry report on immediate and 30 day follow-up results. Circulation 85:448–461, 1992.
10. Popma J, Dick R, Handenschild C, et al: Atheretomy of right coronary ostial stenosis: Initial and long-term results, technical features and histologic findings. Am J Cardiol 67:431–433, 1991.
11. Savage MP, Goldberg S, Hirshfield, et al: Clinical and angiographic determinants of primary coronary angioplasty success. J Am Coll Cardiol 17:22–28, 1991.
12. Topol EJ (ed): Textbook of Interventional Cardiology. Philadelphia, W.B. Saunders, 1990.
13. Zijlestra F, De Boer MJ, Hoorntje KCA, et al: A comparison of immediate coronary angioplasty with intravenous streptokinase in acute myocardial infarction. N Engl J Med 328:680–684, 1993.

III. Arrhythmias

13. SUPRAVENTRICULAR TACHYCARDIAS

Stuart W. Adler, M.D.

1. What is the most common supraventricular arrhythmia?

Excluding simple atrial premature depolarizations, atrial fibrillation is the most commonly encountered supraventricular arrhythmia. Its incidence rises dramatically after the fifth decade for both men and women, and it reaches an estimated prevalence of 9–12% in elderly men. As many as 1 million Americans may have chronic nonvalvular atrial fibrillation.

2. What cardiovascular diseases are likely to coexist in patients with atrial fibrillation?

Hypertensive heart disease is the most common preexisting condition; however, congestive heart failure (of various etiologies—ischemic, cardiomyopathic, etc.) and rheumatic heart disease are more potent risk factors for the development of atrial fibrillation. Patients without identifiable cardiovascular disease or other conditions associated with atrial fibrillation are said to have "lone atrial fibrillation." An estimated 3–25% of all patients with chronic atrial fibrillation have "lone atrial fibrillation."

3. Which agents are effective in slowing the ventricular response in acute atrial fibrillation?

Although frequently used as a first-line drug, digoxin is much less effective in acute rate control than other drugs. The onset of action for digoxin is slow, and it exerts its acute rate-slowing effects largely by an indirect vagotonic activity. Digoxin's effect tends to vanish when patients increase their circulating catecholamine levels during exercise. Digoxin, however, does continue to be the agent of choice for rate control in patients with congestive heart failure or severe impairment of left ventricular function.

In contrast to digoxin, intravenous diltiazem (bolus of 20–25 mg and maintenance of 5–15 mg/hr) has an onset of action within minutes and is generally not associated with significant hypotension. Intravenous beta blockers (e.g., esmolol, 500 µg/kg/min load, then 100 µg/kg/min; or propranolol, 1 mg over 1 min repeated 3–5 times, then start oral) are also effective and are the treatment of choice in atrial fibrillation associated with elevated catecholamine levels (i.e., postoperative patients).

4. What heart rate range is appropriate in patients with chronic atrial fibrillation?

The average ventricular response over a 24-hour period should be similar to that in a patient of comparable age without atrial fibrillation. A resting heart rate of 70–90 bpm is generally appropriate. The ventricular response associated with exertion should be appropriate for the level of exercise (i.e., rates of 90–100 bpm for modest activity, 100–120 bpm for more vigorous exertion, and 120–170 bpm for very vigorous exertion).

Many elderly patients are sedentary and may require digoxin only for control of the ventricular response at rest and with modest exertion. However, in more active patients of all ages, a combination of digoxin with a beta blocker or a long-acting calcium channel blocker will result in better 24-hour heart rate control.

5. What techniques are used to evaluate heart rate in patients with chronic atrial fibrillation?
The heart rate response can be evaluated by two techniques. The use of 24-hour Holter monitoring allows for the assessment of ventricular response during the activities of daily living. The formal graded exercise treadmill test yields information about the rate of rise for the ventricular response as well as peak heart rate at maximal exercise. Both forms of evaluation are helpful in establishing the efficacy of chronic medical therapy.

6. Can thromboembolic risk in patients with atrial fibrillation be predicted from clinical variables? Echocardiographic variables?
The risk of stroke in patients with chronic atrial fibrillation (nonvalvular) is approximately 4–5% per year. The recent SPAF (Stroke Prevention in Atrial Fibrillation) studies as well as earlier studies (Copenhagen Atrial Fibrillation Trial, AFASAK; Canadian Atrial Fibrillation Anticoagulation Study, CAFA; and Boston Area Anticoagulation Trial in Atrial Fibrillation, BAATAF) suggest that a history of hypertension, congestive heart failure, and previous stroke all are significant clinical predictors of stroke in patients with chronic atrial fibrillation. Additional clinical risk factors may include age > 65 years and diabetes mellitus. The SPAF study identified echocardiographic variables, including increased left atrial size and left ventricular dysfunction, as significant risk factors. Additionally, mitral stenosis, prosthetic mitral valves, rheumatic heart disease, and severe mitral regurgitation with marked left atrial enlargement all appear to be associated with increased risk of stroke.

7. In patients with chronic atrial fibrillation, does the benefit of anticoagulation outweigh the risk of bleeding?
Many randomized studies have looked at the use of warfarin or aspirin as therapies to reduce the risk of systemic embolism. These studies have all demonstrated efficacy of warfarin therapy with stroke risk reduction of approximately 60% in treated patients. The level of anticoagulation varied (target international normalized ratio [INR] ranged from 1.5–4.2), and no increased benefit appears when more aggressive anticoagulation is used. In two studies, aspirin (80 or 325 mg/day) reduced the risk of thromboembolism by approximately 35%. The risk of a serious bleeding complication while on warfarin therapy is about 1.5% per year, which means virtually all patients with atrial fibrillation should be considered for antithromboembolic therapy.

8. Which antiarrhythmic drugs are effective in maintaining normal sinus rhythm and preventing recurrence of atrial fibrillation?
Each of the antiarrhythmic drugs in class Ia (quinidine, disopyramide, procainamide), class Ic (flecainide, propafenone), and class III (sotalol, amiodarone) have some efficacy in treating atrial fibrillation. Unfortunately, there is a paucity of prospective data on the long-term efficacy of antiarrhythmic drugs in maintaining sinus rhythm, but one can generalize that the likelihood of maintaining sinus rhythm for 1 year is approximately 50% for each of the drugs, excluding amiodarone. The class Ic and class III drugs have an added advantage of slowing the ventricular response when atrial fibrillation does recur. Amiodarone therapy probably has a higher likelihood of maintaining sinus rhythm, although even low-dose therapy (200 mg/day) increases the risk of pulmonary toxicity. The class Ia drugs as well as sotalol prolong repolarization, which is manifest as an increase in the QT interval. Consequently, all these drugs can provoke torsade de pointes. Individualized care will allow for the selection of patients who may benefit from antiarrhythmic therapy for maintaining sinus rhythm and reducing the risk of thromboembolism.

9. Do other therapeutic options exist for rate control and/or maintenance of sinus rhythm in patients with atrial fibrillation?
In patients with chronic atrial fibrillation refractory to rate-control drugs or those who are intolerant to those drugs, **radiofrequency catheter ablation** of the atrioventricular (AV) node can be performed to permanently interrupt conduction between the atria and ventricle. This procedure is followed by implantation of a rate-responsive single-chamber ventricular pacemaker

to achieve an adequate resting heart rate as well as appropriate heart rate increase in response to activity.

Two surgical approaches (both considered investigational) may prove helpful for patients with chronic atrial fibrillation. The first is the **"corridor" procedure** which isolates a narrow band of atrial tissue between the sinus and AV nodes. Theoretically, this allows the sinus node to maintain chronotropic control of the ventricle, while the remainder of the right and left atrium continues to fibrillate. The disadvantage of this approach is the high incidence of sinus node dysfunction and the continued requirement for life-long anticoagulation. A second surgical approach, **"maze" procedure,** uses multiple incisions precisely placed in the right and left atrium to effectively form "electrical channels" such that reentrant atrial fibrillation excitatory wave fronts can no longer propagate. In the maze procedure, sinus node input into the AV node is preserved, and theoretically both right and left atrial systolic activity is restored. Both surgical procedures are currently considered useful in a very small subset of carefully selected patients.

10. What is a PSVT?

Paroxysmal supraventricular tachycardia (PSVT) is a broad label that encompasses arrhythmias of several different causes. Patients with PSVT describe their episodes of palpitations as having both abrupt onset as well as termination. Individual patients' symptoms may vary markedly but include shortness of breath, chest discomfort, lightheadedness, weakness, diaphoresis, or generalized sense of anxiety during an episode of palpitations.

Several different pathophysiologic substrates account for the specific types of tachycardia grouped under PSVT. The most common is **AV node reentry tachycardia,** which manifests as a regular narrow QRS complex tachycardia with individual rates that can vary widely but usually have a mean of approximately 160–180 bpm. Typically, the P wave is not discernible, as it is "buried" within the QRS complex. If it is visible, the P-wave vector is negative in the inferior leads and it usually follows the QRS complex by ≤ 120 ms. The second most common form of PSVT is due to accessory connections between the atrium and ventricle (**Wolff-Parkinson-White syndrome**). The accessory connection has electrical characteristics similar to atrial or ventricular muscle and allows for the development of reentry tachycardias with the two limbs of the circuit being the accessory connection and the AV node. Again, the individual tachycardia rate can be quite variable and in general does not help distinguish between tachycardias due to AV node reentry and those due to accessory connections. Frequently, a discrete P wave that is different in morphology from the sinus P wave can be seen following shortly after the QRS complex.

Other forms of PSVT, although less common, may arise from various conditions, including sinus node reentry (P wave during tachycardia identical to sinus P wave) or ectopic atrial tachycardia (due to intraatrial reentry, enhanced automaticity, or triggered activity). Typically, the latter form of tachycardia has a stable P-wave morphology that differs from that seen in sinus rhythm. The PR interval is usually > 120 ms and tends to prolong if the tachycardia accelerates.

11. What maneuvers and medications are effective in terminating regular, narrow QRS complex PSVT?

Vagal stimulation (Valsalva maneuver or carotid sinus massage) may affect the tachycardia and, in some cases, bring about termination. These maneuvers at times can slow or transiently interrupt conduction through the AV node, thereby disturbing the reentry circuit and stopping the tachycardia. Several intravenous medications also can be used to terminate sustained supraventricular tachycardias by achieving the same result in the AV node. Intravenous adenosine (6–12 mg), verapamil (5–10 mg), diltiazem (20–25 mg), and esmolol (0.5 mg/kg) are all effective in slowing and/or blocking AV node conduction and thereby terminating the tachycardia. It is useful to record the rhythm during these maneuvers or drug administration, as the tracings can provide insight into the tachycardia mechanism.

12. What is the delta wave in patients with the Wolff-Parkinson-White syndrome?

The delta wave represents the portion of ventricular muscle (left or right ventricle) that is activated before normal ventricular activation via the His-Purkinje system. Depending on the location of the accessory connection and the conduction of the AV node at a given time, the delta wave may be more or less apparent. The delta wave is manifest in the first portion of the QRS, and the vector may be positive (upright), negative (pseudo-Q wave), or isoelectric (inapparent), depending on the location of the accessory connection. The delta wave vector on the 12-lead ECG is frequently helpful in making a first approximation of the accessory connection location.

13. Is there a treatment of choice for patients with the Wolff-Parkinson-White syndrome who present in atrial fibrillation?

These patients will typically have an ECG with an irregularly irregular rhythm and a QRS that varies in width (depending on the ratio of AV node to accessory pathway penetration). In patients who are hemodynamically stable, AV nodal-blocking drugs (verapamil, adenosine, beta blockers, and digoxin) should *not* be used. These drugs can slow conduction through the AV node and paradoxically accelerate the ventricular response by increasing the conduction over the accessory connection. Furthermore, hypotension resulting from drug-induced vasodilation may result in increased catecholamine release which can directly enhance accessory connection conduction. It is in this setting that ventricular fibrillation is most likely to occur. Intravenous procainamide is the drug of choice, as it slows accessory pathway conduction and frequently converts the atrial fibrillation to normal sinus rhythm. In patients who are hemodynamically compromised, the use of direct current cardioversion is recommended.

14. How is PSVT with aberrancy distinguished from ventricular tachycardia?

In the hemodynamically stable patient with wide-complex tachycardia, always obtain a 12-lead ECG to help distinguish between different tachycardia mechanisms. Supraventricular tachycardias most frequently occur in young patients without any structural heart disease. Patients with aberrant conduction typically manifest either a right or left bundle branch block with the QRS characteristics typical for these conditions, and AV dissociation is *never* seen. Patients with ventricular tachycardia are usually older and have significant structural heart disease, such as prior myocardial infarction. The defining characteristic is the presence of AV dissociation, but other features which favor the diagnosis of ventricular tachycardia include QRS > 0.14 second, right bundle branch block with a far left axis vector, and concordance of QRS vector in the precordial leads. If in doubt, assume the rhythm is ventricular tachycardia and treat accordingly.

15. Can a definitive diagnosis of the exact PSVT mechanism be made?

Although the 12-lead ECG and response to vagal maneuvers or medical interventions are frequently helpful in distinguishing causes of PSVT, the exact mechanism may remain unclear, even in cases of overt preexcitation (Wolff-Parkinson-White syndrome). A diagnostic electrophysiologic study can be very accurate in reproducing the arrhythmia and elucidating the underlying pathophysiologic substrate. These studies employ three to four temporary transvenous pacing electrode catheters placed in the right atrium, right ventricle, His bundle region, and coronary sinus to pace and record local electrical signals.

16. Does the patient with PSVT require treatment once an episode is terminated?

Except for patients with the Wolff-Parkinson-White syndrome in whom there is very rapid conduction over their accessory connection (manifest during atrial fibrillation or electrophysiologic study), most episodes of PSVT are not life-threatening. The frequency of arrhythmia recurrence and the need for medical intervention to terminate episodes influence the decision to treat individual patients. Medical therapies (digoxin, calcium channel blockers, beta blockers, and antiarrhythmic agents) are all associated with relatively high failure rates (often 40% in the first year). Patients with frequent arrhythmia recurrence or patients at risk for a more serious arrhythmia should be evaluated by a cardiac electrophysiologist so that risk and treatment strategies can be discussed.

17. What is radiofrequency ablation?

Ablative therapies, either direct current (100–200 joules) or radiofrequency (400–500 Hz), use intracardiac electrode catheters to map and then permanently destroy the local tissue (atrial or ventricular) that plays a critical role in the maintenance of a reentrant circuit or automatic rhythm. The cardiac electrophysiologist first performs a diagnostic electrophysiologic study to uncover the underlying tachycardia mechanism. Then, at the same or a separate setting, specialized mapping catheters are used to locate precisely and destroy the patient's abnormal electrical connection (i.e., the accessory connection in patients with Wolff-Parkinson-White syndrome). Radiofrequency ablation is generally regarded as the safer of the two procedures because the lesions created are smaller and more discrete. Radiofrequency ablation can be used to cure patients with the Wolff-Parkinson-White syndrome (accessory connection ablation), AV node reentry tachycardia ("slow" or "fast" pathway ablation), primary atrial tachycardia (automatic or "triggered" activity focus), as well as other, rarer forms of supraventricular tachycardia. The success rate in the first two conditions is > 90% and the procedure can be used in the very young to the elderly.

BIBLIOGRAPHY

1. Akhtar M, Shenasa M, Jazayeri M, et al: Wide QRS complex tachycardia: Reappraisal of a common clinical problem. Ann Intern Med 109:905, 1988.
2. Antman EM, Beamer AD, Cantillon C, et al: Therapy of refractory symptomatic atrial fibrillation and atrial flutter: A staged care approach with new antiarrhythmic drugs. J Am Coll Cardiol 15:698, 1990.
3. Becker AE, Anderson RH, Durrer D, et al: The anatomic substrates of Wolff-Parkinson-White syndrome. Circulation 57:870, 1978.
4. The Boston Area Anticoagulation Trial for Atrial Fibrillation Investigators: The effect of low-dose warfarin on the risk of stroke in patients with nonrheumatic atrial fibrillation. N Engl J Med 323:1505, 1990.
5. Connelly SJ, Laupacis A, Gent M, et al: Canadian Atrial Fibrillation Study (CAFA). J Am Coll Cardiol 18:349, 1991.
6. DiMarco PJ, Sellers TD, Lerman BB, et al: Diagnostic and therapeutic use of adenosine in patients with supraventricular tachyarrhythmias. J Am Coll Cardiol 6:417, 1985.
7. Falk RH, Podrid PJ (eds): Atrial Fibrillation: Mechanisms and Management. New York, Raven Press, 1992.
8. Jackman WM, Wang X, Friday KJ, et al: Catheter ablation of accessory atrioventricular pathways (Wolff-Parkinson-White syndrome) by radiofrequency current. N Engl J Med 324:1605, 1991.
9. Jackman WM, Beckman KJ, McClelland JH, et al: Treatment of supraventricular tachycardia due to atrioventricular nodal reentry by radiofrequency catheter ablation of slow pathway conduction. N Engl J Med 327:313, 1992.
10. Kannel W, Abbott R, Savage D, McNamara P: Epidemiologic features of chronic atrial fibrillation: The Framingham Study. N Engl J Med 306:1018, 1982.
11. Kay GN, Chong F, Epstein AE, et al: Radiofrequency ablation for treatment of primary atrial tachycardias. J Am Coll Cardiol 21:901, 1993.
12. Kopecky S, Gersh B, McGoon M, et al: The natural history of lone atrial fibrillation. N Engl J Med 317:669, 1987.
13. Morganroth J, Horowitz LN, Anderson J, et al: Comparative efficacy and tolerance of esmolol to propranolol for control of supraventricular tachyarrhythmia. Am J Cardiol 56:33F, 1985.
14. Pritchett E: Management of atrial fibrillation. N Engl J Med 326:1264, 1992.
15. Salerno DM, Dias VC, Kleiger RE, et al: Efficacy and safety of intravenous diltiazem for treatment of atrial fibrillation and atrial flutter. Am J Cardiol 63:1046, 1989.
16. Scheinman MM, Olgin JE: Comparison of high energy direct current and radiofrequency catheter ablation of the atrioventricular junction. J Am Coll Cardiol 21:557, 1993.
17. The Stroke Prevention in Atrial Fibrillation Investigators: Predictors of thromboembolism in atrial fibrillation: I. Clinical features of patients at risk. Ann Intern Med 116:1, 1992.
18. The Stroke Prevention in Atrial Fibrillation Investigators: Predictors of thromboembolism in atrial fibrillation: II. Echocardiographic features of patients at risk. Ann Intern Med 116:6, 1992.

14. VENTRICULAR TACHYCARDIA

William Bailey, MD

1. What is the differential diagnosis of a wide complex tachycardia?
Ventricular tachycardia
Supraventricular tachycardia with aberration
Supraventricular tachycardia using an accessory pathway (Wolff-Parkinson-White
  syndrome)
Hyperkalemia

2. What are the clinical characteristics of patients with ventricular tachycardia?
The majority of patients with recurrent sustained ventricular tachycardia have a history of ischemic coronary artery disease associated with previous infarction and aneurysm. The next largest group of patients have an underlying congestive or hypertrophic cardiomyopathy. The remainder have a primary electrical disorder (with or without a normal structural heart), valvular disorder, congenital heart disease (repaired or nonrepaired), metabolic disorder, or drug toxicity.

3. What presenting symptoms and features on physical exam may help to make the diagnosis of ventricular tachycardia?
The presenting symptoms of ventricular tachycardia in large part depend on the rate of the rhythm and the extent of underlying cardiac disease. The presenting symptoms can be modulated by coronary artery narrowing, carotid and peripheral vascular disease, ejection fraction, and even relative hydration of the patient. Concomitant medications also may play a role in the initial symptoms. Symptoms vary from minor palpitations, chest heaviness, and lightheadedness to frank syncope and cardiac arrest; most patients experience a constellation of symptoms between the two extremes.

The classic findings on physical exam depend on the interrelationship between atrial and ventricular contraction. If the patient is not capable of conducting an electrical impulse retrograde from the ventricle to the atrium, the classic findings of atrioventricular (AV) dissociation are present: variable intensity of the first heart sound, inconsistent relationship between the jugular a wave and the v wave, and occasional cannon a waves when the atrium and the ventricle contract simultaneously. Retrograde conduction is associated with a regularity to the cannon a waves, and the signs of AV dissociation are absent.

4. What three features of the rhythm strip of a wide complex tachycardia establish it as ventricular tachycardia?
The three classic features are fusion beats, capture beats, and AV dissociation. Fusion beats are an intermediate form between the wide complex rhythm and the narrow rhythm of sinus and represent simultaneous depolarization of the ventricle by both a supraventricular impulse and an impulse originating in the ventricle. This is best understood by mentally combining the wide ventricular beat with the narrow sinus beat. Capture beats are interspersed narrow complex beats that generally occur at a shorter interval than the tachycardia. P waves identical to P waves seen during sinus rhythm may precede. AV dissociation is the finding of independent atrial and ventricular activity at differing rates. Careful measurement with calipers shows differing rates for ventricular and atrial rhythms. These findings are uncommon but highly specific. AV dissociation is present in about 25% of patients with ventricular tachycardia, whereas fusion beats and capture beats are found in about 5%.

5. Which electrocardiographic characteristics help to differentiate ventricular tachycardia from supraventricular tachycardia with aberration?

Although rate has been proposed as a potential way to differentiate the two rhythms, it is highly unreliable in individual patients. A QRS width of greater than 140 msec strongly favors ventricular tachycardia, especially in the setting of a normal QRS during sinus rhythm. A leftward QRS axis strongly favors ventricular tachycardia. Concordance (identical QRS direction) in the precordial leads (V1–V6), especially negative concordance, is highly specific for the diagnosis of ventricular tachycardia. Certain QRS morphologic features also may be helpful. An atypical right bundle pattern (R > R'; in classic right bundle-branch block, R < R'), a monophasic or biphasic QRS in lead V1, and a small R wave coupled with a large deep S wave or a Q-S complex in V6 support the diagnosis of ventricular tachycardia of right bundle branch block morphology. The presence in V1 of an R wave of > 30 msec, notching of the downstroke of the S wave, a time > 60 msec from the onset of the R wave to the bottom of the S wave, and in lead V6 the presence of any small Q wave with a large R wave strongly favor the diagnosis of ventricular tachycardia with left bundle branch block morphology. The longest R-S interval also may be measured. The finding of a longest R-S interval in any precordial lead of > 100 msec is highly specific for the diagnosis of ventricular tachycardia.

Slowing or termination of a rhythm with vagal maneuvers strongly supports the diagnosis of supraventricular tachycardia with aberrancy. Clear linkage of the atrial and ventricular rhythm, presence of a classic bundle branch pattern, and a very short R to P interval (time from the onset of the QRS to the next P wave) characterize supraventricular tachycardia with aberrancy.

6. What critical decisions must be made in the management of ventricular tachycardia?
The critical decision in the management of a patient with sustained ventricular tachycardia is the urgency with which to treat the rhythm. In a patient who is hemodynamically stable, treatment should be delayed until a 12-lead electrocardiogram has been obtained. During the delay, a brief medical history and baseline laboratory values can be obtained. Specific attention should be paid to a history of myocardial infarction and potentially proarrhythmic drugs. If you are not sure about a drug, look it up. Levels of potassium and magnesium and appropriate drugs must be checked. Toxicologic screens should be obtained immediately on arrival in the emergency department.

7. Why is it important to obtain a 12-lead electrocardiogram?
The axis and morphology help to make the diagnosis of ventricular tachycardia, as well as shed light on the potential mechanism and origin of the rhythm. For example, a rhythm with a right bundle branch block morphology generally originates from the left ventricle and implies that the rhythm is secondary to ischemic heart disease with scar formation and/or aneurysm. Rhythms with left bundle branch block morphology generally originate from the right ventricle. Once the initial electrocardiographic data are obtained, a decision has to be made about the best way to terminate the rhythm. If there is any question about the patient's stability or if the clinical situation deteriorates, it is best to terminate the rhythm by cardioversion.

8. After the baseline data have been obtained, what method is used to terminate the rhythm?
With any question of hemodynamic instability, termination should be done immediately with synchronized DC electrical cardioversion. Hemodynamic instability is defined as hypotension resulting in shock; congestive heart failure; myocardial ischemia (infarction or angina); or signs or symptoms of inadequate cerebral perfusion. It is important to ensure that the energy is delivered in a synchronized fashion before cardioversion. Failure to do so may introduce the energy in a vulnerable period (into the T wave—late phase 3 in repolarization) and accelerate the rhythm or induce ventricular fibrillation.

Energy levels as low as 10 watt-seconds may be successful, but at the risk of ventricular fibrillation due to incomplete defibrillation of a critical mass of the myocardium sufficient to extinguish the rhythm. It is therefore wise to begin at a level of 100 watt-seconds. If the patient is conscious, adequate intravenous sedation should always be provided.

9. How is hemodynamically stable ventricular tachycardia terminated?

Termination of hemodynamically stable ventricular tachycardia may be attempted medically. Treatment is begun with intravenous lidocaine or procainamide, followed by a maintenance infusion if the drug is successful. Levels of the drug should be checked and used to guide maintenance infusion rates. Bretylium may be used if the rhythm is refractory to first-line drugs. Bretylium is associated with a high incidence of orthostatic hypotension. Although quinidine is available, its use is limited to the oral and intramuscular routes of administration because of the hypotension associated with intravenous use.

Other intravenous drugs that are still investigational include amiodarone and several class III agents.

10. How is medically unresponsive ventricular tachycardia treated?

Stable medically refractory ventricular tachycardia may be terminated by insertion of a temporary transvenous pacing wire and ventricular pacing. This method is most useful for patients who have frequent recurrences of a hemodynamically stable ventricular rhythm. There is a small risk (about 5%) of acceleration of the rhythm and/or inducing ventricular fibrillation. Provisions for immediate defibrillation should be in place when attempting pace termination. Pace termination should be done only by physicians with adequate training and experience. There is inadequate experience with transcutaneous pacing to recommend its use to terminate sustained ventricular tachycardia. Rhythms that are refractory to medical therapy also may be electrically cardioverted with synchronized DC shock and appropriate patient sedation.

11. Once the acute episode is terminated, how is recurrence prevented?

Any potentially reversible cause should be sought and treated—specifically, ischemia or electrolyte abnormalities. Antiarrhythmic drugs have been the mainstay of preventive therapy. Appropriate drug therapy has been guided by Holter monitor or electrophysiologic testing. When single-drug therapy has failed, combination regimens have been tried. The long-term clinical success of medical regimens is low. Sotalol and amiodarone are the most effective medications.

Recent technologic advances have given patients the option of an implantable antitachycardia cardioverter-defibrillator. Such devices are capable of sensing the rhythm continuously and responding with an appropriate algorithm (either pacing or defibrillation), as previously programmed by the physician. The success rate for rhythm termination is high. Studies are under way to determine if such devices prolong long-term survival. Additional options include ablation of the arrhythmia focus either with catheter or surgical ablation. Ablation and device therapy demand specialized training on the part of the physician.

BIBLIOGRAPHY

1. Ahktar M, Shensa M, Jazayeri M, et al: Wide QRS complex tachycardia: Reappraisal of a common clinical problem. Ann Intern Med 109:905–912, 1988.
2. Ahktar M: Clinical spectrum of ventricular tachycardia. Circulation 82:1561–1573, 1990.
3. Echt D, Liebson P, Mitchell B, et al: Mortality and morbidity in patients receiving encainide, flecanide, or placebo. N Engl J Med 324:781–788, 1991.
4. Mason J, ESVEM investigators: A comparison of electrophysiologic testing with holter monitoring to predict antiarrhythmic-drug efficacy for ventricular tachyarrhythmias. N Engl J Med 329:445–451, 1993.
5. Shensa M, Borggrefe M, Haverkamp W, et al: Ventricular tachycardia. Lancet 341:1512–1519, 1993.
6. Surawicz B: Ventricular arrhythmias: Why is it so difficult to find a pharmacologic cure? J Am Coll Cardiol 14:1401–1416, 1989.

15. CARDIAC PACING IN ATRIOVENTRICULAR BLOCK

William Bailey, M.D.

This chapter deals with the indications for pacing in the setting of atrioventricular (AV) block. Decisions about pacing arise in one of three settings: (1) acquired AV block, (2) AV block associated with myocardial infarction, and (3) bifascicular and trifascicular block. The indications presented are those for which there is widespread agreement that pacing is indicated and for which survival benefit is expected. Indications for which there is not a consensus are excluded.

1. What are the three types of acquired AV block?
There are three degrees of AV block: first, second, and third (complete). This classification is based on the electrocardiogram.

First-degree block refers to prolongation of the PR interval to > 200 msec and represents delay in conduction in the AV node. There are no accepted indications for pacing in isolated first-degree block.

Second-degree block is divided into two types. Type I (Wenckebach) exhibits progressive prolongation of the PR interval before an impulse fails to stimulate the ventricle. Anatomically this form of block occurs above the bundle of His in the AV node. Type II exhibits no prolongation of the PR interval before a dropped beat and anatomically occurs at the level of the bundle of His. This rhythm may be associated with a wide QRS complex. Advanced second-degree block refers to the block of two or more consecutive P waves.

Third-degree or complete block refers to complete dissociation of the atrial and ventricular rhythms, with a ventricular rate less than the atrial rate. The width and rate of the ventricular rhythm help to infer an anatomic location for the block: narrow QRS results in minimal slowing of the rate, generally at the AV node, and wide QRS in considerable slowing of rate at or below the bundle of His.

2. What is the most important clinical feature that establishes the need for cardiac pacing?
The most important clinical feature consists of symptoms clearly associated with bradycardia secondary to AV block. Reversible causes such as digoxin or beta blockers should be sought, and, when possible, the offending agents should be discontinued. This is not always possible, especially if a medication is necessary for the control of tachyrhythmia. Symptomatic bradycardia is the cardinal feature in the placement of a permanent pacemaker in acquired AV block in adults. The many clinical manifestations of symptomatic bradycardia include lightheadedness, dizziness, near syncope, frank syncope, manifestations of cerebral ischemia, dyspnea on exertion, decreased exercise tolerance, and even congestive heart failure.

3. In what clinical settings is placement of a pacemaker indicated in acquired AV block?
Pacing is indicated for third-degree (complete) block that is either permanent or paroxysmal when it is associated with symptoms that are clearly related to (1) bradycardia, (2) congestive heart failure, (3) treatment to suppress other rhythms or to control medical conditions (digitalis for congestive heart failure with agents that suppress automaticity of pacemaker tissue, (4) an escape rhythm < 40 beats/min or asystole for > 3.0 seconds (may be symptom free), (5) mental cloudiness that clearly resolves with temporary pacing, (5) ablation of the AV node, and (6) myotonic dystrophy.

Pacing is indicated in second-degree block, regardless of the site, when symptoms are clearly related to heart block.

Pacing is also indicated in the setting of atrial fibrillation or flutter when it is associated with complete third-degree block or advanced second-degree block resulting in bradycardia and any of the above conditions (1–6).

4. Does pacing in the setting of AV block and myocardial infarction require the presence of symptoms?

No. Symptoms related to the form of block are not a requirement. The indications in large part are treated to the intraventricular conduction defects that result from infarction. The prognosis of patients requiring pacing is influenced more by the extent of the infarction than by symptoms. Pacing in the setting of an acute myocardial infarction may be temporary rather than long-term or permanent.

5. What are the indications for pacing after myocardial infarction?

Indications in this setting do not require the presence of symptoms. Pacing is indicated in the setting of acute myocardial infarction for (1) complete third-degree block or advanced second-degree block that is associated with block in the His-Purkinje system (wide complex ventricular rhythm) and (2) transient advanced (second- or third-degree) AV block with a new bundle-branch block.

6. What is the anatomic location of bifascicular or trifascicular block?

Bifascicular or trifascicular block is located below the AV node and involves a combination of either two or three of the fascicles of the right or left bundle (divided into the left anterior and left posterior fascicle).

7. Are symptoms required for permanent pacing in the setting of bifascicular and trifascicular block?

Yes. Symptoms must be present in the setting of bifascicular and trifascicular block, just as in acquired AV block.

8. What are the indications for permanent pacing in bifascicular and trifascicular block?

Pacing is indicated when bifascicular or trifascicular block is associated with (1) complete block and symptomatic bradycardia or (2) intermittent type II second-degree block with or without related symptoms.

BIBLIOGRAPHY

1. Dreifus LS, Fisch C, Griffin JC, et al: Guidelines for implantation of cardiac pacemakers and antiarrhythmic devices. A Report of the American College of Cardiology/American Heart Association Task Force on Assessment of Diagnostic and Therapeutic Cardiovascular Procedures (Committee on Pacemaker Implantation). J Am Coll Cardiol 18:1–16, 1991.
2. Frye RL, Collins JJ, DeSanctis RW, et al: Guidelines for permanent cardiac pacemaker implantation, May 1984. A Report of the Joint American College of Cardiology/American Heart Association Task Force on Assessment of Cardiovascular Procedures (Subcommittee on Pacemaker Implantation). Circulation 70:331A–339A, 1984.
3. Frye RL, Collins JJ, DeSanctis RW, et al: Guidelines for permanent cardiac pacemaker implantation, May 1984. A Report of the Joint American College of Cardiology/American Heart Association Task Force on Assessment of Cardiovascular Procedures (Subcommittee on Pacemaker Implantation). J Am Coll Cardiol 4:434–442, 1984.
4. Pacemaker Study Group, Parsonnet V, Furman S, Smyth NPD, Bilitch M: Optimal resources for implantable cardiac pacemakers. Circulation 68:226A–244A, 1983.

IV. Symptoms and Disease States

16. CHEST PAIN

Howard D. Weinberger, M.D.

1. What is angina and what is it caused by?
Angina is a discomfort in the chest or adjacent area that is associated with myocardial ischemia without myocardial necrosis. Angina is due to an imbalance in myocardial oxygen supply and demand.

2. What factors contribute to myocardial oxygen supply and demand?
Myocardial oxygen supply may be decreased by hypoxia, coronary arterial vasoconstriction, atherosclerotic narrowing of one or more coronary arteries, a nonocclusive intracoronary thrombus, or a combination of two or more of these conditions. Myocardial oxygen demand may be increased by physical exertion, eating (by shunting blood to the gut for digestion), emotional stress (by increasing sympathetic stimulation), and increased metabolic demands (fever, tachycardia, thyrotoxicosis, etc.). Cold weather increases myocardial oxygen demand by increasing peripheral vascular resistance, causing the heart to work harder to maintain adequate peripheral perfusion.

3. Can the history provide any helpful clues in establishing the diagnosis of angina?
Yes. With a careful history and physical examination, the etiology of the patient's symptoms can be determined most of the time. The key features of the history that can help in making the diagnosis of angina are:
- Character and quality of the chest pain
- Location and radiation (if any) of the chest pain
- Precipitating, exacerbating, and relieving factors
- Duration of the chest pain
- Associated symptoms

4. What conditions increase the likelihood of a patient's chest pain being angina?
There are five major risk factors for coronary artery disease. The more risk factors present, the greater is the likelihood that any one patient's symptoms may be due to myocardial ischemia (angina). The risk factors are:
1. Smoking cigarettes
2. Hypertension
3. Elevated cholesterol
4. Diabetes mellitus
5. Family history of premature coronary artery disease (before age 60)

Not only are these factors important in helping to establish the diagnosis of angina (and therefore coronary artery disease), but all except family history can be modified to reduce the chances of developing (or of having progression of currently existent) coronary artery disease.

5. Besides myocardial ischemia, are there other conditions that cause angina-like chest pain?
Yes. Many entities may cause chest pain, several of which may produce symptoms similar to angina. The differential diagnosis of angina-like chest pain includes, but is not limited to:

Angina
Myocardial infarction
Pericarditis
Aortic dissection
Mitral valve prolapse
Pulmonary hypertension

Acute pulmonary embolus
Esophageal spasm
Chest wall pain
Peptic ulcer disease
Pancreatitis

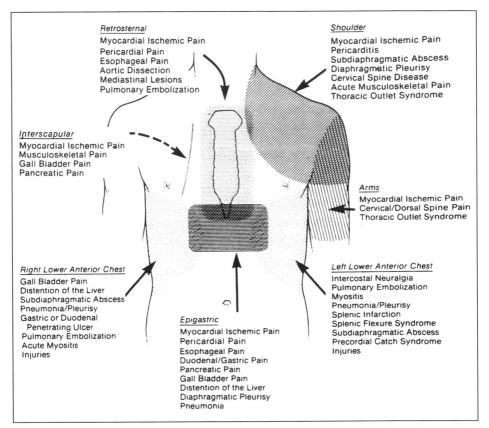

Retrosternal
Myocardial Ischemic Pain
Pericardial Pain
Esophageal Pain
Aortic Dissection
Mediastinal Lesions
Pulmonary Embolization

Shoulder
Myocardial Ischemic Pain
Pericarditis
Subdiaphragmatic Abscess
Diaphragmatic Pleurisy
Cervical Spine Disease
Acute Musculoskeletal Pain
Thoracic Outlet Syndrome

Interscapular
Myocardial Ischemic Pain
Musculoskeletal Pain
Gall Bladder Pain
Pancreatic Pain

Arms
Myocardial Ischemic Pain
Cervical/Dorsal Spine Pain
Thoracic Outlet Syndrome

Right Lower Anterior Chest
Gall Bladder Pain
Distention of the Liver
Subdiaphragmatic Abscess
Pneumonia/Pleurisy
Gastric or Duodenal
  Penetrating Ulcer
Pulmonary Embolization
Acute Myositis
Injuries

Epigastric
Myocardial Ischemic Pain
Pericardial Pain
Esophageal Pain
Duodenal/Gastric Pain
Pancreatic Pain
Gall Bladder Pain
Distention of the Liver
Diaphragmatic Pleurisy
Pneumonia

Left Lower Anterior Chest
Intercostal Neuralgia
Pulmonary Embolization
Myositis
Pneumonia/Pleurisy
Splenic Infarction
Splenic Flexure Syndrome
Subdiaphragmatic Abscess
Precordial Catch Syndrome
Injuries

Differential diagnosis of chest pain according to location where pain starts. (From Miller AJ: Diagnosis of Chest Pain. New York, Raven Press, 1988, p 175; with permission.)

6. How do patients describe anginal chest pain?

Patients may not refer to their symptoms as true "pain." They may describe a deep discomfort or unpleasant sensation that is hard to define, often as a pressure sensation, tightness, squeezing, or "weight on the chest." Angina is *not* pleuritic or positional.

7. How long does an episode of angina last?

Angina may last from 2–5 minutes after cessation of exercise or taking nitroglycerin. If symptoms last longer than 20 minutes, they are usually due to myocardial necrosis (myocardial infarction) or are noncardiac in etiology. Brief, fleeting pains are rarely cardiac in origin.

8. What factors may induce or exacerbate angina, and what may relieve it?

Anything that increases cardiac work (myocardial oxygen demand) and/or decreases myocardial oxygen supply may precipitate or worsen angina. Rest, by decreasing myocardial work and oxygen demand, often relieves angina. Nitroglycerin, which dilates coronary arteries, allowing increased blood flow and oxygen delivery to the myocardium, also relieves angina.

9. Where is anginal pain felt and where may it radiate?

Anginal chest pain may occur anywhere between the diaphragm and mandible, but it is most often substernal or on the left side of the chest. It tends to be diffuse and not localized to a small discrete area. It may radiate to the neck, throat, mandible, shoulder, or arm (usually the inner aspect of the arm and more commonly the left arm).

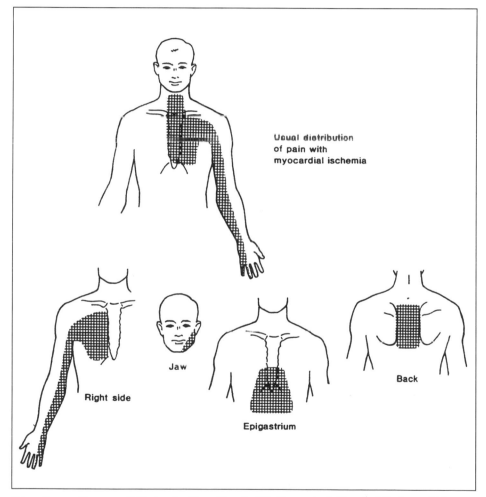

Pain patterns with myocardial ischemia. (From Horwitz LD: Chest pain. In Horwitz LD, Groves BM, (eds): Signs and Symptoms in Cardiology, Philadelphia, J.B. Lippincott, 1985, p 9; with permission.)

10. What are the classic associated symptoms for myocardial ischemia?

In addition to typical anginal chest pain, one or more of the following may be observed:
- Shortness of breath
- Diaphoresis
- Nausea and emesis

Differential Diagnosis of Episodic Chest Pain Resembling Angina

	DURATION	QUALITY	PROVOCATION	RELIEF	LOCATION	COMMENT
Effort angina	5–15 min	Visceral (pressure)	Effort or emotion	Rest, nitroglycerin	Substernal, radiates	First episode vivid
Rest angina	5–15 min	Visceral (pressure)	Spontaneous (? with exercise)	Nitroglycerin	Substernal, radiates	Often nocturnal
Mitral prolapse	Minutes to hours	Superficial (rarely visceral)	Spontaneous (no pattern)	Time	Left anterior	No pattern, variable character
Esophageal reflux	10 min to 1 hr	Visceral	Recumbency, lack of food	Food, antacid	Substernal, epigastric	Rarely radiates
Esophageal spasm	5–60 min	Visceral	Spontaneous, cold liquids, exercise	Nitroglycerin	Substernal, radiates	Mimics angina
Peptic ulcer	Hours	Visceral, burning	Lack of food "acid" foods	Foods, antacids	Epigastric, substernal	—
Biliary disease	Hours	Visceral (waxes and wanes)	Spontaneous food	Time, analgesia	Epigastric, ? radiates	Colic
Cervical disc	Variable (gradually subsides)	Superficial	Head and neck movement, palpation	Time, analgesia	Arm, neck	Not relieved by rest
Hyperventilation	2–3 min	Visceral	Emotion, tachypnea	Stimulus removal	Substernal	Facial paresthesia
Musculoskeletal	Variable	Superficial	Movement, palpation	Time, analgesia	Multiple	Tenderness
Pulmonary	30 min +	Visceral (pressure)	Often spontaneous	Rest, time, bronchodilator	Substernal	Dyspneic

From Christie LG Jr, Conti CR: Systematic approach to the evaluation of angina-like chest pain. Am Heart J 102:897, 1981; with permission.

11. What findings on the physical examination may be seen with myocardial ischemia?
The physical findings may be normal. An **S₄gallop** (4th heart sound) is due to atrial contraction against a stiff or noncompliant ventricle. If an S_4gallop is heard with symptoms and disappears as the symptoms resolve, this suggests transient ventricular noncompliance (from ischemia) and is strong evidence for myocardial ischemia. An S_4gallop may be present before symptoms develop (and then will likely be present after symptoms resolve) due to other causes of ventricular noncompliance (left ventricular hypertrophy, hypertension, aortic stenosis, previous myocardial infarction, etc.). Evidence of **congestive heart failure** may exist (elevated jugular venous pressure, pulmonary râles, S_3gallop). There may be a visible and/or palpable **dyskinetic bulge** of the chest wall during active ischemia or infarction. **Murmurs,** especially if new, may suggest ischemic-related processes. Papillary muscle ischemia may lead to mitral regurgitation. Rupture of the interventricular septum will produce a ventricular septal defect and its associated murmur. Aortic stenosis and hypertrophic obstructive cardiomyopathy have characteristic murmurs and can cause myocardial ischemia and symptoms of angina.

12. What changes on the 12-lead electrocardiogram (ECG) may be seen with myocardial ischemia?
The classic ECG changes of myocardial ischemia are horizontal ST-segment depression in leads corresponding to the anatomic regions of the heart. ST depression is neither 100% sensitive (there can be myocardial ischemia and angina without ST depression) nor 100% specific (not all ST depression represents myocardial ischemia). ECG changes associated with symptoms that resolve as the symptoms resolve more strongly suggest myocardial ischemia.

13. How do you differentiate between angina and myocardial infarction?
The symptoms of an acute myocardial infarction are usually more intense, longer in duration (1–8 hours), and more often associated with shortness of breath, diaphoresis, nausea, and emesis. In addition, the 12-lead ECG shows ST-segment elevation rather than depression and may show T-wave inversion and/or pathologic Q waves.

BIBLIOGRAPHY

1. Braunwald E (ed): Heart Disease: A Textbook of Cardiovascular Medicine, 4th ed. Philadelphia, W.B. Saunders, 1992.
2. Donat WE: Chest pain: Cardiac and noncardiac causes. Clin Chest Med 8:241–252, 1987.
3. Hammermeister KE: Cardiac and aortic pain. In Bonica JJ (ed): The Management of Pain. Philadelphia, Lea & Febiger, 1990, pp 1001–1042.
4. Lee MG, Sullivan SN, Watson WC, Melendez LJ: Chest pain—esophageal, cardiac, or both? Am J Gastroenterol 80:320–324, 1985.
5. Nevens F, Janssens J, Piessens J, et al: Prospective study on prevalence of esophageal chest pain in patients referred on an elective basis to a cardiac unit for suspected myocardial ischemia. Dig Dis Sci 36:229–235, 1991.

17. ANGINA

Stephen T. Crowley, M.D., FACC

1. What are the characteristics features of angina?

Angina is chest discomfort associated with myocardial ischemia. Typically, it is described as substernal discomfort, pressure, heaviness, or a weight-like sensation that often radiates across the mid-thorax, into the left arm (ulnar aspect), neck, or jaw. It is also associated with shortness of breath, diaphoresis, and nausea. Angina is often related to precipitating causes, the most common of which is exertion. Other precipitating factors include stress or emotion and secondary conditions such as anemia, tachycardia, or aortic stenosis. Angina discomfort usually occurs for at least 30 seconds and < 15 minutes and is typically relieved with rest or nitroglycerin. Because angina is a visceral sensation, it is poorly localized, and patients therefore rarely point to the location of their discomfort with one finger.

2. What is the differential diagnosis of a patient presenting with chest pain?

Differential Diagnosis of Chest Pain

CONDITION	QUALITY OF PAIN
Cardiac causes	
Aortic stenosis	Angina-like chest pain
Hypertropic cardiomyopathy	Angina-like chest pain associated with dyspnea
Acute periocarditis	Sharper in quality, lasts for hours, not affected by effort, positional
Aortic aneurysm	Localized, radiates to back, severe
Mitral valve prolapse	Variable in character
Syndrome X	Angina-like chest pain
Noncardiac causes	
Esophageal disorders (reflux or spasm)	Often spontaneous, rarely radiates, relieved by food or antacids
Peptic ulcer or gastritis	More epigastric, lasts for hours, related to food ingestion
Costochondritis and musculoskeletal syndromes	Exacerbated with inspiration, movement, or palpation; superficial
Pulmonary hypertension	Frequently spontaneous and associated with dyspnea

3. What is the relationship between clinical presentation and coronary anatomy in patients with chest pain?

Patients who present with chest pain can be divided into three subsets:
- Typical angina
- Atypical angina
- Nonanginal chest pain.

The incidence of coronary artery disease in these patient subsets is approximately 90%, 50%, and 16%, respectively. In many instances, the clinical-pathologic correlation is poor, such as in patients with advanced coronary artery disease who have silent ischemia or those with Prinzmetal's angina (vasospastic) who have severe angina but usually minimal or no coronary atherosclerosis.

4. Compare underlying pathophysiologic mechanisms in angina and unstable angina.

Stable angina is most commonly related to an increase in myocardial oxygen demand triggered by physical activity. Invariably, a fixed coronary artery obstruction is present, which limits oxygen delivery during times of increased metabolic demands. The severity of the obstruction determines the threshold for cardiac ischemia.

Recently, it has become apparent that angina also can be caused by transient decreases in oxygen delivery due to coronary vasoconstriction. Nonocclusive intracoronary thrombi are usually present in patients with **unstable angina** and cause acute impairment in oxygen delivery. Intracoronary thrombi and platelet aggregation occur in unstable or "ruptured" coronary artery plaques. The local release of vasoactive compounds, such as serotonin and thromboxane A_2, is thought to mediate acute vasoconstriction in patients with unstable angina.

5. What role does exercise ECG have in the diagnosis of coronary artery disease (CAD)?

In patients with a chest pain syndrome of uncertain etiology and a normal resting ECG, a standard exercise test is useful in the diagnosis of CAD.

1. Exercise ECG testing *adds little* in detecting the presence or absence of CAD in patients with a *high pretest probability* of CAD (i.e., history of typical angina with one or more risk factors).

2. Exercise testing is *most valuable* in confirming or excluding the diagnosis of CAD in patients with an *intermediate pretest probability* of CAD. Typically, these are patients with some atypical anginal features and a normal ECG, who may or may not have risk factors for CAD. In such patients, if typical anginal discomfort occurs during exercise and is associated with ≥ 1-mm ST-segment depression (horizontal or downsloping in nature), the predictive value for the diagnosis of CAD is > 90%. If a ≥ 2-mm ST-segment depression occurs with typical angina, this finding is virtually diagnostic of CAD. An exercise ECG test associated with a hypotensive blood pressure response carries an 80% predictive value for significant CAD.

A negative exercise test in a patient with a *low pretest probability* of CAD is *highly reliable* in excluding the diagnosis of significant CAD.

6. How is prognosis assessed in patients with angina?

Prognosis of patients with angina is most easily assessed by an exercise stress test. Performance on an exercise test is strongly dependent on left ventricular function and the severity of CAD. Exercise duration or capacity during exercise testing is independently predictive of survival. Patients who exercise to stage 4 of a Bruce protocol have an 8-year survival rate of 93%, compared to a survival of only 45% in those who stop in stage 1. Exercise-induced hypotension correlates with left main or multivessel CAD and indicates a threefold increase in risk for subsequent death or myocardial infarction. Likewise, early-onset ST-segment depression during exercise is associated with a worse outcome. Patients with multivessel disease and impaired left ventricular function have a poor prognosis with medical therapy and strongly benefit from coronary artery bypass surgery. Multiple thallium-201 redistribution defects are also highly predictive of multivessel or left main artery disease and therefore predictive of a worse prognosis.

7. How effective is risk factor modification in improving the prognosis of patients with angina?

Risk factor modification is effective in reducing risk for cardiac events in patients who are asymptomatic or do not carry a diagnosis of CAD. Once symptoms of angina have appeared, there are still benefits of risk factor modification are less. Risk factor modification is a vital part of the management of patients with angina.

- Control of **hyperlipidemia** in patients with CAD and prior myocardial infarction can reduce the risk of nonfatal myocardial infarction by 27% and fatal infarction by 15%.
- **Smoking** increases the relative risk for myocardial infarction 2.8-fold, and this risk is substantially reduced after patients quit smoking. Cessation of smoking after coronary artery bypass grafting also improves graft patency and prognosis.
- How effective **blood pressure control** is on preventing subsequent cardiac mortality in patients with known CAD has not been well studied. Hypertension is a well-established major risk factor for the development of CAD, but numerous trials have indicated a lack of

effect of antihypertensives on CAD mortality, which may reflect the adverse effects of certain drugs on glucose tolerance, lipid levels, and insulin resistance.

8. What is the optimal medical management for patients with angina?

Aspirin has been shown to reduce the risk of myocardial infarction by 87% during a 5-year follow-up in men with chronic stable angina. It should be given to all patients with angina who are without contraindications to the drug.

Aspirin and β-**blockers** have both been shown to improve survival in patients with prior myocardial infarction and to reduce the incidence of reinfarction. If tolerated, β-blockers should be used in these patients. Whether β-blockers improve survival in patients with chronic stable angina is not clear, yet they are clearly indicated for patients with hypertension and angina and are primary therapy for effort-induced stable angina.

Nitroglycerin administered sublingually is the drug of choice for treatment of acute angina episodes. Sublingual nitroglycerin is also very effective as a prophylactic to prevent an anticipated angina attack.

Because of problems with marked variations in plasma concentration and tolerance, long-acting oral **nitrates** are often used as secondary therapy.

In patients with variable-threshold angina, in whom anginal episodes can occur due to increased oxygen demand or concomitant coronary vasoconstriction, a **calcium channel blocker** is the treatment of choice. Such patients have anginal patterns that vary considerably due to presumed vasoconstriction acting on a fixed obstructive lesion. Calcium channel blockers are also preferable in patients with variant or Prinzmetal's angina. β-Blockers and verapamil should be avoided in patients with overt congestive heart failure and a left ventricular ejection fraction of < 30%.

9. Define unstable angina.

Unstable angina is a poorly defined syndrome but includes patients with either: (1) crescendo angina (more severe or frequent) superimposed on chronic stable angina; (2) angina at rest or with minimal activity; or (3) new-onset angina (within 1 month) which is brought on by minimal exertion. Unstable angina describes a very heterogenous population with single or multivessel disease, with or without prior myocardial infarction, and an uncertain outcome. Unstable angina can be classified according to severity (accelerating angina versus angina at rest, acute), clinical circumstances (secondary to other extrinsic conditions or primary), and intensity of treatment.

10. What clinical markers predict adverse outcomes in patients with unstable angina?

Although left ventricular function and the extent of CAD ultimately determine long-term prognosis, recognition of certain clinical markers in patients with unstable angina is of value in defining management strategies:

- Recurrence of chest pain within 48 hours after admission carries a reduction in survival by 20% in patients with crescendo angina.
- ECG changes consistent with ischemia on admission predict recurrence of ischemia, myocardial infarction, or need for revascularization in 80% of patients.
- Postinfarction angina within 24 hours confers a 10% reduction in survival during the next year compared to asymptomatic patients.
- Rapidly accelerating symptoms of angina are the main determinant of prognosis in new-onset angina.

Aggressive medical management and early coronary angiography are indicated in these patient subsets.

11. What is the approach to management in patients with unstable angina?

Unstable angina is a potentially dangerous condition, and management should be tailored to prevent adverse outcomes. Patients should be admitted to the cardiac care unit, placed at bedrest, and begun on antianginal therapy with either β-blockers or calcium channel blockers, aspirin, and intravenous nitrates. β-Blockers, when added to nitrates, have been shown to reduce symptoms of recurrent ischemia and the occurrence of myocardial infarction. Intravenous heparin should be added to the regimen of patients who present with rest angina within 48 hours or those with chest pain and ischemic ECG changes on admission. Heparin significantly reduces in-hospital cardiac events, including myocardial infarction. Aspirin also decreases recurrent ischemia and infarctions in patients with unstable angina, although neither aspirin nor heparin taken as sole therapy appears to be better than the other. Long-term aspirin therapy should be given to all patients with unstable angina without contraindications, because it reduces the incidence of nonfatal myocardial infarction and death. Most patients with unstable angina will stabilize on this regimen of medical therapy.

A small percentage of patients will develop medically refractory rest angina. Treatment with intraaortic balloon counterpulsation is usually effective in stabilizing patients with refractory symptoms or poor hemodynamic profiles. This technique is useful to stabilize patients before and during cardiac catheterization.

Although most patients with unstable angina have nonocclusive intracoronary thrombi, to date the use of thrombolytic agents has not demonstrated a benefit in recurrent ischemia, myocardial infarction, or mortality when compared to heparin or aspirin. A large-scale randomized trial addressing this issue is in progress.

12. How useful is the resting ECG in evaluating patients with angina?

A resting ECG should be obtained in all patients who complain of chest discomfort. In patients with chronic stable angina, the ECG is normal in one-third of patients and, if abnormal, most often shows nonspecific ST-T changes without evidence for myocardial infarction.

The presence of left bundle branch block in patients with angina is often associated with significant left ventricular dysfunction and may reflect multivessel CAD. The presence of Q waves is usually a specific but insensitive indicator of myocardial infarction. Ischemic ST-segment deviations (depressions or elevations) and/or T-wave inversions occur commonly in patients with unstable angina; these changes usually resolve with relief of pain. New persistent symmetric T-wave inversion in the anterior precordial leads is a marker for high-grade left anterior descending or left main artery disease, and it should be recognized that these patients are at increased risk for infarction. Persistence of ST and T-wave changes may also suggest a non-Q wave infarction.

There is a fairly close correlation between ischemic ECG lead abnormalities and the anatomic site of coronary obstruction. Ischemic changes in the inferior leads (II, III, aVF) indicate right coronary or circumflex artery disease. Abnormal changes in the anterior precordial leads suggest left anterior descending artery disease, and changes in the left lateral (V_2–V_4) or high lateral leads (I, aVL) imply either diagonal or circumflex artery disease.

13. What are the indications for cardiac catheterization in patients with angina?

Cardiac catheterization and coronary angiography should be performed if the diagnosis of CAD cannot be reliably made by noninvasive diagnostic tests. Whether all patients with unstable angina need catheterization is controversial. Clearly, those patients with unstable angina who carry high-risk clinical markers need coronary angiography. An argument can be made to assess those patients with low-risk clinical profiles and who respond quickly to medical therapy with a noninvasive test such as a stress thallium scan. Catheterization is indicated for patients with chronic stable angina who begin to "break through" or fail medical therapy. Patients under age 50 who present with angina may also benefit from coronary angiography, since some of these patients may have advanced multivessel CAD or significant coronary anomalies. Patient age, in itself, is not a contraindication to catheterization, but patients who are not candidates for either angioplasty or bypass grafting and who have another life-threatening illness usually do not need cardiac catherterization.

BIBLIOGRAPHY

1. Braunwald E: Unstable angina: A classification. Circulation 80:410–414, 1989.
2. Conti CR, Hill JA, Mayfield WR: Unstable angina pectoris: Pathogenesis and management. Curr Probl Cardiol 14:549–624, 1989.
3. Kannel WB: Detection and management of patients with silent myocardial ischemia. Am Heart J 117:221–226, 1989.
4. Munger TM, Oh JK: Unstable angina. Mayo Clin Proc 65:384–406, 1990.
5. Ridker PM, Manson JE, Gaziano JM, et al: Low dose aspirin therapy for chronic stable angina: A randomized, placebo-controlled clinical trial. Ann Intern Med 114:835–839, 1991.
6. Shah PK: Pathophysiology of unstable angina. Cardiol Clin 9:11–26, 1991.
7. Vane JR, Anggard EE, Botting RM: Regulatory functions of the vascular endothelium. N Engl J Med 323:27–36, 1990.
8. Yasue H, Takizawa A, Nagao M, et al: Long-term prognosis for patients with variant angina and influential factors. Circulation 78:1–9, 1988.

18. MYOCARDIAL INFARCTION

Nelson P. Trujillo, M.D., and JoAnn Lindenfeld, M.D.

1. What are the known risk factors for coronary artery disease?

The known risk factors for coronary artery disease include:

1. Dyslipidemias (total cholesterol > 200 mg/dL, low density lipoprotein cholesterol > 160 mg/dL, increased triglycerides, and high density lipoprotein cholesterol < 35 mg/dL
2. Age
3. Male sex
4. Tobacco use
5. Hypertension
6. Sedentary lifestyle
7. Obesity
8. Family history (first myocardial infarction in a first-degree relative at < 55 years)
9. Diabetes mellitus.

Other more controversial risk factors include elevated apoprotein a, alcohol use, stress, hyperinsulinemia, elevated fibrinogen levels, left ventricular hypertrophy, type A personality behavior, angiotensin-converting enzyme (ACE) genotype, and cocaine use.

2. What is the pathophysiology of acute myocardial infarction?

The pathophysiology of acute myocardial infarction is currently based on observations made in 1912 by Herrick and reconfirmed in 1980 by Dewood. They described occlusion of stenotic coronary arteries by thrombus in the setting of acute myocardial infarction. Thrombus formation most often results in the setting of a ruptured atherosclerotic plaque. The degree of obstruction and thrombus is variable and due of multiple factors including dysfunctional coronary endothelium, extent of obstruction, platelet aggregation, and altered vasomotor tone. These mechanisms are believed to be responsible for at least 85% of all myocardial infarctions.

Other mechanisms of myocardial infarction include coronary artery vasculitis, embolic phenomena, coronary artery spasm, congenital abnormalities, and increased blood viscosity. Cocaine-induced myocardial infarction is thought to be multifactorial since severe vasospasm and acute thrombus have been described in both stenotic and normal coronary arteries.

In most patients, no precipitating cause for ruptured plaques resulting in myocardial infarction can be found. A modest relationship to heavy exercise, emotional stress, trauma, and neurologic disturbances has been described. Early-morning predilection for acute myocardial infarction has also been demonstrated and may be related to circadian rises in catecholamines and platelet aggregation.

3. Describe the typical signs and symptoms of acute myocardial infarction.

The classic symptoms of myocardial infarction include dull substernal chest pain, dyspnea, nausea, diaphoresis, palpitations, or sense of impending doom. The chest pain typically lasts at least 15–30 minutes and may radiate into the arms, jaw, or back. The elderly often have atypical presentations, such as dyspnea, confusion, vertigo, syncope, and abdominal pain. Approximately 25% of myocardial infarctions are either asymptomatic or unrecognized and are termed *silent*.

General examination findings include pallor, diaphoresis, and anxiety. Abnormalities in blood pressure, heart rate, and respiratory rate are variable, depending on the type and extent of infarction. A low-grade fever may be present. A fourth heart sound is almost always present. Jugular venous distention and a third sound may occur, depending on the site and extent of infarction. Precordial friction rubs and peripheral edema may be present later but are not usually present in the first few hours after infarction. In the setting of papillary muscle dysfunction or rupture, the murmur of mitral regurgitation may be present, although it is often much shorter and softer than expected.

4. How is the diagnosis of acute myocardial infarction made?

The diagnosis of myocardial infarction is made on the basis of clinical presentation, electrocardiographic (ECG) findings, and elevated serum enzymes. Classic ECG findings of acute **Q-wave myocardial infarction** initially include hyperacute T waves and ST-segment elevation. T-wave inversion and the development of Q waves follow over hours to days. In **nontransmural infarction,** ECG findings are less specific and include T-wave inversion and ST-segment depression. It is important to note that the ECG is normal in 20% of acute myocardial infarctions. **Right ventricular infarction** can be diagnosed using right-sided precordial ECG leads. ST elevation of 0.5 mm or more in V_3R-V_6R is diagnostic. Precordial lead V_4R is the most sensitive. Right-sided ECG leads should be obtained routinely in the setting of inferior ischemia.

Creatinine kinase (CK), lactate dehydrogenase (LDH), and serum glutamic oxaloacetic transferase (AST, SGOT) are enzymes used in making the diagnosis of infarction. **CK** rises within 6–8 hours of infarction, peaks at 24 hours, and normalizes by 48–96 hours. **CK-MB** is an isoenzyme of CK found almost exclusively in myocardium and is the cornerstone of enzymatic diagnosis. Elevations in CK-MB have also been reported with myocarditis, cardiac defibrillation, cardiac surgery, cardiac contusions, and prolonged ischemia without infarction. It may be falsely elevated in renal failure and hypothyroidism. **LDH** and its isoenzymes also rise in myocardial infarction, beginning at 24–48 hours, peaking in 3–5 days, and normalizing in 7–10 days. A ratio of isoenzymes LDH_1/LDH_2 of > 1.0 is sensitive for myocardial infarction. **SGOT** levels usually peak in 48–72 hours, although this enzyme is not specific for myocardial infarction and has been replaced by CK measurements.

Echocardiography may have a limited role in the diagnosis of myocardial infarction by demonstrating new wall-motion abnormalities when the ECG is nondiagnostic. This tool is essential in diagnosing mechanical complications and will be discussed later.

5. What are the differences between Q-wave and non-Q-wave myocardial infarction?

Q-wave infarction (once called *transmural* infarction) represents 60–70% of all acute myocardial infarctions and generally occurs when the ECG initially shows ST elevation and there is no intervention. Non–Q-wave infarction (once referred to as *subendocardial* infarction) represents 30–40% of all acute infarctions. Pathologically, non–Q-wave infarctions may exhibit complete transmural involvement. Thus, the terms transmural and subendocardial infarction have been replaced by the terms Q-wave and non–Q-wave infarction as defined by the development of Q waves postinfarction.

Non–Q-wave infarction	*Q-wave infarction*
Nonspecific ST or T-wave changes or ST depression	ST-segment elevation
10–20% early total occlusion rate in infarct-related vessels	90% early total occlusion rate in infarct-related vessels
Lower CK peaks	Higher CK peaks
Higher ejection fractions	Lower ejection fractions
Less wall-motion abnormalities	Wall-motion abnormalities more frequent
Higher early reinfarction rate (40%)	Higher early morbidity (1.5–2 times increased)

The 3-year mortality is the same in the two groups. Up to 60% of patients with non–Q-wave myocardial infarction have significant two- or three-vessel coronary artery disease. In light of this, many physicians suggest early angiography to stratify the risk in these patients. Calcium channel blockers may affect the short-term reinfarction rate in non–Q-wave infarction but have not been shown to improve mortality. In non–Q-wave infarction, the benefit of routine acute therapy with thrombolytic agents or percutaneous transluminal angioplasty has not been definitively proven.

6. What is the initial management of acute myocardial infarction?

The cornerstone of management of acute myocardial infarction is prompt emergency care. Initial therapy in the field should include oxygen, nitroglycerin, morphine (if hypotension is not present), rapid transport to an emergency department, and evaluation for thrombolytic therapy. On arrival at the hospital, assessment should focus on hemodynamic stability and eligibility for thrombolytic therapy or emergency angioplasty. All patients should be given aspirin if there are no contraindications.

7. What forms of therapy can result in reperfusion?
1. Prompt use of thrombolytic agents
2. Percutaneous transluminal coronary angioplasty (PTCA)
3. Coronary artery bypass surgery (CABG)

8. Explain the recommendations for thrombolytic therapy.
Thrombolytic therapy should be considered in all patients with presumed acute myocardial infarction and ST elevation or new left bundle branch block. The benefit of thrombolytic therapy in these patients has been demonstrated in numerous studies, where it routinely decreased mortality, improved left ventricular function, was associated with fewer arrhythmias, and improved long-term survival. Thrombolytic therapy accelerates the conversion of plasminogen to plasmin, an enzyme which dissolves fibrin clots, enhancing endogenous fibrinolysis. Nearly 80% of thrombosed arteries can be opened with thrombolytic therapy; however, there is a 15–20% reocclusion rate. The choice of thrombolytic agents is controversial. Currently approved agents and regimes are shown in the accompanying table.

Timely use of thrombolytic therapy seems to be the most important factor in predicting who will benefit. The use of thrombolytic agents within 6 hours of presentation confers the most survival benefit, although effectiveness has been shown up to 12 hours. More recent data suggest the accelerated tPA may provide some survival benefit over other regimens. Adjunctive therapy for thrombolysis includes aspirin and heparin to prevent reocclusion. Heparin is necessary in conjunction with tPA but is probably not necessary with streptokinase or APSAC. Better agents are being developed and include thrombin-specific inhibitors (hirudin) and other platelet inhibitors.

Thrombolytic Regimens for Acute Myocardial Infarction

Streptokinase	1.5 million units IV over 1 hr
APSAC*	30 units IV over 2–5 min
Tissue plasminogen activator (tPA)†	
Standard	IV: 10-mg bolus, 50 mg in first hour, 20 mg each in second and third hours (+ heparin)
Accelerated	IV: 15-mg bolus, 0.75 mg/kg over 30 min up to 50 mg, then 0.5 mg/kg up to 35 mg over the next 1 hr (+ heparin)

*APSAC = anisoylated plasminogen–streptokinase activator complex.
†Heparin is generally recommended for both tPA regimens as a 5000-U bolus, followed by an IV (intravenous) infusion of 1000 U/hr (1200 U/hr in patients >80 kg), with dose adjustments to raise the activated partial thromboplastin time (aPTT) to 60–85 seconds.

9. Are there contraindications to thrombolytic therapy?
1. Absolute contraindications
Active bleeding
Puncture of a noncompressible vessel
Possible aortic dissection
Active intracranial malignancy
Recent major surgery (< 1 wk)
Acute pericarditis
Previous drug allergy (to streptokinase or APSAC)

2. Relative contraindications
Major trauma or surgery in last 6–8 wks   Severe uncontrolled hypertension
Recent stroke or brain tumor   Pregnancy
Prolonged cardiopulmonary resuscitation   History of bleeding diathesis
History of peptic ulcer disease   Cancer
Diabetic retinopathy   Severe hepatic dysfunction

10. What are the possible complications?
Both minor and major complications with thrombolytic therapy have been reported. Allergic reactions have been described with streptokinase and APSAC secondary to streptokinase antibodies. Hypotension is more frequent with streptokinase than tPA. The major complications of thrombolytic therapy are directly related to impairment of hemostasis and are far more common in the presence of a vascular procedure. In the absence of a vascular procedure, major bleeding occurs in 0.1–0.3% of patients and hemorrhagic cerebral infarctions occur in up to 0.6%.

11. How do you reverse thrombolytic therapy?
Bleeding complications occur in 5% of patients receiving thrombolytic therapy and may be divided into major and minor events. Intracranial bleeding is the most severe and occurs in 0.2–0.6% of cases, with a 50–75% mortality. Fortunately, 70% of all bleeding complications occur at the site of an invasive procedure and can be controlled locally. Treatment of bleeding complications should be tailored to the individual.

In the initial evaluation of the bleeding patient, all vascular sites should be inspected and pressure applied as needed. Blood should be sent for crossmatch testing. Heparin and any antiplatelet drugs therapies should be discontinued. If necessary, protamine may be given to reverse the heparin effect (1 mg protamine/100 U heparin not to exceed 50 mg in 10 min). For severe bleeding, cryoprecipitate and fresh frozen plasma should be given, especially if the fibrinogen level is < 100 mg/dL. Platelets can be given when the bleeding time is prolonged. If life-threatening bleeding continues, antifibrinolytic drugs may be considered.

12. What are the indications for primary and secondary use of percutaenous transluminal coronary angioplasty (PTCA)?
Indications for the use of PTCA in myocardial infarction are evolving. At present, PTCA should be considered in patients with contraindications to thrombolytic therapy, when lytic therapy has failed, and in high-risk patients (age >70 years, anterior myocardial infarction, persistent sinus tachycardia, or cardiogenic shock).

Primary PTCA for myocardial infarction has been demonstrated to be safe and effective. Patency rates exceed 90%, and lower rates of serious bleeding, recurrent ischemia, and death have been reported compared to thrombolytic therapy in high-risk patients. However, primary PTCA should be considered instead of thrombolytic therapy only if it can be performed quickly. Unfortunately, at present only 18% of U.S. hospitals can perform PTCA, and surgical back-up should be available in case of emergency. The overall goal in patients with myocardial infarction is safe, prompt restoration of antegrade flow in the occluded artery with whatever method is available. There is no role for early and routine PTCA in patients who have received successful thrombolytic therapy.

13. Is there a role for surgery in acute myocardial infarction?
Coronary artery bypass graft surgery (CABG) can be used in acute myocardial infarction as both primary and secondary therapy. Patients with recurrent ischemia uncontrolled by medical therapy who are ineligible for PTCA may require emergent CABG. Operative mortality is increased in the peri-infarction period, primarily in patients with poor hemodynamics, congestive heart failure, and advanced age.

14. What arrhythmias occur in acute myocardial infarction?
Both supraventricular and ventricular arrhythmias are seen in acute myocardial infarction. Of **supraventricular arrhythmias,** sinus bradycardia is present most commonly with inferior infarction and suggests a better prognosis. Sinus tachycardia (heart rate > 100 bpm) in acute myocardial infarction may be caused by pain, anxiety, left ventricular dysfunction, hypovolemia, pericarditis, or atrial infarction; it is a marker of poor prognosis because it generally signals a significant amount of left ventricular dysfunction. Premature atrial contractions (PACs) are also common and may result from increased atrial pressure with congestive heart failure. Atrial fibrillation occurs in 15% of infarctions and is a marker of poor prognosis. Other supraventricular tachycardias are infrequent in myocardial infarction but should be treated promptly if symptomatic.

Ventricular arrhythmias are the leading cause of prehospital mortality in acute myocardial infarction. Ventricular fibrillation (VF) is believed to be responsible for 60% of infarction-related prehospital mortality and occurs predominantly in the first 12 hours. Primary VF (without heart failure) should be distinguished from secondary VF (with significant heart failure). Primary VF occurs predominantly in the first few hours after myocardial infarction and rarely results in death if the patient is hospitalized and defibrillation is available early. Secondary VF may occur at any time during the hospitalization, and defibrillation is not always successful. Premature ventricular beats (PVCs) occur in 90% of patients with acute myocardial infarction and do not predict VF. However, in the immediate postinfarction period, PVCs that occur frequently or in pairs or groups of three do predict risk of VF.

Although prophylactic lidocaine is no longer recommended for all patients with acute infarction, it may be indicated in those with very frequent or complex ectopy in the first 24 hours post infarction. Treatment of chronic but asymptomatic PVCs with antiarrhythmic drugs in the late postinfarction period leads to higher mortality and is not recommended. Accelerated idioventricular rhythm is a nonspecific marker for myocardial reperfusion and should not be treated unless symptoms exist.

15. How is the risk for sudden death assessed in postinfarction patients?
The signal-averaged ECG may be useful in predicting risk for sudden death in postinfarction patients as well as for guiding medical management or placement of an automatic implantable defibrillator. Electrophysiologic studies may be useful in assessing risk of late sudden death postinfarction and are usually performed if the patient has an episode of ventricular tachycardia or ventricular fibrillation after the first 48 hours of infarction or if the signal-averaged ECG is positive in patients with complex ventricular ectopy.

16. When are pacemakers useful in acute myocardial infarction?
Abnormalities of atrioventricular (AV) conduction occur in as many as 25% of patients with myocardial infarction. Often these progress to third-degree heart block and are associated with a 50% increase in acute mortality. In general, patients with inferior myocardial infarction have block in the AV nodal area, and there is often a junctional escape rhythm with a rate of 40–60 beats per minute. These patients usually have an associated right ventricular infarction. In patients with anterior infarction, the block occurs in the His-Purkinje system, and there is often an unreliable ventricular escape rhythm with a rate of less than 40 beats per minute. Temporary pacing is required whenever any bradyarrhythmia or conduction disturbance results in significant symptoms, hypotension, or shock. In asymptomatic patients with inferior myocardial infarction, prophylactic pacing is rarely required. In asymptomatic patients with anterior myocardial infarction, indications for prophylactic pacing are controversial but generally include two or more of the following: first-degree AV block, new bundle branch block, or bifascicular bundle branch block.

The only absolute indication for permanent pacing in acute myocardial infarction is high-degree AV block that persists. In patients with acute inferior myocardial infarction, high-degree AV block almost always resolves within 2 weeks and permanent pacing is not indicated. There is controversy surrounding the use of prophylactic permanent pacing in patients with first-degree AV block combined with fascicular blocks in whom high-degree AV block has resolved.

17. Explain the potential mechanisms for hypotension in acute myocardial infarction.
The differential diagnosis for hypotension in the patient with myocardial infarction is important because treatment depends on the etiology.

1. **Cardiogenic shock** is categorized as hypotension (systolic blood pressure <90 mmHg) with a cardiac index of < 1.8 L/min/m^2 and elevation of left ventricular filling pressures (generally measured by the capillary wedge pressure). Clinical signs of hypoperfusion are also present, including oliguria, mental status changes, pulmonary edema, tachycardia, and pallor. Commonly, massive left ventricular myocardial damage (> 40% of left ventricular myocardium) is the etiology of shock in acute myocardial infarction. Another potential etiology of cardiogenic shock is right ventricular infarction which occurs in an inferior infarction. In this situation, the right

ventricle may not be able to pump sufficient blood through the pulmonary circulation to support cardiac output. This should be suspected in patients with inferior infarction, hypotension, clear lung fields, and elevated neck veins with Kussmaul's sign. The diagnosis can be confirmed with right-sided ECG leads or echocardiography. Right atrial pressures will be elevated out of proportion to pulmonary capillary wedge pressure in this situation, and invasive monitoring may be indicated. Hypovolemia should also be considered early in these patients, since fluid resuscitation alone may reverse the shock state. Pulmonary emboli, sepsis, aortic dissection, and tamponade must also be considered.

2. Symptomatic **mechanical complications** occur in < 1% of patients with myocardial infarction and result from rupture of necrotic cardiac tissue. These complications usually occur from days 3–7 following acute infarction and include rupture of the ventricular free wall (often seen in first transmural anterior infarctions in hypertensive women), ventricular septal rupture, and acute papillary muscle rupture causing acute mitral regurgitation. Often presenting with hypotension and shock, patients with these complications approach 90% mortality if managed medically. Surgical repair of these mechanical complications is the only option if the patient can be stabilized using intraaortic balloon pumping and vigorous vasodilator therapy. The diagnosis can be established with the use of echocardiography and invasive hemodynamic monitoring. Mild to moderate mitral regurgitation is common in acute infarction and is managed medically.

18. What are the indications for invasive hemodynamic monitoring in acute myocardial infarction?
Use of invasive hemodynamic monitoring should be reserved for those patients with clear indications, including diagnosis of suspected left or right ventricular failure with hypotension and pulmonary edema, acute mitral regurgitation, acute ventricular septal defects, or persistent oliguria and azotemia in the patient with unclear volume status. Invasive monitoring may also be useful when initiating treatment with inotropic or vasoactive agents.

19. What techniques are used to risk stratify patients with myocardial infarction?
Postinfarction risk stratification and assessment of prognosis are important in planning long-term therapy. In patients with postinfarction angina, heart failure, or late arrhythmias, urgent angiography should be performed to evaluate the need for PTCA or CABG. In patients with uncomplicated myocardial infarction, noninvasive means may be used to assess ventricular function and residual ischemia, including a symptom-limited exercise test and assessment of left ventricular function by echocardiography or gated blood pool scan. Other tests available for special problems include exercise thallium testing, stress echocardiography, dipyridamole thallium scanning, positron emission tomography, and ambulatory Holter monitoring. These tests can be performed in most patients 1–4 weeks after myocardial infarction to determine high and low risk groups. High-risk groups are identified by low exercise capacity, hypotension, ST-segment depression at low heart rates, and angina during traditional exercise testing. Evidence of ischemia in addition to the infarction visualized on echocardiography or radionuclide imaging may also be useful in assessing risk after myocardial infarction. These principles should be applied to those who have received thrombolytic therapy as well as those who have had a non–Q-wave myocardial infarction. There is controversy surrounding the use of noninvasive tests for risk stratification following non–Q-wave infarctions, and some recommend routine angiography in all these patients.

20. What agents or interventions are used in secondary prevention of myocardial infarction?
Secondary prevention of myocardial infarction should focus on modification of risk factors. In particular, smoking cessation should be encouraged. Lipid-lowering agents in combination with diet modification in certain subsets of patients can reduce mortality by 20% and should be instituted in the appropriate settings. Exercise should be encouraged and supplemented by a rehabilitation program. β-blockers have been extensively studied and, in the postinfarction patient with moderate to high risk, have been shown to reduce mortality and risk of reinfarction by as much as 33%. Aspirin decreases the rates of reinfarction and should be used in all postinfarction

patients. Calcium channel blockers may have a role in secondary prevention of non–Q-wave infarctions, particularly reinfarction, but no mortality benefit has been shown. Angiotensin-converting enzyme (ACE) inhibitors decrease reinfarction rates and incidence of sudden death and improve mortality, and they should be standard in postinfarction patients with ejection fractions < 40%, especially those with symptoms of heart failure.

21. Is there a role for free radical scavengers?

In animal models, free radical scavengers have been shown to limit reperfusion injury in myocardial infarction. Such drugs may have a role in the future, although currently none are approved for clinical use. Most recently, the use of vitamin E has been suggested to benefit patients in primary prevention of myocardial infarction, but further study is necessary.

22. What is ventricular remodeling?

Remodeling of the heart is defined as a change in the mass and shape of the heart in response to damage caused by myocardial infarction and is characterized by hypertrophy and progressive dilatation. Depending on the extent of damage, subsequent wall stress, and local tissue environment, remodeling may result in late pump failure, instability of electrical activity, and reinfarction. Factors that favorably modify this process include prevention of reinfarction, reperfusion, afterload reduction, and possibly prevention of reperfusion injury by free radicals. Therapy should aim to prevent complications of ventricular remodeling by ventricular unloading with ACE inhibitors and resolving chronic ischemia by PTCA or CABG.

BIBLIOGRAPHY

1. ACC/AHA guidelines for the early management of patients with acute myocardial infarction. Circulation 82:664–707, 1990.
2. DeWood MA, Spores J, Notske R, et al: Prevalence of total coronary occlusion during the early hours of transmural myocardial infarction. N Engl J Med 303:897 902, 1980.
3. Falk E: Why do plaques rupture? Circulation Suppl 3:30–42, 1992.
4. Forrester JH, Diamond G, Chatterjee K, et al: Medical therapy of acute myocardial infarction by application of hemodynamic subsets. N Engl J Med 295:1356–1362, 1976.
5. Fuster V, Badiman L, Badiman JJ, Chesebro JH: The pathogenesis of coronary artery disease and the acute coronary syndromes. N Engl J Med 326:242–250, 310–318, 1992.
6. Gibson RS: Non-Q wave myocardial infarction: Diagnosis, prognosis, and management. Curr Probl Cardiol 13:1–72, 1988.
7. GISSI Investigators: Effectiveness of intravenous thrombolytic treatment in acute myocardial infarction. Lancet i:397–401, 1986.
8. Grines CL, Brorone KF, Marco J, et al: A comparison of immediate angioplasty with thrombolytic therapy for acute myocardial infarction. N Engl J Med 328:673–679, 1993.
9. GUSTO Investigators: An international randomized trial comparing four thrombolytic strategies for acute myocardial infarction. N Engl J Med 329:673–682, 1993.
10. Hindman MC, Wagner GS, JaRo M, et al: The clinical significance of bundle branch block complicating acute myocardial infarction: I. Clinical characteristics, hospital mortality, and one year follow-up. Circulation 58:679–688, 1978.
11. Hindman MC, Wagner GS, JaRo M, et al: The clinical significance of bundle branch block complicating acute myocardial infarction. 2. Indications for temporary and permanent pacemaker insertion. Circulation 58:689–697, 1978.
12. ISIS-2 (Second International Study of Infarct Survival) Collaborative Group: Randomized trial of intravenous streptokinase, oral aspirin, both, or neither among 17,187 cases of suspected acute myocardial infarction: ISIS-2. Lancet ii:349–60, 1988.
13. Kulbertus HE, Rigo P, Legrand V: Right ventricular infarction: Pathophysiology, diagnosis, clinical course and treatment. Mod Concepts Cardiovasc Dis 54:1–5, 1985.
14. TIMI Study Group: Comparison of invasive and conservative strategies after treatment with intravenous tissue plasminogen activator in acute myocardial infarction. N Engl J Med 320:618–627, 1989.
15. Tofler GH, Brezinski D, Shafer AL, et al: Concurrent morning increase in platelet aggregability and the risk of myocardial infarction and sudden cardiac death. N Engl J Med 316:1514–1518, 1987.
16. Vatterott PJ, Hammill SC, Bailey KR, et al: Signal averaged electrocardiography: A new non-invasive test to identify patients at risk for ventricular arrhythmias. Mayo Clin Proc 63:931–942, 1988.

19. COMPLICATIONS AND CARE FOLLOWING MYOCARDIAL INFARCTION

Raul Mendoza, M.D.

1. What are the causes of a new pansystolic murmur following myocordial infarction?
The development of a new systolic murmur following myocardial infarction often may be catastrophic due to the hemodynamic instability that usually accompanies this murmur. The etiologies include:
- Rupture and/or dysfunction of a left papillary muscle causing severe mitral regurgitation
- Rupture of the interventricular septum
- Right ventricular infarction and tricuspid regurgitation
- False aneurysm and rupture of the external wall

2. What is the clinical presentation of right ventricular infarction?
Right ventricular (RV) infarction is observed in 29–36% of patients presenting with acute inferoposterior or true posterior myocardial infarction. Isolated RV infarctions are rare. Ischemia or infarction of the RV may lead a range of disorders, from minimal hemodynamic abnormalities to its most severe presentations, which include jugular venous distention, clear lung fields and hypotension, a positive Kussmaul's sign, and RV third and fourth sounds.

3. How is RV infarction diagnosed and what is its recommended management?
The electrocardiogram (ECG) demonstrates the features of acute inferior myocardial infarction (direct posterior or lateral infarction also may be present) and ST elevation in leads $V_4R–V_6R$. Hemodynamic evaluations with a pulmonary artery catheter usually demonstrate an elevated right atrial or RV end-diastolic pressure, a normal or minimally elevated pulmonary artery pressure, and usually normal or low pulmonary capillary wedge pressure.

The mainstay of therapy is fluid administration in order to maintain a wedge pressure of 18–20 mmHg. Inotropic support may be needed and, rarely, intra-aortic balloon pump insertion is indicated in patients with refractory hypotension. Vasodilator drugs should be strictly avoided.

4. What is the difference between true and false aneurysms that develop after myocardial infarction?
A **true ventricular aneurysm** is a circumscribed noncontractile outpouching of the left ventricle and develops in 8–14% of patients who survive myocardial infarction. The wall of the true aneurysm usually is composed of fibrous tissue as well as necrotic and viable myocardium. In contrast, a **psuedoaneurysm** results from rupture of the left ventricle free wall and is concealed by the adjacent pericardium. The wall of the pseudoaneurysm is composed of fibrous tissue and no myocardial elements. Rupture is frequent with pseudoaneurysms but rarely seen in true aneurysms.

5. Is mitral regurgitation following myocardial infarction of clinical concern?
Murmurs of mitral regurgitation are common (55–80%), especially in the early phase of myocardial infarction (MI). However, they are transient and are related to the dynamic nature of the ischemic process. A more serious form of ischemic mitral regurgitation may develop post-MI, though fortunately with a low incidence ranging from 0.9–5%. This complication may lead to severe mitral regurgitation frequently associated with pulmonary edema, hypotension, and death. Three etiologies have been described: (1) papillary muscle dysfunction. (2) generalized left ventricular dilatation, and (3) papillary muscle rupture.

Complete transection of a left ventricular papillary muscle is uniformly fatal because of sudden massive mitral regurgitation that is usually hemodynamically intolerable. Mitral regurgitation post-MI has a wide clinical spectrum, ranging from minimal hemodynamic consequences to a catastrophic syndrome, frequently fatal unless aggressive medical and surgical management is rapidly implemented.

6. Why does severe mitral regurgitation occur following myocardial infarction?
Blood supply to the anterolateral papillary muscle is dual, with branches from both the left anterior descending and circumflex arteries. In contrast, the posteromedial papillary muscle has a single blood supply, either the posterior branches of the dominant right coronary artery or the dominant circumflex artery. Therefore, inferoposterior and posterolateral MIs are the ones most commonly associated with severe mitral regurgitation. Ischemic mitral regurgitation is seen mostly in women and the elderly. Its prognosis depends on the degree of rupture, severity of mitral regurgitation, and previous left ventricular function.

7. How often does rupture of the interventricular septum occur?
This complication occurs in 1–3% of all infarctions and accounts for approximately 12% of all cardiac ruptures. It usually occurs early, 2–6 days after MI, with 66% occurring in the first 3 days. It is commonly seen in patients with hypertension and those with anteroseptal MI (60%), the rest occurring usually in patients with inferior wall MI with rupture of the posterobasilar septum.

8. Is rupture of the ventricular free wall always fatal?
Rupture of the ventricular free wall is a most feared complication and accounts for 8–15% of all infarct deaths and up to 10% of hospital deaths post-MI. Most ruptures (84%) occur in the first week and 32% in the first day. The most common presentation is sudden hemodynamic collapse followed by rapid demise with or without clinical signs of tamponade.

This complication is more commonly seen in the anterior or lateral wall of the left ventricle and usually is preceded by infarct expansion. In some instances, rupture may be heralded by episodes of recurrent pericardial pain, at times with features of pericardial effusion, hypotension, and tamponade. If treatment is to be successful, diagnosis must be prompt and management aggressive. Interventions include infarctectomy, closure of viable myocardial wall, and bypass surgery.

9. Is surgical intervention required immediately in patients with papillary muscle rupture or interventricular septal rupture?
These two complications post-MI have an abrupt onset, with rapid development of a new systolic murmur, pulmonary edema, and shock. Prognosis depends on the degree of rupture, severity of mitral regurgitation, and previous left ventricular function. Initial therapy usually consists of hemodynamic support, including inotropic and vasodilator therapy, guided arterial and pulmonary artery catheterization, and on occasion, the use of an intraaortic balloon pump. If hemodynamic stability is not achieved with these measures and if the patient remains hypotensive, then surgical intervention is required immediately. However, perioperative mortality is high, ranging from 35–50%. In patients who achieve hemodynamic stability with medical therapy, surgery is usually delayed 6–12 weeks in an attempt to improve healing around the infarct margins, thus facilitating surgery as well as lowering the mortality rate.

10. What are the clinical and hemodynamic features of cardiogenic shock?
Cardiogenic shock is profound circulatory failure, usually due to cumulative myocardial loss of 40% or more. Cardiogenic shock is most often secondary to acute myocardial infarction, but other etiologies exist which include primary myocardial disease (myocarditis or end-stage cardiomyopathy).
    1. **Clinical findings**
    Peak systolic blood pressure of < 90 mmHg
    Peripheral vasoconstriction with cool, clammy, and often cyanotic skin

Oliguria or anuria

Altered mental status (confusion, lethargy, obtundation, coma)

Persistence of shock after correction of contributory factors (e.g., hypovolemia, drug side effect or toxicity, arrhythmias, acid-base imbalance)

   2. **Hemodynamic findings**

Low cardiac index of < 1.8 L/min/m^2

Blood pressure of < 90 mmHg systolic and 60 mmHg diastolic

Elevated pulmonary capillary wedge pressure of ≥ 18 mmHg

Tachycardia

Increased systemic vascular resistance

Low stroke volume index of < 20 ml/m^2.

11. Can cardiogenic shock be predicted?

Approximately 7–9% of patients admitted with acute MI develop cardiogenic shock. The average time from admission to onset of this complication is 3.4 ± 0.8 days. The following factors, present at the time of admission, are related to the inhospital development of cardiogenic shock:

   1. Age > 65 years
   2. Poor left ventricular function (LV ejection fraction $< 35\%$)
   3. Large infarct size
   4. History of diabetes mellitus
   5. Previous MI
   6. Female gender

The probability for development of cardiogenic shock depends on the number of these factors present: when 3 are present, there is an 18% probability of shock, and when 5 are present, it is 54%.

12. What other complications can develop in patients with cardiogenic shock?

Patients with cardiogenic shock have a significantly higher incidence of atrioventricular block, intraventricular conduction defects, congestive heart failure, cardiac arrest, cardiac arrhythmia, ventricular septal rupture, and significant mitral regurgitation. The inhospital mortality rate among these individuals is approximately 65%. In patients who have increased risk factors for cardiogenic shock, initiation of early aggressive therapy, including a specific invasive intervention, may be warranted to prevent further myocardial damage.

13. Do all patients who develop hypotension post-MI require inotropic support or/and a pulmonary artery catheter?

Hypotension that develops post-MI has many causes and is not necessarily secondary to left ventricular dysfunction. RV infarction is a common cause of hypotension post-MI. Hypovolemia (absolute or relative) is frequent in the setting of acute MI; patients may be fluid-depleted due to anorexia, vomiting, diaphoresis, or fever, as well as the common use of many drugs that have hypotensive effects. These drugs include narcotic analgesics or tranquilizers, nitrates, diuretics, and most antianginal and antiarrhythmic drugs that tend to be used in patients with acute MI. Recognition and treatment of these reversible causes of hypotension often improve the hemodynamic status of the patient without the need of inotropic drug support or invasive monitoring procedures.

14. Why do patients with complete heart block and acute MI have a higher mortality?

Acute heart block complicates MI in 5–8% of all cases. Most of the cases of complete heart block occur with inferior wall MI; however, mortality is higher with anterior wall MI. This increased mortality is due to the fact that heart block developing during MI signifies increased infarct size, which explains the higher incidence of congestive heart failure, cardiogenic shock, and cardiac arrest in this group of patients.

15. What is the clinical implication of left ventricular mural thrombus formation post-MI?

Left ventricular mural thrombi are common, occurring in 20–40% of patients with anterior infarcts, usually are well visualized by echocardiography, and are mainly seen in anteroseptal and apical MI. Unfortunately, embolism occurs in these patients with a highly variable incidence of 0–25%, usually in the first 10 days post-MI, although thrombus formation may persist during the first 1–3 months. Infarct size is directly related to the thromboembolic risk. The clinical problem is how to prevent emboli rather than how to treat "left ventricular thrombus." It is not entirely clear whether heparinization or combined thrombolytic–heparin therapy prevents emboli. Recommendations for anticoagulation vary, but a reasonable approach is to recommend anticoagulation for 3–6 months with warfarin in patients with demonstrable mural thrombi, particularly if the thrombus is mobile, and in patients in whom an embolic event has already occurred.

16. Differentiate the kinds of pericarditis that develop post MI.

Two kinds of pericarditis occur in the post-MI period. **Early pericarditis** usually develops 24–72 hours after the onset of MI and is seen in patients with transmural MI and congestive heart failure. **Delayed pericarditis** (Dressler syndrome) is characterized by fever, persistent and recurrent pericarditis, and pericardial and pleural effusions and usually appears days to weeks after MI.

Early pericarditis is a marker of extensive myocardial damage and frequently is seen in anterior infarction that may be complicated by the development of atrial and ventricular arrhythmias. Despite a frequently stormy hospital course, patients with early pericarditis usually do not have increased early mortality, however, their 12-month mortality is higher than that of patients who do not develop this complication (18% vs 12%).

17. What are the indications for using an intra-aortic balloon pump post-MI?

The intra-aortic balloon pump is used as adjunctive therapy in acute MI in several groups of patients:

1. Patients whose conditions are hemodynamically unstable and in whom circulatory support is required to perform cardiac catheterization and assessment of potentially correctable lesions.

2. Patients with cardiogenic shock unresponsive to medical therapy, including those who develop mechanical complications (i.e., ventricular septal rupture or papillary muscle rupture).

3. Patients with persistent ischemic pain despite all medical therapy, including beta and calcium channel blockers, nitrates, full anticoagulation, and oxygen.

18. Does temporary pacing improve survival in patients with conduction disturbances in MI?

Patients who develop significant conduction disturbances in acute MI usually have increased morbidity and mortality, mainly because this conduction defect occurs in larger MIs regardless of the coronary artery occluded. Temporary pacing will not improve prognosis in these patients despite the resumption of a physiologic heart rate, since the extent of the myocardial damage is directly related to mortality.

19. What are the indications for temporary and permanent pacing post-MI?

Temporary pacing is recommended in patients with MI who have high-grade atrioventricular (AV) block (second or third degree) or are at risk of developing these conduction disturbances. Indications include:

- Second-degree Mobitz II block
- Second-degree Mobitz I block and hemodynamic instability
- Third-degree heart block
- New left bundle branch block
- New right bundle branch block with either left anterior or left posterior hemiblock
- Asystole

Pacing is rarely necessary with inferior MI unless associated with hemodynamic instability. The indications for **permanent pacing** post-MI remain controversial; the aim of this therapy is to prevent sudden death, but not all sudden deaths are due to high-grade AV block. Also, the timing for implantation of a permanent pacemaker is debatable. Indications for permanent pacing include:

- Persistent advanced AV block (usually > 7–10 days duration), located at either the AV node or His-Purkinje system
- Transient advanced AV block in association with bundle branch block
- Paroxysmal AV block

BIBLIOGRAPHY

1. ACC/AHA Task Force Report: Guidelines for implantation of cardiac pacemakers and antiarrhythmia devices. J Am Coll Cardiol 18:1–13, 1991.
2. Berger PB, Ryan TJ: Inferior myocardial infarction: High risk subgroups. Circulation 81:401–411, 1990.
3. Braunwald E (ed): Heart Disease: A Textbook of Cardiovascular Medicine, 4th ed. Philadelphia, W.B. Saunders, 1992, pp 1239–1291.
4. Goldstein TA: Right heart ischemia. Choices in Cardiology 7: 292–296, 1993.
5. Gunnar RM: Cardiogenic shock complicating acute myocardial infarction. Circulation 78:1508–1510, 1988.
6. Halperin JL, Fustes V: Left ventricular thrombus and stroke after myocardial infarction: Towards prevention or perplexity? J Am Coll Cardiol 14:912–914, 1989.
7. Hands ME, et al: The in-hospital development of cardiogenic shock after myocardial infarction: Incidence, predictors of occurrence, outcome and prognostic factors. J Am Coll Cardiol 14:40–46, 1989.
8. Held CA, et al: Rupture of the interventricular septum complicating acute myocardial infarction: A multicenter analysis of clinical findings and outcome. Am Heart J 116(5 pt I):1330–1336, 1988.
9. Kostuk WJ, Beanlands DS: Complete heart block associated with acute myocardial infarction. Am J Cardiol 26:380–384, 1970.
10. Lehmann KG, et al: Mitral regurgitation in early myocardial infarction. Ann Intern Med 117:10–17, 1992.
11. Meltzer RS, Visser VA, Fuster V: Intracardiac thrombi and systemic embolization. Ann Intern Med 104:689–698, 1986.
12. Pappas DJ, et al. Ventricular free-wall rupture after myocardial infarction. Chest 99:892–895, 1991.
13. Radford MJ, et al: Ventricular septal rupture: A review of clinical and physiologic features and an analysis of survival. Circulation 64:545–553, 1981.
14. Shapira I, et al: Cardiac rupture in patients with acute myocardial infarction. Chest 92:219–223, 1987.
15. Tcheng JE, et al: Outcome of patients sustaining acute ischemic mitral regurgitation during myocardial infarction. Ann Intern Med 117:18–24, 1992.
16. Tcheng JE, et al: Managing myocardial infarction complicated by mitral regurgitation. Prim Cardiol 19(10):40–48, 1993.
17. Tofler GH, et al: Pericarditis in acute myocardial infarction: Characterization and clinical significance. Am Heart J 117:86–90, 1989.

20. CORONARY RISK FACTORS AND MODIFICATION

Gumpanart Veerakul, M.D.

1. What is the purpose of identifying coronary risk factors in patients with and without coronary artery disease (CAD)?

CAD is multifactorial with a long latent period. Despite a 24% decline in its mortality since 1980, CAD remains a leading cause of death in Western society and has a high morbidity. Since its pathophysiologic mechanisms remain undefined, epidermiologic data have verified a number of CAD risk factors which are statistically associated with its development, although there may not necessarily be a causal relationship. Therefore, it is desirable to normalize all potential modifiable risk factors in order to prevent or delay disease progression in a high-risk asymptomatic subgroup (**primary prevention**) or to postpone or regress well-established lesions in patients with preexisting CAD (**secondary prevention**).

2. What characteristics make people high risk?

Risk Factors for Coronary Artery Disease

Major risk factors	Minor risk factors
Unmodifiable	Obesity
Increasing age	Sedentary lifestyle
Family history of CAD before age 55	Psychological stress
Male gender	Type A personality
Postmenopause (in women)	Gout
White race	Hyperuricemia
Modifiable	Oral contraceptive use
Hypertension	Impaired glucose tolerance
Hypercholesterolemia	
Diabetes mellitus	
Cigarette smoking	

Combinations of risk factors are additive and perhaps synergistic, as combinations greatly increase the probability of CAD.

3. When should hypercholesterolemia be treated?

The positive association between elevated serum total cholesterol levels and CAD is primarily due to the high level of low density lipoprotein cholesterol (LDL-C). The current guideline provided through the National Cholesterol and Hypertension Education Program in 1993 defined a total cholesterol > 240 mg/dl and LDL-C > 160-170 mg/dl as a high-risk level requiring medication. Total cholesterol between 200 and 239 mg/dl and LDL-C between 130 and 159 mg/dl are considered as borderline-high, and diet control should be tried with a close follow-up. A total cholesterol < 200 and LDL-C < 100 mg/dl are desirable. In patients with CAD, LDL-C < 100 is desirable.

4. What is the clinical impact of a high density lipoprotein cholesterol (HDL-C)?

HDL-C has been shown epidemiologically to have an inverse relationship to CAD. People with borderline-high total cholesterol but low HDL-C were also considered at risk for CAD, whereas those with high HDL-C (especially if the ratio of total cholesterol/HDL-C was < 4.5) achieved a protective effect against atherosclerosis. Although its exact role is unclear, HDL-C is believed to work by removing cholesterol from the peripheral tissues and arterial wall, transporting it back to the liver for further degradation. Increasing the level of HDL-C can be aided by halting smoking, reducing body weight (in obese persons), controlling hypertriglyceridemia, reducing carbohydrate intake, continuing aerobic exercise, and taking estrogen supplement and nicotinic acid.

5. Will reduction in serum cholesterol help in primary prevention of CAD?

Evidence from three major randomized, double-blinded, placebo-controlled trials confirm the beneficial effects of cholesterol-lowering agents:

    1. **World Health Organization Trial (1978):** Clofibrate, 1.6 gm/day, reduced the incidence of ischemic events 20% in the treated group compared to the control group after 5 years.

    2. **Lipid Research Clinics Coronary Primary Prevention Trial (1984):** With cholestyramine, 14–24 gm/day, patients showed a 19% reduction of coronary death/nonfatal myocardial infarction rates over a 7-year period. Roughly, reducing the cholesterol level by 1% resulted in a reduction of CAD risk of about 2%.

    3. **Helinski Heart Study (1988):** Gemfibrozil, 600 mg twice a day for 5 years, resulted in a 34% reduction of coronary events.

6. Will those who achieve a cholesterol reduction live longer?

Despite a statistically significant decline in ischemic events, the overall mortality in these studies was the same or slightly higher than that with placebo. The causes of death were mainly noncardiovascular and primarily due to motor vehicle accidents and other violent deaths. Criticisms of the studies are that it would require longer time and a larger sample size to show a reduction in total mortality. However, the overall mortality may not be a suitable goal to evaluate the effect of cholesterol treatment. Because the nonfatal infarction rate had been reduced, the sequelae of CAD, such as ischemic cardiomyopathy, were simultaneously prevented, and therefore the quality of life was improved.

7. How promising is cholesterol reduction in people with known CAD?

Secondary prevention is very promising. In the Coronary Drug Project, nicotinic acid effectively reduced LDL and very low density lipoprotein (VLDL) levels and increased HDL-C in male heart attack victims, resulting in a 29% lower rate of myocardial infarction recurrence than with placebo. The overall mortality in the treated group was not initially significant but later showed an 11% reduction at the end of 9 years. In the Stockholm Ischemic Heart Study, a combination of clofibrate and nicotinic acid showed a 36% reduction of CAD-related mortality in most myocardial infarction victims compared to the control group.

8. How important is diet in cholesterol management?

In the Japan–Honolulu–San Francisco Study, Japanese persons who moved to Hawaii or California, where they were exposed to a cholesterol-rich diet, had a higher incidence of CAD accompanied by a rise in serum cholesterol levels compared to a matched Japanese population remaining in Japan. These findings emphasize the influence of dietary cholesterol in the same genetic background.

9. Is hypertriglyceridemia an independent CAD risk factor?

Despite many recent epidemiologic and clinical studies suggesting a positive correlation between an elevated triglyceride level and CAD, the role of triglycerides as an independent risk factor remains controversial.

    1. In persons with CAD, an elevated triglyceride level was usually associated with a low HDL or a high LDL-C, well-established major CAD risk factors.

    2. Multivariate analysis failed to document the independent relation between hypertriglyceridemia and the CAD.

    3. Hypertriglyceridemia is frequently found in various disease states (ie., diabetes mellitus, chronic renal failure, obesity) that are already prone to CAD development.

10. To what degree does smoking cessation truly reduce CAD and major cardiovascular events?

In general, stopping smoking resulted in a 50–70% reduction in CAD risk at the end of 5 years. When combined with lowering of dietary cholesterol in the Oslo study, the incidence of myocardial infarction (fatal and nonfatal) and the CAD death rate were 47% and 55% lower than those in the control group. Similar results were observed in the Multiple Risk Factor Intervention Trial (MRFIT), in which hypertensive treatment was combined with smoking cesation.

11. With control of hypertension, is there a reduction in myocardial infarction?

Meta-analysis of 14 randomized trials showed that a reduction of 5–6 mmHg in diastolic pressure was associated with a 42% reduction in stroke incidence but only a 14% decrement in myocardial infarction incidence. The reason for this difference remains to be defined.

The target goal in reducing the elevated blood pressure also remained unestablished. The second US Joint National Committee provided an initial goal to maintain the diastolic pressure under 90 mm Hg. Recent studies have found that a myocardial infarction risk reduction was achieved if the diastolic pressure was reduced to 84 mmHg.

BIBLIOGRAPHY

1. Badimon JJ, Fuster V, Chesebro JH, Badimon L: Coronary atherosclerosis: A multifactorial disease. Circulation (Suppl 87): II-3–II-16, 1993.
2. Canner PL, Berge KG, Wenker NK, et al: Fifteen year mortality in Coronary Drug Project patients: Long-term benefit with niacin. J Am Coll Cardiol 8:1245–1255, 1986.
3. Carlson LA, Rosenhamer G: Reduction of mortality in the Stockholm Ischemic Heart Disease Secondary Prevention Study by combined treatment with clofibrate and nicotinic acid. Acta Med Scand 223:405–418, 1988.
4. Casper M: Trends in ischemic heart disease mortality—United States, 1980–1988. MMWR 41:548–549, 1992.
5. Collins R, Peto R, MacMahon S, et al: Blood pressure, stroke, and coronary heart disease: Part 2. Short-term reductions in blood pressure: overview of randomised drug trials in their epidemiological context. Lancet 335:827–838, 1990.
6. Committee of Principal Investigators: A cooperative trial in the primary prevention of ischemic heart disease using clofibrate. Br Heart J 40:1069–1118, 1978.
7. Farmer LA, Gotto AM: Risk factors for coronary artery disease. In American Heart Association: 1991 Heart and Stroke Facts. Dallas, American Heart Association, 1991.
8. Gotto AM, LaRossa JC, Hunningghake D, et al: The cholesterol facts, a special report: AHA medical/scientific statement. Circulation 81:1721–1733, 1990.
9. Hjermann I, Holme I, Byrek V, Leren P: Effect of diet and smoking intervention on the incidence of coronary heart disease: Report from the Oslo Study Group of a randomised trial in healthy men. Lancet ii:1303–1310, 1981.
10. Kagan A, Harris BR, Winkelstein MJ, et al: Epidemiologic studies of coronary heart disease and stroke in Japanese men living in Japan, Hawaii and California: Demographic, physical, dietary and biochemical characteristics. J Chronic Dis 27:345–364, 1974.
11. Kannel WB: Some lessons in cardiovascular epidemiology from Framingham. Am J Cardiol 37:269–282, 1976.
12. Keys A (ed): Coronary heart disease in seven countries. Circulation 41(suppl I):I-1–I-211, 1970.
13. Lipid Research Clinics Program: The Lipid Research Clinics' Coronary Primary Prevention Trial results: I. Reduction in incidence of coronary heart disease; II. The relationship of reduction in incidence of coronary heart disease to cholesterol lowering. JAMA 251:351–364, 1984.
14. Mannienn V, Elo MO, Frick L, et al: Lipid alterations and decline in the incidence of coronary heart disease in the Helsinki Heart Study. JAMA 260:641–651, 1988.
15. Manson JE, Tosteson H, Ridker PM, et al: The primary prevention of myocardial infarction. N Engl J Med 326:1406–1416, 1992.
16. McCloskey LW, Psaty BM, Koepsell ID, Ragard GN: Levels of blood pressure and risk of myocardial infarction among treated hypertensive patients. Arch Intern Med 152:513–520, 1992.
17. Multiple Risk Factor Intervention Trial Research Group: Relationship between baseline risk factors and coronary heart disease and total mortality in the Multiple Risk Factors Intervention Trial. Prev Med 15:254–273, 1986.

21. CONGESTIVE HEART FAILURE

Edward P. Havranek, M.D.

1. What is heart failure?
Believe it or not, heart failure is somewhat difficult to define. It is best thought of as a condition in which the heart cannot meet the demands of the peripheral circulation in all situations.

2. How is it diagnosed?
No single test is diagnostic for congestive heart failure. The diagnosis is usually not difficult to make and is based on an assessment of the history, physical examination, and chest x-ray. It is important to use these data to decide if the patient has **left ventricular failure, right ventricular failure,** or a combination of both, since the causes and treatments differ. Occasionally, it is necessary to call on more sophisticated testing to make the diagnosis.

3. What are the four determinants of cardiac output?
Afterload, preload, heart rate, and myocardial contractility.

4. Which of these is abnormal in heart failure?
Actually, all four are abnormal. In most cases of heart failure, the initial event is a decline in myocardial contractility from any one of a number of causes.

5. What happens to afterload?
In response to decreased peripheral perfusion caused by a decline in cardiac output, systemic vascular resistance rises. Although there are several mechanisms for this, the most important are a rise in circulating catecholamines and activation of the sympathetic nervous system. Initially, this rise in afterload helps to maintain organ perfusion. When more advanced, it can become counterproductive and lead to a further reduction in cardiac output.

6. What happens to preload?
In response to decreased renal perfusion, intravascular volume rises. Again, several mechanisms contribute. Activation of the renin-angiotensin system is the most important. The dilated, poorly contractile left ventricle becomes less compliant. This means that small increases in volume produce a relatively large increase in pressure. The net result is an increase in preload. Initially, this helps to maintain cardiac output via the Starling mechanism. As with the changes in afterload, more severe rises are counterproductive, and cause pulmonary vascular congestion, and edema.

7. What happens to heart rate?
It rises. With decreased stroke volume caused by decreased contractility, an increase in heart rate helps preserve cardiac output. The rise in heart rate is due in part to the increased sympathetic tone noted above.

8. What are the symptoms?
The hallmark of heart failure is **exercise intolerance.** This is most commonly experienced as dyspnea on exertion, but some patients report easy fatigue. When **left heart failure** is more severe, patients may complain of orthopnea or paroxysmal nocturnal dyspnea. With this latter symptom, patients are awakened by a severe sensation of shortness of breath, often described as a ''smothering'' feeling. It is relieved by sitting on the edge of the bed or walking around; some patients get relief from sitting by an open window.

With **right heart failure,** patients most frequently notice edema of the feet and ankles.

Sometimes, they are aware only of their shoes getting tighter. When edema involves the liver and gut, they notice right upper quadrant discomfort and abdominal fullness.

9. What are the signs?

Jugular venous distention is the most specific indicator of right heart failure. The examination is most reproducible if patients are examined sitting upright. The jugular venous pressure can then be measured as the distance from the top of the pulsation to the clavicle or manubrium. In almost all patients, if the jugular pulsation cannot be seen above the clavicle, the jugular venous pressure is normal.

Rales are usually, but not universally, present in left heart failure. They are, however, nonspecific.

The **precordial examination** is of key importance. Lateral displacement of the apical impulse indicates left ventricular enlargement. With systolic dysfunction, the impulse is enlarged, sustained, and not forceful. An atrial filling wave (corresponding to S_4) or a late diastolic filling wave (corresponding to S_3) is sometimes palpable. On auscultation, one should listen for S_3 and S_4. A soft holosystolic murmur from mitral or tricuspid insufficiency may be heard when the left or right ventricles are enlarged.

Hepatomegaly is common in right heart failure. The liver edge is soft to slightly firm and frequently tender. Sustained pressure on the liver may cause sustained elevation of the jugular venous pressure (hepatojugular reflux).

Pitting edema is present in dependent body parts, usually the feet and ankles. Edema should be graded by how deeply pitting is noted and by how far up the lower extremity it extends.

10. Are there other diagnosis I should consider?

Pulmonary disease and congestive heart failure share many signs and symptoms, and it can be difficult to differentiate the two disease states. Patients with pericardial tamponade frequently present with dyspnea, jugular venous distention, and an enlarged heart on x-ray. Constrictive pericarditis may mimic many conditions, including heart failure. Some forms of valvular heart disease or congenital heart disease may be confused with heart failure.

Differential Diagnosis of Congestive Heart Failure

ISOLATED RIGHT HEART FAILURE	LEFT OR BIVENTRICULAR FAILURE
Pulmonary embolus	Aortic stenosis
Tricuspid stenosis	Aortic insufficiency
Tricuspid regurgitation	Mitral stenosis
Right atrial tumor	Mitral regurgitation
Cardiac tamponade	Most cardiomyopathies
Constrictive pericarditis	Restrictive cardiomyopathy
Pulmonic insufficiency	Acute myocardial infarction (MI)
Right ventricular (RV) infarction	Myxoma
Intrinsic lung disease	Hypertensive heart disease
Ebstein's anomaly	Myocarditis
	Supraventricular arrhythmias
	Left ventricular (LV) aneurysm
	Cardiac shunts
	High cardiac output states (anemia, systemic fistulae, beriberi, Paget's disease, carcinoid, thyrotoxicosis, etc.)

11. What are the chest x-ray findings?

The chest x-ray is important in diagnosing left heart failure. The x-ray shows signs of interstitial edema or alveolar filling. The cardiac shadow is usually enlarged. A pleural effusion may be present.

12. What is pulmonary edema?

This term refers to the presence of extracellular fluid in the alveolar spaces. In heart failure, it occurs when pulmonary venous pressure rises acutely and hydrostatic forces push fluid out of capillaries faster than it can be removed by the lymphatic system. This fluid accumulates in the alveoli, and pulmonary edema is present.

13. What other studies are useful?

More specialized studies may help establish the diagnosis or assess the course of the disease. Echocardiography is the most useful test when there is diagnostic uncertainty, because it can exclude the cardiac diseases similar to heart failure, assess left ventricular contractility, and give physiologic data such as estimates of pulmonary artery pressure. The radionuclide ventriculogram is best at quantifying ejection fraction. Right heart catheterization is useful in assessing response to therapy in some situations.

An exercise treadmill test, particularly when combined with expired gas analysis, is a useful functional test for determining the degree of heart failure and response to therapy. In difficult cases, it can separate cardiac disease from pulmonary disease.

14. Define "diastolic dysfunction."

The term diastolic dysfunction refers to cardiac dysfunction that results from excessive stiffness of the heart, resulting in an inability of the heart to fill properly. It contrasts with systolic dysfunction, which is an impairment of contractility. Diastolic dysfunction may be severe enough to cause congestive heart failure. This occurs through two mechanisms. First, the noncompliant left ventricle develops a high pressure during diastole, causing an elevation in pulmonary capillary wedge pressure. Second, less blood fills the ventricle during diastole, reducing preload, which in turn reduces cardiac output. Heart failure from diastolic dysfunction is seen in a wide variety of cardiac diseases.

15. What are some causes of diastolic dysfunction?

1. Familial hypertrophic obstructive cardiomyopathy (also known as asymmetric septal hypertrophy or idiopathic hypertrophic subaortic stenosis)
2. Severe hypertrophy (as in hypertensive heart disease or aortic stenosis)
3. Restrictive cardiomyopathies (such as amyloidosis or endomyocardial fibroelastosis)

Although not usually classified with diastolic heart failure, constrictive pericarditis represents the same pathophysiology. Occasionally, ischemic heart disease may cause intermittent heart failure in the absence of systolic dysfunction.

16. How is diastolic dysfunction recognized clinically?

It is sufficient to identify the combination of left heart failure (by symptoms, physical examination, and chest x-ray) and normal systolic function (by echocardiogram or radionuclide ventriculogram). One should also look for the more specific findings for some of the disease states causing diastolic dysfunction, such as Kussmaul's sign seen in restrictive cardiomyopathy or the characteristic decrease in murmur intensity during Valsalva maneuver in hypertrophic obstructive cardiomyopathy. More sophisticated tests of diastolic function using echocardiography or radionuclide ventriculography have been described in research studies but are of limited usefulness in individual patients and may not be well done in all laboratories.

17. What drugs are used in patients with heart failure?

In patients with **systolic dysfunction,** treatment with angiotensin-converting enzyme (ACE) inhibitors should receive first consideration, since these agents decrease mortality. It is important to use the maximum tolerated dose. These drugs are almost always used in combination with a diuretic. In patients with left ventricular enlargement, especially if an S_3 is present, digoxin is added. Although there are no definitive studies to support their use, most specialized centers use anticoagulants in patients with severe systolic dysfunction to decrease the risk of stroke from left ventricular thrombi.

In patients with **diastolic dysfunction,** treatment is aimed at the underlying cause, such as valve replacement in aortic stenosis. In hypertensive or obstructive disease states, β-blockers or verapamil should receive first consideration.

18. If a patient's symptoms of heart failure persist despite appropriate use of these medications, what can be done?
Patients who have unacceptable symptoms despite use of adequate doses of ACE inhibitors, diuretics, and digitalis should be considered for admission. Further adjustment of drug dosing based on data obtained from a pulmonary artery catheter is often useful. Short-term infusion of dobutamine for 48–72 hours has benefit that may last up to a month. When drug treatment fails, heart transplantation is an option in selected patients.

CONTROVERSY

19. Are beta blockers useful in the treatment of heart failure?
Because the negative inotropic properties of beta blockers are so well known, it seems odd to suggest that they might be useful in the treatment of heart failure. Yet, over the past 20 years, a number of small-scale studies have done exactly that. Both laboratory and clinical studies have shown that advancing heart failure is accompanied by increasing levels of activation of the sympathetic nervous system. Although this activation starts as a consequence of the physiologic abnormalities in heart failure, it leads to excessive peripheral vasoconstriction which increases afterload and to down-regulation of cardiac β-receptors. These latter two actions contribute to a downward spiral of declining contractility. Some have speculated that this spiraling might be interrupted by blockading the peripheral effects of catecholamines with β-blockers.

For: In one recent study, 383 patients with heart failure were randomized to receive either placebo or a carefully titrated dose of metoprolol. After 12 months, fewer patients in the metoprolol group required heart transplantation than in the placebo group, but there was no difference between the two groups in mortality or in the combined endpoint of death or need for transplantation.

Against: Although some argue that a decrease in need for heart transplantation (as in the above study) is reason enough to initiate β-blockade in all patients with heart failure, others argue that such a recommendation must be based on a decrease in mortality.

BIBLIOGRAPHY

1. Abrams J: Essentials of Cardiac Physical Diagnosis. Philadelphia, Lea & Febiger, 1987.
2. Bonow RO, Udelson JE: Left ventricular diastolic dysfunction as a cause of congestive heart failure: Mechanisms and management. Ann Intern Med 117:502–510, 1992.
3. Captopril-Digoxin Multicenter Research Group: Comparative effects of therapy with captopril and digoxin in patients with mild to moderate heart failure. JAMA 259:539–544, 1988.
4. Leier CV, Huss P, Lewis RP, Unverferth DV: Drug-induced conditioning in congestive heart failure. Circulation 65:1382–1387, 1982.
5. SOLVD Investigators: Effect of enalapril on survival in patients with reduced left ventricular ejection fractions and congestive heart failure. N Engl J Med 325:293–302, 1991.
6. SOLVD Investigators. Effect of enalapril on mortality and the development of heart failure in asymptomatic patients with reduced left ventricular ejection fractions. N Engl J Med 327:685–691, 1992.
7. Smith TW: Digoxin in heart failure [editorial]. N Engl J Med 329:51–53, 1993.
8. Waagstein F, Bristow MR, Swedberg K, et al: Beneficial effects of metoprolol in idiopathic dilated cardiomyopathy. Lancet 342:1441–1446, 1993.

22. ENDOCARDITIS

Arnold Einhorn, M.D.

1. Discuss the incidence and mortality rate of infective endocarditis (IE).
Although the mortality rate of IE has declined from almost 100% to 5–15% with the use of antibiotics, the incidence probably has increased. The reason for this increase is multifactorial: an aging population, increased number of patients with prosthetic valves, adults surviving with congenital heart disease, improved detection, recurrence in survivors of endocarditis, virulence of pathogens, poor compliance or inadequate prophylaxis, and intravenous drug use. The majority of cases involve patients with prosthetic cardiac valves, users of illicit intravenous drugs, and patients with mitral valve prolapse or other nonrheumatic abnormalities. Underlying anatomy, clinical situation, and infecting organism serve as the basis for prognosis and management.

2. What are the predisposing risk factors for endocarditis of native valves in adults?
Native valve endocarditis in nonintravenous drug users has an identifiable predisposing cardiac lesion in 60–80% of patients, including mitral valve prolapse, degenerative lesions of the aortic and mitral valves, congenital heart disease, and rheumatic heart disease. Rheumatic heart disease was the most common underlying lesion in the past (37–76%) but now accounts for approximately 30% of lesions in adults with endocarditis. Other important risk factors are advanced age, male gender, and diabetes mellitus.

3. Which congenital heart diseases (CHD) are associated with IE?
CHD accounts for the underlying cardiac lesion in 10–20% of adults with IE. The most common lesions are patent ductus arteriosus, ventricular septal defect, bicuspid aortic valve, coarctation of the aorta, and pulmonic stenosis. With improvement in echocardiographic technology, isolated IE of the pulmonic valve has been increasingly recognized, especially in patients with atrial and ventricular septal defects, patent ductus arteriosus, and tetralogy of Fallot. Additional risk factors for IE are bucuspid aortic valve, especially in men older than 60 years; hypertrophic obstructive cardiomyopathy, which accounts for 5% of adults who develop endocarditis; and Marfan syndrome associated with aortic insufficiency.

4. What organisms are associated with IE of native valves in patients who are not intravenous drug users?
In patients who are not intravenous drug users the majority of cases of IE are due to
- Streptococci (50–70%) (alpha-hemolytic and *S. viridans* account for the majority)
- Staphylococci (25%) (especially *S. aureus*)
- Enterococci (10%)

Native valve infections due to *Staphylococcus epidermidis*, enteric bacilli, or fungi are uncommon.

5. Intravenous drug users are at high risk for IE. Describe the course of IE in this subgroup of patients.
Bacteremias in intravenous drug users are common, and the organisms most frequently originate on the skin. *Staphylococcus aureus* is the most common organism in IE (50–60%), whereas various species of streptococci and enterococci account for approximately 20% of cases; gram-negative bacilli, especially *Pseudomonas* and *Serratia* spp., for 10–15%; and fungi, usually culture-negative, for approximately 5% of cases. Infection still shows a slightly higher preference for the tricuspid valve (44%), followed by the mitral (43%), aortic (40%), and pulmonic (3%) valves; infection also may involve both right- and left-sided valves (16%) or both left-sided valves (13%). The majority of patients with IE of the tricuspid valve (70–100%) have pneumonia or multiple septic emboli, and the majority of intravenous drug users with *S. aureus* (70–80%) have isolated IE of the tricuspid valve.

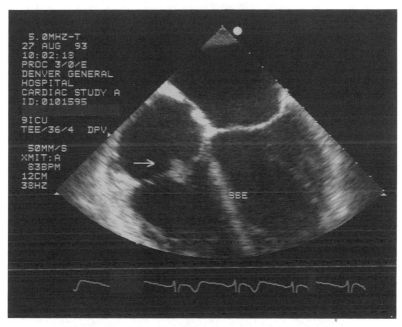

Endocarditis of the tricuspid valve with large mobile vegetation.

6. What are the most common organisms found in prosthetic valve endocarditis (PVE)?

PVE is divided into early (within 60 days of valve insertion) and late disease. Early PVE reflects perioperative contamination, either directly or through catheters (especially central lines). Staphylococcal infection accounts for 45–50% of cases, with *S. epidermidis* the most commonly isolated agent in early PVE (25–30%), followed by *S. aureus* (20–25%), gram-negative aerobic organisms (20%), and fungi (10–20%). Late PVE reflects seeding of the valve by transient bacteremia, especially from dental, genitourinary, or gastrointestinal manipulation; thus the organisms resemble those in native valve IE, with *Streptococcus viridans* being the most commonly isolated (25–30%), followed by *Staphylococcus epidermidis* and *S. aureus* (25% and 10%, respectively).

7. Which prosthetic valve is more likely to acquire IE?

The rate of PVE is approximately the same for mechanical and tissue valves, but the aortic valve is 2–5 times more likely to be involved than the mitral valve.

8. What is the most common cause of culture-negative endocarditis?

The most common cause is inadequate therapy of prior endocarditis; culture-negative IE accounts for 5% of total cases.

9. What are the HACEK gram-negative organisms?

Haemophilus aphrophilus
Actinobacillus actinomycetemcomitans
Cardiobacterium hominis
Eikenella corrodens
Kingella kingae

10. Why is echocardiography important in the management of IE?

Echocardiography, especially transesophageal echocardiography (TEE) for patients with prosthetic valves, is important for both diagnosis and management decisions. A positive finding of vegetation constitutes a major criterion for diagnosis, second only to blood cultures. Echocardiography also provides important information about other valvular abnormalities, abscesses, leaflet perforation, pericarditis, and ventricular function; serial studies are important in medically unresponsive patients to change management or to consider surgery. Outcome is markedly affected by complications. Sensitivity for detecting vegetation is 50–70% by transthoracic echocardiography and >95% with TEE. A negative study has some negative prognostic indicators but does not exclude IE. Because of the numerous complications of PVE, patients with suspected IE should have TEE; the high mortality rate (up to 50% in late PVE and 40–80% in early PVE) is best countered with aggressive management.

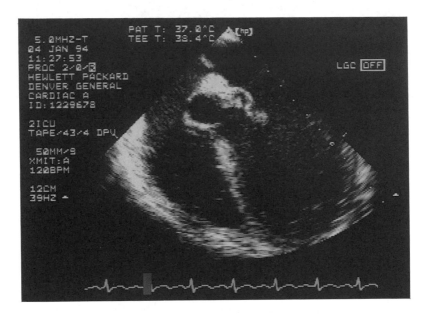

Aortic valve endocarditis with a ring abscess on TEE.

11. What are the definite indications for surgery in IE?
- Acute valvular dysfunction (i.e., severe mitral regurgitation or aortic insufficiency)
- Myocardial invasion
- Antibiotic-resistant organism and persistent sepsis
- Continuing (intractable) congestive heart failure
- Nonfatal emboli

12. If a clinical diagnosis of IE of a native valve is certain, which empirical therapy should be used while blood cultures are being incubated, barring regional-specific modifications?
Vancomycin and gentamicin should be used in suspected drug users, as *S. aureus* is resistant to beta-lactam antibiotics. If the clinical picture is acute endocarditis with methicillin-susceptible staphylococci, nafcillin or oxacillin plus gentamicin may be used.

13. In 1990 the American Heart Association changed its *Recommendations for Infectious Endocarditis Prevention* to replace penicillin as the primary dental agent. With what drug was penicillin replaced? What other change was made?
Amoxicillin, 3.0 gm orally 1 hour before the procedure and 1.5 gm 6 hours after the initial dose, replaces penicillin as the standard antibiotic for routine dental procedures (for patients allergic to amoxicillin and penicillin, erythromycin or clindamycin should be used). Also of significance

were the deletion of gastrointestinal endoscopy from the list of procedures for which protection is warranted, regardless of accompanying biopsy procedures, and provisions for routine use of oral regimens in high-risk patients (e.g., those with prosthetic valves) for dental, oral, or upper respiratory procedures.

14. What is the empirical therapy for prosthetic valve endocarditis?
Ampicillin, vancomycin, and gentamicin.

15. Name four peripheral stigmata of IE.
1. Janeway lesions
2. Roth's spots
3. Splinter hemorrhages
4. Osler's nodes

16. What is Osler's or Austrian triad?
Osler's or Austrian triad consists of endocarditis, pneumonia, and meningitis. The most common organism is *Streptococcus pneumoniae,* which is especially prevalent in alcoholic (40%), elderly, and diabetic patients. The course is fulminant, with rapid valve destruction and abscess formation. The aortic valve is most often involved, followed by the tricuspid valve. Infection is usually responsive to penicillin, but resistant strains that require vancomycin are becoming more common.

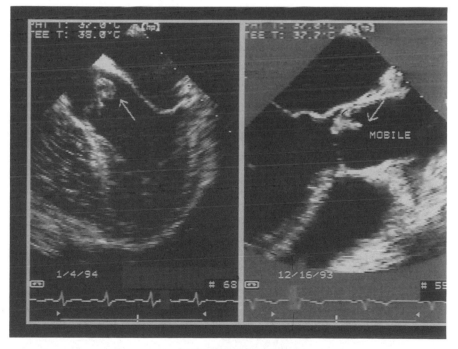

Aortic valve endocarditis.

17. Is anticoagulation helpful in the management of IE?
Although the vegetation is basically a thrombotic lesion and may embolize, no evidence suggests that anticoagulation is helpful in reducing embolization or preventing growth of vegetation. In fact, negative results, including increased rates of fatal intracerebral hemorrhage from mycotic

aneurysms, cerebral embolus, and infarction, have been associated with use of heparin. However, recent data show that use of warfarin with antibiotic therapy is safe in patients with prosthetic valve IE. The suggested protocol is to avoid heparin entirely unless there is a major indication (e.g., massive pulmonary embolism) and to use warfarin anticoagulation as necessary at the low range (international normalized ratio 2.5–3.5).

18. What are the common complications of IE?

1. **Heart failure:** more common in IE of the aortic valve (75%) than in mitral valve (50%) or tricuspid valve disease (14%); poor prognostic sign (death rate with vs. without heart failure, 85% vs. 37%).

2. **Embolization:** clinically seen in up to 35% of patients; pathologic evidence in up to 65%.

3. **Neurologic manifestations:** 40–50% of patients.

4. **Mycotic aneurysm:** 3–15% of patients; highest incidence in the proximal aorta.

5. **Renal failure:** approximately 5%; dialysis can maintain the patient until bacterial antigens are cleared.

19. What is the prognosis of IE?

The prognosis depends on organism, type of valve, location, patient age, and complications. Adverse prognostic indicators are heart failure, renal failure, culture-negative disease, gram-negative or fungal infection, prosthetic valve, and abscess. Favorable factors are young age, early diagnosis and treatment, penicillin-sensitive streptococcal infection, and young intravenous drug users with *Staphylococcus aureus* infection of the tricuspid valve (90% cure rate). Cure is 90% for native valve streptococcal infection, approximately 75–90% for enterococcal infection, and 30–60% for infection with *S. aureus*. Multiple valve involvement also has a higher mortality rate, as does aortic vs. mitral and left-sided vs. right-sided disease. Left-sided IE due to *S. aureus* carries a mortality rate of 25–40%. PVE has a worse prognosis; early PVE has a mortality rate of 41–80% and late PVE of 20–50%.

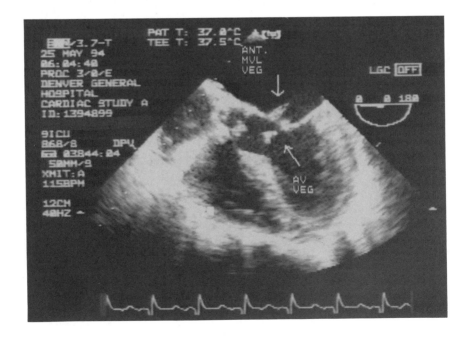

IE involving both aortic and mitral valve.

20. What does the electrocardiogram (ECG) show in patients with IE? How often should the EKG be repeated?

An ECG should be done at admission for patients in whom IE is suspected and repeated according to response to treatment, initial findings, and echocardiographic data. Findings include possible silent myocardial infarction or ischemia secondary to vegetation embolism involving a coronary artery. A prolonged P-R interval also may suggest extension into the conduction system, focal myocarditis, or abscess close to the conduction system. Other disturbances in conduction also may involve major complications, need for surgery, and worse prognosis.

BIBLIOGRAPHY

1. Birmingham GD, Rahko PS, Ballantyne F III: Improved detection of infective endocarditis with transesophageal echocardiography. Am Heart J 123:774–781, 1992.
2. Bisno AL, Dismukes WE, Durack DT, et al: Antimicrobial treatment of infective endocarditis due to viridans streptococci, enterococci and staphylococci. JAMA 261:1471–1477, 1989.
3. Dajani AS, Bisno AL, Chung KJ, et al: Prevention of bacterial endocarditis. Recommendations by the American Heart Association. JAMA 264:2919–2922, 1990.
4. Daniel WG, Mugge A, Martin RP, et al: Improvement in the diagnosis of abscesses associated with endocarditis by transesophageal echocardiography. N Engl J Med 324; 795–800, 1991.
5. Durack DT: Infective and noninfective endocarditis. In Hurst JW (ed): The Heart, vol. 2, 8th ed 1994, pp 1681–1704.
6. Korzeniowski OM, Kay D: Infective endocarditis. In Braumwald E (ed): Heart Disease: A Textbook of Cardiovascular Medicine. Philadelphia, W. B. Saunders, 1992, pp 1078–1105.
7. Pavlides GS, Hauser AM, Stewart JR, et al: Contributions of transesophageal echocardiagraphy to patient diagnosis and treatment: A prostpective analysis. Am Heart J 120:910–914, 1990.

23. AORTIC DISSECTION AND DISEASES OF THE AORTA

Mark Keller, M.D.

1. What are the typical symptoms of aortic dissection?

Pain is generally described as severe ("tearing" pain) and of maximum severity at onset. It often radiates to the back or will follow the course of the dissection with its radiation, i.e., dissection of the distal aorta will radiate down to the abdomen.

2. What are the classic physical findings?

There are many clues in the physical examination that enable the diagnosis of aortic dissection to be made. The blood pressure is often elevated, as this disease is associated with hypertension. However, patients can present in shock if the dissection is large. Other physical findings are the result of the dissection itself, mainly pulse deficit, aortic insufficiency, or neurologic manifestation associated with carotid artery occlusion. Aortic regurgitation is present in over 50% of patients.

3. What is the best available laboratory test for detecting aortic dissection?

There is some controversy as to the best test for the detection of aortic dissection. Frequently, the dissection will be apparent on chest x-ray; it is imperative to obtain adequate upright posteroanterior and lateral chest views in patients.

More specialized tests that will aid the diagnoses include computed tomography (CT), magnetic resonance imaging (MRI), transesophageal echocardiography, and arteriography. MRI and transesophageal echocardiography are the best tests for detection. The sensitivity and specificity for both are over 90%. If MRI is available, it is the better test for detection, but one must keep in mind that the patient must be put into a large magnet and it is difficult to follow such patients carefully. Transesophageal echocardiography is performed with a cardiologist in close proximity; it does provide information regarding left ventricular function and aortic insufficiency which is not as readily obtainable from an MRI scan.

4. What is appropriate initial therapy for patients with suspected aortic dissection?

All patients should be admitted to the intensive care unit for close monitoring. Initial therapy should consist of (1) lowering the blood pressure in hypertensive patients, and (2) decreasing the rate of change in aortic pressure. Blood pressure is best lowered with an intravenous effusion of sodium nitroprusside. The change in aortic pressure should be lowered with intravenous beta blockers (i.e., metoprolol or propranolol). These two maneuvers will help decrease extension of the dissection.

5. Which patients should be treated with surgery?

Patients who have dissection involving the ascending portion of the aorta extending into the aortic arch are the ones best treated with surgery. In addition, surgery should be considered in those with distal aortic dissection if there is an unsatisfactory response to medical treatment, compromise of vital organs, or threat of impending rupture.

6. Which patients are best treated medically?

Medical treatment is a treatment of choice for uncomplicated dissection of the descending aorta. It also appears to be superior to surgical therapy for patients with stable isolated dissection of the aortic arch in which none of the great vessels is compromised. Finally, if a dissection is detected 2 weeks after its proposed onset, then it is considered to be a stable chronic dissection and is best treated medically. Long-term medical therapy should focus on the control of hypertension.

7. What diseases or syndromes predispose patients to aortic dissection?

Patients often have long-standing high blood pressure which produces stress on the aortic wall. In addition, hereditary disease, such as Marfan syndrome, can cause cystic medial degeneration of the aortic wall, predisposing to the dissection. There is also a relationship with pregnancy and dissection.

8. What is the most common site for an atherosclerotic aneurysm involving the aorta?

The abdominal aorta (abdominal aortic aneurysm).

9. What are the best tests for following an abdominal aortic aneurysm?

Repeat abdominal ultrasound is the best because it allows accurate and simple evaluation of the size of the aortic aneurysm. Other tests that can successfully resolve this are MRI, CT, aortography, and digital subtraction angiography.

10. When should abdominal aneurysms be repaired?

All patients with abdominal aortic aneurysms > 6 cm in diameter should have surgical repair. However, the management of patients with smaller aneurysms is controversial and is a subject of ongoing research. Some advise earlier operation to improve long-term prognoses, but no study has yet adequately defined how "early."

11. How does cardiovascular syphilis affect the aorta?

A rare disease in the present day, cardiovascular syphilis, or lues disease, was once prevalent, accounting for 10% of all cardiac deaths. This disease typically presents as an aneurysm of the ascending aorta. The cornerstone of diagnosis is a history of syphilis and serologic confirmation that the patient has the disease.

BIBLIOGRAPHY

1. Cooke JP, Kazmier FJ, Orszulak TA: The penetrating aortic ulcer: Pathologic manifestations, diagnosis, and management. Mayo Clin Proc 63:718–725, 1988.
2. Crawford, ES: The diagnosis and management of aortic dissection. JAMA 264:2537–2541, 1990.
3. Huang HK, Aberle DR, Lufkin R, et al: Advances in medical imaging. Ann Intern Med 112:203–220, 1990.
4. Karalis DG, Chandrasekaran K, Victor MF, et al: Recognition and embolic potential of intraaortic atherosclerotic debris. J Am Coll Cardiol 17:73–78, 1991.
5. Marsalese DL, Moodie DS, Vacante M, et al: Marfan's syndrome: Natural history and long-term follow-up of cardiovascular involvement. J Am Coll Cardiol 14:422, 1989.
6. Nevitt MP, Ballard DJ, Hallet JW Jr: Prognosis of abdominal aortic aneurysms: A population-based study. N Engl J Med 321:1009–1014, 1989.
7. Pyeritz RE: Genetics and cardiovascular disease. In Braunwald E (ed): Heart Disease, 4th ed. Philadelphia, W. B. Saunders, 1992.

24. PERICARDIAL DISEASE

Paul D. Sherry, M.D.

1. What are the basic anatomic features and functions of the pericardium?
The pericardium consists of two layers of tissue: an outer fibrous layer (parietal pericardium) composed of collagen and elastin fibers, and an inner serous membrane (visceral pericardium) composed of a thin layer of mesothelial cells. The space between the two pericardial layers normally contains 15–50 ml of clear fluid.

There are ligamentous attachments from the pericardium to the sternum, veterbral column, and diaphragm which help to keep the heart fixed in place during changes in body position. The tough outer layer serves as a barrier to the spread of infection and neoplastic processes to the heart. In dog studies, the pericardium appears to provide a restraining effect during acute volume loading. Studies in humans who have undergone pericardiectomy also support the concept of a volume-restraining effect provided by the pericardium.

2. What are the most common causes of acute pericarditis?
In the outpatient setting, pericarditis is usually idiopathic. It is thought that viral infection probably comprises many of the cases categorized as idiopathic. The coxsackie A and B viruses are highly cardiotropic and are two of the most common viruses to lead to pericarditis and myocarditis. Other viruses associated with pericarditis include mumps, varicella-zoster, influenza, Epstein-Barr, and human immunodeficiency virus (HIV).

In the inpatient setting, some of the more common etiologies can be recalled with the mnemonic TUMOR. "Tumor" also serves as a useful reminder that metastatic cancer is a frequent cause of pericarditis and pericardial effusion in hospitalized patients.

T = **T**rauma
U = **U**remia
M = **M**yocardial infarction (acute and post), **M**edications (e.g., hydralazine and procainamide)
O = **O**ther infections (bacterial, fungal, tuberculous)
R = **R**heumatoid arthritis and other autoimmune disorders, **R**adiation.

3. How does the pain of pericarditis differ from the pain of myocardial infarction?
It is important to understand how pericarditis pain differs from that of myocardial infarction because the two processes may share some of the same features and can be confused. Both pericarditis and myocardial infarction may produce retrosternal or precordial chest pain with radiation to the neck, back, left shoulder, or left arm. However, pericarditis pain differs in that it is far more likely to be sharp and pleurtic, becoming worse with coughing or inspiration. Usually, thoracic motion does not change the intensity of ischemic pain. In contrast, pericarditis pain is often worsened by lying supine and relieved by sitting forward. Another important historical point is that some patients report exacerbation of pericarditis pain with swallowing.

4. Which auscultatory finding is pathognomonic for pericarditis?
The pericardial friction rub is pathognomonic for pericarditis. Rubs often have a characteristic scratching or grating sound that is heard best with the diaphragm of the stethoscope. Classically, rubs are described as having three components:
1. A presystolic rub during atrial filling
2. A ventricular systolic rub (the loudest component and the one almost always present)
3. A ventricular diastolic rub following the second heart sound.
A rub in the same patient may vary from faint to loud and may sometimes transiently disappear.

5. What are the typical findings of acute pericarditis on the electrocardiogram (ECG)?

Conventionally, acute pericarditis causes ST-segment elevation in most ECG leads, particularly the ones reflecting the epicardium (since the inflammation involves the epicardial surface of the heart)—leads I, II, aVL, aVF, and V_3–V_6. Lead aVR usually shows ST depression. Unlike the ST elevation of acute myocardial infarction, which may concave downward like a "cat's back," the ST elevation of pericarditis is concave upward. Depression of the PR segment occurs in the earlier stages of pericarditis and usually involves the limb and precordial leads. Another important distinguishing feature of pericarditis is that the T-wave inversion occurs *after* the ST segment returns to baseline. In myocardial infarction there is often some degree of T-wave inversion accompanying the ST elevation.

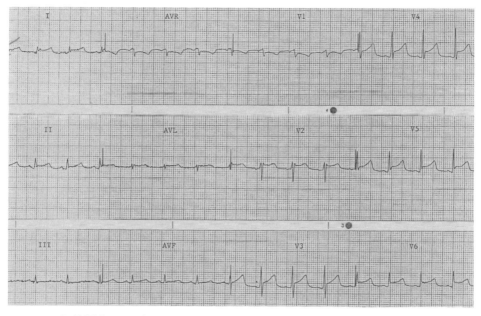

An ECG from a patient with purulent pericarditis shows some of the classic features.

6. When does cardiac tamponade occur?

Cardiac tamponade occurs when the accumulation of fluid in the pericardial space increases pericardial pressure and thus decreases cardiac output. As the intrapericardial pressure rises, there is a progressive elevation and usually equalization of intracardiac chamber pressures. Ventricular diastolic filling becomes progressively limited, leading to a reduction in stroke volume. Compensatory adrenergic activation leads to tachycardia and increased myocardial contractility. If tamponade is unrelieved, the compensatory mechanisms are unable to keep the systemic arterial pressure from falling and hemodynamic collapse occurs.

7. What is Beck's triad?

Described in 1935 by thoracic surgeon Claude S. Beck, these three features are typical of acute cardiac tamponade developing from trauma or invasive cardiac procedures:

- Decline in systemic arterial pressure
- Elevation in systemic venous pressure (e.g., distended neck veins)
- A small, quiet heart

The syndrome described by Beck is likely to occur when the pericardium is suddenly filled with blood from an injury. When there is no time for pericardial stretching, less than 200 ml of fluid can rapidly raise the intrapericardial pressure. In contrast, slowly developing effusions may become very large before signs of tamponade develop, as there is more time for the pericardium to stretch. Most slowly developing effusions do not manifest the quiet heart of Beck's triad.

8. Generally, how much pericardial fluid must be present to alter the appearance of the cardiac silhouette on chest x-ray?
Enlargement of the cardiac silhouette in adults usually is not manifest until at least 250 ml of fluid is present. Therefore, a normal chest x-ray does not exclude the possibility of cardiac tamponade.

9. What is pulsus paradoxus, and how is it measured?
Pulsus paradoxus is an exaggerated response from the normal physiologic drop in blood pressure that occurs with inspiration. Normally, up to a 10-mmHg drop in systolic blood pressure can occur with inspiration. In cardiac tamponade, multiple factors lead to a larger-than-usual drop in systolic blood pressure with inspiration. Right ventricular filling is augmented over left ventricular filling, causing the interventricular septum to bulge into the left ventricle with a resultant drop in stroke volume. The lower stroke volume with inspiration is then reflected in lower blood pressure.

Pulsus paradoxus is measured in the following manner: With the patient breathing normally, the cuff is inflated and then deflated very slowly until Korotkoff sounds are first heard intermittently (representing the sound during expiration). Then, the cuff is further slowly deflated until all beats are heard (representing the sound during inspiration). The difference between the two pressures is defined as the pulsus paradoxus. On physical examination, pulsus paradoxus also can be detected by a decrease in the amplitude of the palpated carotid or femoral pulse during inspiration.

10. Is tamponade always associated with pulsus paradoxus?
No. Tamponade may occur without pulsus paradoxus when there is coexistent atrial septal defect, aortic insufficiency, or preexisting elevated left ventricular diastolic pressure (as in left ventricular hypertrophy). Also, pulsus paradoxus may occur without tamponade as in chronic obstructive pulmonary disease, right ventricular infarction, and pulmonary embolism.

11. What are two of the classic ECG changes of pericardial effusion?
Diffuse low voltages and **electrical alternans** may be seen with pericardial effusions. Changes in the QRS voltage is not only due to the amount of fluid but also the electrical conductivity of the fluid. In canine studies, saline introduced into the pericardial space produced a greater voltage reduction than blood.

Electrical alternans is a repetitive alternating change in the P, QRS, and T-wave amplitudes that occasionally occurs with cardiac tamponade. Most commonly, the QRS alone shows the alternating amplitude. The swinging motion of the heart in a relatively large volume of pericardial fluid is thought to produce electrical alternans. Sometimes electrical alternans is noticeable in only one lead and could therefore be missed on a bedside cardiac monitor. It should be noted that electrical alternans may occur in other conditions, such as paroxysmal supraventricular tachycardia, hypertension, and acute episodes of ischemia.

12. Outline the treatment of acute pericarditis.
1. **Treat the underlying cause** whenever possible. For example, treatment of rheumatoid arthritis or systemic lupus erythematosus may help lead to the resolution of associated pericarditis.
2. **Analgesic agents.** Codeine, 15–30 mg every 4–6 hours, usually provides adequate pain relief.
3. **Anti-inflammatory agents.** Aspirin, 650 mg every 3–4 hours, may be tried initially. Indomethacin, 25–50-mg doses four times/day, is a very effective form of treatment either initially or when aspirin has not provided adequate relief. The use of corticosteroids is controversial; many authors consider steroid use as an absolute last resort, as it may become very difficult to withdraw the therapy without precipitating relapses.

13. What is the role of echocardiography in the diagnosis of pericarditis and cardiac tamponade?

The echocardiogram is the most sensitive test for the detection of pericardial effusion. As little as 15 ml of fluid can be detected by two-dimensional echocardiography. Pericardial fluid appears as an echo-free space between the walls of the heart and pericardium (*see* figure). In tamponade, the cardiac chambers may appear underfilled and contracted. Collapse of the right atrium and right ventricle during diastole is virtually diagnostic of cardiac tamponade. Right atrial collapse tends to occur earlier and may be detected at a time when no clinical signs of tamponade exist, making it less specific for diagnosing tamponade than right ventricular collapse. The echocardiogram can also be used to guide placement of the needle used in pericardiocentesis.

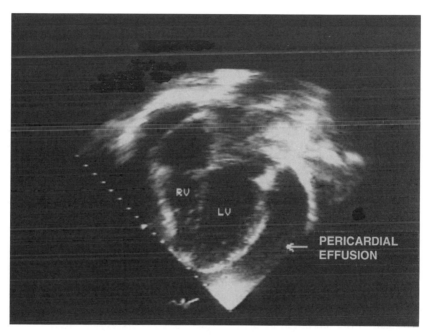

Two-dimensional echocardiogram from a patient with pericardial effusion (LV = left ventricle, RV = right ventricle).

14. What is Dressler's syndrome?

In 1956, Dressler described a syndrome occurring in the first few days to several weeks following myocardial infarction which involved fever, pericarditis, and pleuritis. The incidence of this post-myocardial infarction syndrome is 6–25%. Autopsy studies have shown that it is very common to have a localized area of pericarditis overlying the area of infarcted myocardium. Typically, patients with Dressler's syndrome have a low-grade fever and a pericardial friction rub. When the pain is severe, a short course of high-dose aspirin will usually relieve the pain within 48 hours.

15. Describe the physical findings of constrictive pericarditis.

The neck is the starting point as the jugular venous pattern is the most important part of the examination in this condition.

Jugular veins: The jugular veins are distended with prominent X and Y descents. There is usually an increase in the height of the jugular venous pulsation with inspiration (Kussmaul's sign).

Lungs: The lung fields are usually clear. Sometimes, a pleural effusion may be present and can be a clue to pericardial constriction in patients being evaluated for isolated pleural effusion of unknown etiology.

Heart: The apical impulse is usually soft and diffuse. S_1 and S_2 may be decreased in intensity. A diastolic **pericardial knock** may be heard along the left sternal border. The pericardial knock is a loud sound occurring early in diastole (0.09–0.12 seconds after A_2) and sometimes accentuated with inspiration. Pericardial knocks may be confused with an S_3 but may be distinguished by a higher acoustic frequency and earlier occurrence than an S_3.

Abdomen: There may be distention from ascites. The liver is enlarged and pulsatile. In chronic cases, the spleen may also be enlarged.

Extremities: Peripheral edema is present.

16. How is the diagnosis of constrictive pericarditis made in the cardiac catheterization laboratory?

Arterial and central venous (usually femoral) catheters are placed so that the right and left heart pressures can be measured and recorded simultaneously. When constriction is present, both right and left ventricular diastolic pressures are elevated and virtually identical (≤ 5 mmHg in difference). The right atrial pressure waveform has steep X and Y descents and may show Kussmaul's sign, i.e., rise during inspiration. The right and left ventricular pressure curves may show the classic "square root sign," which represents an early diastolic dip in pressure followed by a plateau. The plateau occurs because the constricting pericardium abruptly limits ventricular filling. The characteristic dip and plateau may be difficult or impossible to see during tachycardia. Restrictive cardiomyopathies may have many of the same hemodynamic findings as constrictive pericarditis, and the distinction between the two processes can sometimes be difficult.

17. How does tuberculous pericarditis present clinically?

Although tuberculosis has become less common in industrialized nations in the last 30 years, it is still seen in patients from developing countries such as Africa and Asia and in association with the acquired immunodeficiency syndrome (AIDS). The incidence of tuberculous pericarditis in patients with pulmonary tuberculosis has ranged from 1–8% in several studies. Common physical findings are fever, pericardial rub, and hepatomegaly. Pulmonary infiltrates have been present in 32–72% of patients in different studies. Tuberculin skin testing is usually positive unless the patient has skin test anergy. Tubercle bacilli are often not found on stained smears of pericardial fluid. Therefore, pericardial biopsy in addition to pericardiocentesis provides a higher probability of definitive diagnosis.

BIBLIOGRAPHY

1. Ameli S, Shah P: Cardiac tamponade, pathophysiology, diagnosis, and management. Cardiol Clin 9:455–476, 1991.
2. Callahan JA, Seward JB, Nishimura RA, et al: Two-dimensional echocardiographically guided pericardiocentesis: Experience in 117 consecutive patients. Am J Cardiol 55:476–479, 1985.
3. Cameron J, et al: The etiologic spectrum of constrictive pericarditis. Am Heart J 113:354–360, 1987.
4. Chou T: Electrocardiography in Clinical Practice. Philadelphia, W. B. Saunders, 1991, pp 219–234.
5. Cimino JJ, Kogan AD: Constrictive pericarditis after cardiac surgery: Report of three cases and review of the literature. Am Heart J 118:1292–1301, 1989.
6. Diamond T: The ST segment axis: A distinguishing feature between acute pericarditis and acute myocardial infarction. Heart Lung 14:629–631, 1985.
7. Fowler N: Tuberculous pericarditis. JAMA 266:99–103, 1991.
8. Lorell BH, Braunwald E: Pericardial disease. In Braunwald E (ed): Heart Disease: A Textbook of Cardiovascular Medicine, 4th ed. Philadelphia, W. B. Saunders, 1992, pp 1465–1527.
9. Soler-Soler J, Permanyer-Miralda G, Sagristà-Sauleda J: A systematic diagnostic approach to primary acute pericardial disease: The Barcelona experience. Cardiol Clin 8:609–620, 1990.
10. Spodick DH: Pericarditis, pericardial effusion, cardiac tamponade, and constriction. Crit Care Clin 5:455–476, 1989.
11. Sternbauch GL: Pericarditis. Ann Emerg Med. 17:214–220, 1988.

25. HYPERTENSION

Arlene Chapman, M.D.

1. How is hypertension defined?

Unfortunately, there is not a simple answer to this question. Abnormal elevation of blood pressure in a given individual best defines the hypertensive state. For example, a blood pressure of 130/80 mmHg in a 10-year-old is considered hypertensive and is greater than the 95th percentile for that age. Generally, physicians accept a blood pressure > 140/90 mmHg in patients older than 30 years and blood pressure > 160/95 mmHg in patients older than 65 years as being hypertensive.

2. What are the two hemodynamic determinants of blood pressure? Which predominates in essential hypertension?

Arterial blood pressure is the product of **cardiac output** and **systemic vascular resistance.** By definition, systemic vascular resistance is elevated in hypertension, but it is unclear if it is the initiating event or response to increases in cardiac output. Relative contributions of both factors to the hypertensive state vary among patients. Both black and elderly hypertensive patients appear to have increased plasma volumes and cardiac output contributing to the hypertensive process, and they may respond more favorably to a diuretic or calcium channel blocker in the treatment of their hypertension.

3. Are there different types of hypertension?

1. **Idiopathic or essential hypertension** is the most common, affecting approximately 40 million American adults. Men are more frequently affected than women until the postmenopausal age; black and Hispanic men and women are more commonly affected than whites.

2. In **labile or intermittent** hypertension, hypertension occurs only in certain circumstances, such as visits to the physician, stress, or exercise. These patients are at increased risk for the development of chronic hypertension.

3. In **isolated systolic hypertension,** systolic blood pressure is elevated but diastolic blood pressure is < 90 mmHg. This type occurs typically in the elderly, in whom large-vessel compliance is decreased secondary to atherosclerosis and age. Systolic blood pressure is usually > 160 mmHg. Recent studies demonstrate that decreasing systolic blood pressure to < 160 mmHg in the elderly results in a significant reduction in the rate of cerebrovascular and cardiovascular accidents.

4. **Borderline hypertension** is defined as elevated blood pressure but not in the hypertensive range. Usually, these patients are in transition from the normotensive to the hypertensive state and are at increased risk for the development of chronic hypertension. Typically they have a family history of essential hypertension.

5. **Malignant hypertension** is a medical emergency requiring immediate therapy. It is characterized by marked elevation in blood pressure, usually > 180/120 mmHg, and is associated with evidence of acute end-organ damage, profound intravascular volume loss, and activation of the renin-angiotensin-aldosterone axis. Patients are usually symptomatic with blurred or decreased vision, headache, confusion, or chest pain. On opthalmologic examination, the presence of papilledema diagnoses malignant hypertension, although grade III neuroretinopathic changes also may be seen. The severe acceleration in hypertension and activation of the renin-angiotensin aldosterone axis result in large- and medium-vessel vasculitis involving the renal vasculature, leading to kidney injury.

6. **Accelerated, urgent, or emergent hypertension** is a milder form of malignant hypertension in which the patient may be symptomatic but papilledema or evidence of renal injury is not present. However, due to the explosive nature of this disorder, these patients also should be treated emergently.

4. Is it important to treat mild or moderate essential hypertension?

Yes. There is good evidence that a reduction in diastolic blood pressure decreases the relative risk for cerebrovascular and cardiovascular events. The data are most convincing with regard to the incidence of cerebrovascular accidents, where the diastolic blood pressure correlates with the risk of cerebrovascular accident. Therefore, patients with diastolic blood pressure < 60 mmHg fare better than patients with diastolic pressure < 80 mmHg with regard to risk for cerebrovascular accident.

5. What is the cause of hypertension?

It is multifactorial. There are good epidemiologic data of a **genetic influence** in offspring of hypertensive parents as well as offspring of parents with extremely low blood pressure, accounting for approximately 25% of the variability of patients' blood pressure measurements. The genetic influences are most likely polygenic and include sodium sensitivity, renal kallikrein excretion, and adrenal sensitivity to angiotensin II and intracellular calcium levels.

Interacting with the genetic contribution are **lifestyle and environmental influences.** Alcohol intake in men and oral contraceptive use in women are the two leading causes of nonessential hypertension. Other factors known to affect blood pressure include caffeine intake, cigarette smoking, dietary potassium, sodium, and calcium intake, as well as obesity.

6. Can essential hypertension be classified?

Yes. The most useful classification system was developed by Dr. Laragh's group, who performed sodium-renin profiling in a large number of hypertensive patients. In sodium-renin profiling, the patient's plasma renin activity is determined in the sitting position without antihypertensive medication while a 24-hour urine collection is obtained to determine the patient's sodium intake. Because sodium intake, postural position, and blood pressure medication all affect plasma renin activity, all variables must be accounted for. Most hypertensive patients demonstrate normal plasma renin activities for a given sodium intake, but approximately 35% have **low-renin hypertension** and 15% have **high-renin hypertension.** Importantly, patients with high-renin hypertension have a greater vasoconstrictor profile than those with low-renin hypertension, who tend to have increased circulating blood volume and a suppressed renin-angiotensin-aldosterone axis.

7. Why is this differentiation important?

Prospective studies have shown that patients with high-renin hypertension are at increased risk for cerebrovascular accidents and there is a trend toward an increased risk for cardiovascular accidents, especially young white men. Not only is renin-sodium profiling important from a prognostic standpoint, but it also allows the physician to choose an antihypertensive medication that will best treat the patient's hypertension. For example, diuretics are most likely an effective antihypertensive agent in patients with low-renin hypertension (most commonly black or elderly) in whom intravascular volume expansion is present. In contrast, in patients with high-renin hypertension (young white men), converting enzyme inhibitors or sympathetic blocking agents are most effective. Clearly, to do renin-sodium profiling, it is necessary to take the patient off antihypertensive medication, which is often impossible to do. As well, the sample must be handled properly for measurement of plasma renin activity.

8. What are some indications that a patient's blood pressure has been poorly controlled for some time?

The three organ systems bear the brunt of end-organ damage in hypertension:

Eyes: The two major circulatory systems involving the optic nerve are the retinal and choroidal vascular systems. Increased vascular reactivity in both is best promoted by the pressor angiotensin II, leading to neuroretinopathy being observed more often in high angiotensin II states.

Kidney: Essential hypertension is the second leading cause of renal failure in the United States. Blacks appear to have an increased renal sensitivity to the effects of hypertension independent of socioeconomic factors. Serum creatinine elevations and proteinuria are clinical markers for end-organ renal damage due to hypertension.

Heart: Left ventricular (LV) hypertrophy and increased LV mass are consequences of the increased cardiac workload imposed by the hypertensive process. M-mode echocardiography is more sensitive than electrocardiography or chest x-ray in demonstrating the presence of LV hypertrophy. The severity of the hypertensive state often correlates with LV mass, which is an early marker of risk for myocardial infarction or sudden death due to hypertension. Patients with LV hypertrophy are at 2- to 5-fold higher risk of sudden cardiac death than patients with normal LV mass (even when accounting for other risk factors). Both systolic and diastolic dysfunction as determined by LV compliance and filling are also markers of end-organ damage due to hypertension.

9. What guidelines are useful in the treatment of hypertension?
The most noninvasive way of treating hypertension should be attempted first:
- Dietary sodium restriction and calcium or potassium supplementation
- Removal of alcohol or cigarette use
- Increased physical activity and weight loss in obese patients
- Reduction in dietary saturated fats and cholesterol

More often than not, medication is required.

CONTROVERSIES

10. What are the current recommendations for the medical treatment of uncomplicated mild essential hypertension?
At present, diuretics and sympathetic blocking agents should be used as first-line agents in the treatment of hypertension, due to their lower cost and proven efficacy. Other agents have *not* been shown to be *less* effective, but extended testing has not been performed to demonstrate *equal* benefit. Clearly, some patients may benefit from first-line treatment with calcium channel blockers, converting enzyme inhibitors, as well as alpha or alpha-beta blocking agents.

11. Is there a problem with treating patients' blood pressure too low?
Some investigators seriously believe mortality and blood pressure in treated hypertensive patients are related in a J-shaped curve. In other words, at a certain point, a lower diastolic pressure represents a group of patients who are likely to do worse than their more hypertensive counterparts. Unfortunately, the data to support this view were not collected in a prospective double-blinded fashion and may represent those patients with other medical conditions, such as malignancy or infection.

12. If hypertensive patients with increased LV mass are treated aggressively, will they reduce heart size, return function to normal, or reduce the risk of a fatal arrhythmia or infarction?
Many prospective, blinded antihypertensive trials have demonstrated reversal of LV hypertrophy by echocardiographic measurement. However, whether the increased risk of fatal myocardial infarction is reduced by reversing LV hypertrophy is unknown and debated. Recent work in animal models or hypertension induced by angiotensin II or aldosterone shows an early increase in collagen II levels and induction of myocardial fibrosis that may not be reversible. As well, the increase in collagen synthesis and myocardial fibrosis demonstrated in these studies was inhibited by early application of angiotensin-converting enzyme inhibitors and high doses of spironolactone. Clearly, more work is needed including long-term follow-up studies of cardiovascular mortality in patients with treated and reversed LV hypertrophy.

BIBLIOGRAPHY

1. Alderman MH, Madhavan S, Ooi WL, et al: Association of the renin-sodium profile with the risk of myocardial infarction in patients with hypertension. N Engl J Med 324:1098–1104, 1991.
2. Brilla CG, Matsubara LS, Weber KT: Antifibrotic effects of spironolactone in preventing myocardial fibrosis in systemic arterial hypertension. Am J Cardiol 71:12A–16A, 1993.
3. Duprez DA, Bauwens FR, De Buyzere ML, et al: Influence of arterial blood pressure and aldosterone on left ventricular hypertrophy in moderate essential hypertension. Am J Cardiol 71:17A–20A, 1993.
4. Frohlich ED: Left ventricular hypertrophy, cardiac diseases and hypertension: Recent experiences. J Am Coll Cardiol 14:1587–1594, 1989.
5. Gifford RW, Kirdendall W, O'Connor DT, Weidman W: Office evaluation of hypertension: A statement for health professionals by a writing group of the Council for High Blood Pressure Research, American Heart Association. Hypertension 13:283–293, 1989.
6. Lifton RP, Hopkins PN, Williams RR, et al: Evidence for heritability of non-modulating essential hypertension. Hypertension 13:884–889, 1989.
7. Miller JZ, Weinberger MH, Christian JC, Daugherty SA: Familial resemblance in the blood pressure response to sodium restriction. Am J Epidemiol 126:822–830, 1987.
8. Rostand SG, Brown G, Kirk AK, et al: Renal insufficiency in treated essential hypertension. N Engl J Med 320:684–688, 1989.
9. Rostand SG, Kirk KA, Rutsky EA, Pate BA: Racial differences in the incidence of treatment for end-stage renal disease. N Engl J Med 306:1276–1279, 1982.
10. Samuelsson O, Wikstrand J, Wilhelmsen L, Berglund G: Heart and kidney involvement during antihypertensive treatment. Acta Med Scand 215:305–311, 1984.
11. Sullivan JM, Prewitt RL, Ratts TE: Sodium sensitivity in normotensive and borderline hypertensive humans. Am J Med Sci 295:370–377, 1988.
12. Williams GH, Hollenberg NK: Non-modulating hypertension: A subset of sodium-sensitive hypertension. Hypertension 17(Suppl I):I-81–I-85, 1991.
13. Williams RR, Hunt SC, Hasstedt SJ, et al: Definition of genetic factors in hypertension: A search for major genes, polygenes and homogeneous subtypes. J Cardiovasc Pharmacol 12(Suppl 3):S7–S20, 1988.

26. SHOCK AND CARDIAC ARREST

Richard E. Wolfe, M.D.

1. Define shock.

Shock is the failure of the cardiovascular system to provide adequate blood flow to organs and tissues. It also has been defined as a reduction of cardiac output or a poor distribution of output to a point where potentially irreversible tissue damage occurs.

2. Give a pathophysiologic classification of shock.

Blood flow is determined by three entities: blood volume, vascular resistance, and pump function. Thus, there are three types of shock: hypovolemic, vasogenic, and cardiogenic. Examples of causes of **hypovolemic shock** are gastrointestinal bleeds, ruptured aortic aneurysm, and severe diabetic ketoacidosis. Examples of **vasogenic shock** include septic shock, anaphylactic shock, neurogenic shock, and shock from pharmacologic causes. There was a wide variety of causes of **cardiogenic shock,** although acute myocardial infarction is the most common. Pulmonary embolism can be classified separately as obstructive but has a presentation similar to cardiogenic shock.

3. Which clinical signs are helpful in classifying shock?

The patient's history will usually make the diagnosis, but patients may present with shock of undetermined etiology. The clinician must then rely on the clinical examination to classify the shock state. Feeling the extremities and examining the jugular veins provide vital clues. Warm skin is suggestive of a vasogenic cause; cool, clammy skin reflects enhanced reflex sympatho-adrenal discharge leading to cutaneous vasoconstriction, suggesting hypovolemia or cardiogenic shock. Distended jugular veins, rales, or an S_3 gallop suggest a cardiogenic cause rather than hypovolemia. Measured central venous pressure may aid in differentiating hypovolemia from cardiogenic shock. Subclavian vein cannulation should be avoided if a myocardial infarction is suspected, as thrombolytic agents may be needed.

4. What are the four determinants of central venous pressure?

The normal central venous pressure (CVP) is 5–12 cm H_2O. Intravascular volume, intrathoracic pressure, right ventricular function, and venous tone all affect the CVP. To reduce variability caused by intrathoracic pressure, CVP should be measured at the end of expiration.

5. List 10 causes of cardiogenic shock.

1. Acute myocardial infarction (the most common)
2. Acute myocarditis
3. Chronic congestive cardiomyopathy
4. Valvular heart disease
5. Myocardial contusion
6. Arrhythmias
7. Toxins, drugs
8. Hypothermia
9. Hyperthermia
10. Left atrial myxoma

6. What are the classic changes in systemic vascular resistance and cardiac output in septic shock?

In classic "warm" septic shock, the systemic vascular resistance is reduced and cardiac output is increased. The increase in cardiac output is a compensatory mechanism for the decrease in vascular resistance. It is not completely compensatory because of a circulating myocardial depressant factor released in sepsis. The identity of this factor has not yet been agreed upon.

7. How can septic shock appear like cardiogenic shock?

In hypodynamic or "cold" septic shock, seen more frequently in the elderly, there are two causes for reduced cardiac output. First, the myocardial depressant factor decreases the cardiac index.

Second, in progressive sepsis, there are increases in pulmonary capillary resistance. These factors cause a significant decrease in cardiac output and present clinically like right-sided congestive heart failure. Cold septic shock has a very high mortality.

8. Describe the Killip classification of pump dysfunction in acute myocardial infarction.
The Killip classification is based on clinical criteria that correlate the degree of pump dysfunction with acute mortality in patients with myocardial infarction.
- Class I has no evidence of left ventricular failure and has a 5% mortality.
- Class II has bibasilar rates, an S_3 gallop or heart failure by chest x-ray, and a 15–20% mortality.
- Class III patients are in pulmonary edema. These patients have a 40% mortality.
- Class IV patients are in cardiogenic shock defined by: (1) systolic blood pressure < 90 mmHg, (2) peripheral vasoconstriction, (3) oliguria, and (4) pulmonary vascular congestion. Class IV patients have a mortality of 80%.

9. How significant is a loud holosystolic murmur in a patient with shock and an acute myocardial infarction?
Loud holosystolic murmurs with myocardial infarction indicates either papillary muscle rupture or an acute ventricular septal defect (VSD). These may be indistinguishable, but acute VSD usually occurs with an anteroseptal myocardial infarction and has an associated palpable thrill. Papillary rupture often does not have a thrill and is usually seen in inferior myocardial infarctions. These frequently cause shock on the basis of much reduced forward blood flow and can be differentiated by echocardiography or Swan-Ganz catheterization. Both require emergent cardiothoracic surgery for early repair. In some patients, the murmur may be soft or inaudible.

10. What are the signs and symptoms of massive pulmonary embolism?
Massive pulmonary embolism causes shock on the basis of reduced cross-sectional area of the pulmonary outflow tract. Shock occurs when the cross-sectional area is reduced by 50% or more. In an acute situation, the right ventricle can increase its systolic pressure only to a maximum of about 40 mmHg. This pressure is inadequate to overcome the increased resistance, blood flow is reduced, and shock develops. Massive pulmonary embolism presents with the following signs and symptoms:

Symptoms and Signs of Massive Pulmonary Embolism

SYMPTOMS		SIGNS	
Dyspnea	78%	Tachycardia	90%
Syncope	76%	Cyanosis	74%
Chest pain	72%	Systolic BP < 80 mmHg	87%
		Cardiac arrest	85%

11. What is the emergency treatment of cardiogenic shock?
Supplemental oxygen should be provided. Arrhythmias should be treated by protocols specified in the American Heart Association's textbook of Advanced Cardiac Life Support (ACLS). If the patient is not in pulmonary edema, volume can be administered in aliquots of 200–300 ml of crystalloid. This is particularly true in inferior myocardial infarction or if there is electrocardiographic evidence of right ventricular infarction. Dopamine and dobutamine are the pressors of choice for improvement of hemodynamics. Dobutamine is likely to be a better choice, particularly if there is evidence of pulmonary edema, since dobutamine, unlike dopamine, reduces left ventricular end-diastolic pressure. Dopamine is preferable in patients with a right ventricular infarct. Emergency angioplasty may improve survival in patients with cardiogenic shock from myocardial infarction.

12. What therapeutic measures may improve the condition of a patient with shock from a pulmonary embolism?
Massive pulmonary embolism should be treated similarly to cardiogenic shock from myocardial infarction: oxygen (intubation if necessary), volume, and pressors. Thrombolytics have not been studies well enough in massive pulmonary embolism to show improved survival. However, the use of tissue plasminogen activator, streptokinase, and urokinase has been demonstrated to improve hemodynamics with reduced tricuspid regurgitation, reduced right ventricular dilatation, and improved cardiac output in patients with massive pulmonary embolism, and thus the use of thrombolytics should be considered. Emergency embolectomy can also be considered.

13. What are the causes of traumatic cardiogenic shock?
Pericardial tamponade, myocardial contusion, tension pneumothorax, and air embolism from bronchial tears.

14. In which patients should the clinician suspect pericardial tamponade?
Acute pericardial tamponade occurs in about 2% of penetrating chest trauma cases and is more common with stab wounds than gunshot wounds. Tamponade is rare after blunt trauma. Beck's classic triad of distended neck veins, decreased arterial pressure, and muffled heart sound occurs only in about a third of patients. A high central venous pressure with tachycardia and hypotension in penetrating trauma are reliable signs of tamponade. Examination and chest radiography will exclude tension pneumothorax.

15. Does CPR resuscitate patients in cardiac arrest?
Cardiopulmonary resuscitation (CPR) rarely resuscitates patients from cardiac arrest without early institution of advanced life support interventions: defibrillation, airway management, and administration of appropriate drugs. All cardiac arrest victims should have a monitor placed as soon as possible, as immediate defibrillation is indicated in patients in ventricular fibrillation.

16. How does the blood "flow" with CPR?
Two mechanisms have been proposed to explain blood flow with closed chest compressions.
The **thoracic pump theory** suggests that the heart acts as the passive conduit, with systolic and mean arterial pressures and blood flow to the carotid artery augmented by increased thoracic pressure. Intrathoracic pressure is transmitted into the extrathoracic arteries to a greater extent than into the extrathoracic veins. This is reflected in an extrathoracic arterial–venous pressure gradient. The unequal transmission of intrathoracic pressure into the extrathoracic arteries and veins results from the presence of venous valves and unequal arterial and venous capacitance and collapsibility. Arteries resist collapse and therefore transmit the intrathoracic pressure into the extrathoracic arterial bed.
The **cardiac theory** suggests that the heart itself is compressed, creating a pressure gradient between intracardiac and extracardiac structures. However, there are not enough data at present to determine which mechanism predominates.

17. Describe the common reversible causes of cardiac arrest and their specific treatment.
Cardiac arrest may be successfully resuscitated in a number of cases if the underlying etiology is recognized and promptly treated.
1. **Ventricular fibrillation and ventricular tachycardia.** Immediate defibrillation should be performed before other procedures, as the success rate decreases by 4% with every minute of delay.
2. **Tension pneumothorax.** This condition should be suspected following positive pressure ventilation in a cardiac arrest patient who has a decrease in breath sounds on the affected side, subcutaneous air, or resistance to airflow with bagging. The treatment is needle decompression at the fifth intercostal space, followed by thoracotomy.

3. **Hyperkalemia.** Heralded by wide QRS complexes and the absence of P waves, hyperkalemia should be suspected as the cause of arrest in patients with renal failure. Calcium chloride should be administered immediately, followed by sodium bicarbonate and an insulin-glucose drip.

4. **Anaphylaxis.** This should be suspected whenever cardiac arrest occurs following administration of parenteral medication. As asphyxia or shock is the underlying mechanism, aggressive intervention with endotracheal intubation, fluids, and intravenous epinephrine should be performed immediately.

18. When should intravenous calcium be used in the patient in cardiac arrest?

Overall, patients in cardiac arrest do not appear to benefit from the use of intravenous calcium. Indications are thus limited to three specific causes of cardiac arrest: hyperkalemia, hypocalcemia, and possibly calcium antagonist overdose. Calcium chloride should be administered at a dose of 2–4 mg/kg of a 10% solution intravenously every 10 minutes.

19. Can neurologic outcome be predicted following successful resuscitation of cardiac arrest?

Several reports have attempted to develop prognostic signs for cerebral recovery following CPR. The duration of coma is the most reliable prognostic sign. However, recovery of consciousness has occurred after 10 days of coma. Reactive pupils, oculocephalic reflexes, spontaneous respirations, and purposeful response to painful stimuli are associated with a higher percentage of neurologic recovery. However, a favorable outcome may rarely occur in patients with poor prognostic signs.

BIBLIOGRAPHY

1. Bresler MJ: Future role of thrombolytic therapy in emergency medicine. Ann Emerg Med 18:1331, 1989.
2. Chatterjee K: Myocardial infarction shock. Crit Care Clin 1:563, 1985.
3. Dhainaut JF, et al: Right ventricular dysfunction in patients with septic shock. Intensive Care Med 14:488, 1988.
4. Donahue AM: Central venous pressure measurement. In Roberts JR, Hedges JR (eds): Clinical Procedures in Emergency Medicine. Philadelphia, W. B. Saunders, 1992, pp 332–338.
5. Luce JM: Pathogenesis and management of septic shock. Chest 91:883, 1987.
6. Mannix FL: Hemorrhagic shock. In Rosen P, et al (eds): Emergency Medicine: Concepts and Clinical Practice, 2nd ed. St. Louis, C. V. Mosby, 1988, p 179.
7. Ornato JP, Levine RL, Young DS, et al: The effect of applied chest compression force on systemic arterial pressure and end-tidal carbon dioxide concentration during CPR in human beings. Ann Emerg Med 18:732–737, 1989.
8. Safar P: Effects of the postresuscitation syndrome on cerebral recovery from cardiac arrest. Crit Care Med 13:932–935, 1985.
9. Schmidt RD, Wolfe R: Shock. In Rosen P, et al (eds): Emergency Medicine: Concepts and Clinical Practice, 3rd ed. St. Louis, C. V. Mosby, 1992, p 163.
10. Shamji FM, Todd TRJ: Hypovolemic shock. Crit Care Clin 1:609, 1985.
11. Wilson RF: The pathophysiology of shock. Intensive Care Med 6:89, 1980.

27. MYOCARDITIS

Richard A. Stein, M.D.

1. What are the mechanisms of injury to heart muscle cells thought to play a role in myocarditis due to infectious agents?

1. Direct invasion of the myocardium
2. Production of myocardial toxin
3. Immunologically mediated damage

The main cause of myocarditis in the United States is viral, and the mechanism of injury is thought to be immunologically related. Postulated mechanisms include the viral-related creation of new cell surface antigens, or antigen-antibody complex-related cell damage.

2. What are the major causes implicated in myocarditis?

Major Causes of Myocarditis

Infectious agents
Viral
Rickettsial
Bacterial
Protozoal
Metazoal
Allergic reactions
Pharmacologic agents
Systemic diseases such as vasculitis
Peripartum state (90 days before to 90 days after end of pregnancy)
Toxic agents (alcohol, toxic metals such as cobalt)

3. Describe the patient complaints and clinical findings that frequently accompany myocarditis.

The symptoms vary with the etiology, but most commonly myocarditis is subclinical, especially when it accompanies a generalized infectious processes. Patients may note fatigue, dyspnea, precordial discomfort, or palpitations. Frequently tachycardia is noted; the first heart sound may be muted and an S_4 gallop is often described.

4. What electrocardiographic (ECG) changes are commonly seen in myocarditis?

ST-segment elevation or depression and T-wave inversions are the most frequently noted changes. Atrial arrhythmia are commonly noted, and transient heart block (first, second, or third) may be noted.

5. How are patients with presumed viral myocarditis treated?

Treatment is supportive and responsive to the clinical presentation. Because atrioventricular conduction abnormalities are common in some forms of myocarditis, these patients should be watched carefully for evidence of conduction disturbances. In addition, exercise has been shown in animal models to increase the cell damage in myocarditis, so rest is usually prescribed. When congestive heart failure is noted, the usual treatment is indicated, although digoxin must be used carefully since there may be an increased incidence of digitalis toxic rhythms during active myocarditis. There is no consensus on the use of corticosteroids to decrease the acute inflammation associated with myocarditis; the concern is that they may increase viral replication. Nonsteroidal anti-inflammatory agents, aspirin, and cyclosporine are contraindicated during the first several weeks of an acute viral myocarditis because they increase myocyte damage. In cases possibly caused by atypical pneumonia or psittacosis, antibiotics are indicated.

6. Which viral infections are associated with myocarditis?

1. **Coxsackie B** virus is the most frequent cause of viral myocarditis. There is a presumed myocardial membrane affinity for these viral particles.

2. **Human immunodeficiency virus** (HIV) infection is associated with myocardial involvement in 20–25% of infected patients, but clinical disease is noted in only 10% of HIV-infected patients. Dilated cardiomyopathy presenting as congestive heart failure is the usual presentation, although pericardial effusion is also noted with some frequency. Less commonly noted are marantic endocarditis, ventricular arrhythmia, and right ventricular dilatation or hypertrophy.

3. **Lassa fever** is caused by an arenavirus and is a major cause of death in West Africa. Involvement is usually subclinical with one-half of the patients showing ST changes and low voltage on an ECG.

4. **Myocarditis** was frequently seen in fatal cases of poliomyelitis, especially during epidemics in the past.

7. List the bacterial diseases often associated with myocarditis and their characteristic presentations.

1. *Clostridium perfringens* **infection:** These infections commonly involve the heart, with myocardial changes due to toxin produced by the bacteria. The characteristic pathologic finding is gas bubbles in the myocardium. Abscess formation with resultant rupture into the pericardium and subsequent purulent pericarditis is seen.

2. **Diphtheria:** Myocardial involvement is very common (up to 20% of cases) and is the most common cause of death from this organism. The bacteria-produced toxin, which interferes with protein synthesis, is the basis for the cardiac damage. On pathologic examination, the heart shows "streaks," and microscopic examination reveals fatty infiltration of the myocytes. Clinically the myocarditis usually presents a cardiomegaly and severe congestive heart failure. Antitoxin should be administered as soon as the diagnosis is made, and antibiotic therapy then instituted. Conduction disturbances are common and may require a pacemaker. Some studies indicate that early treatment with carnitine ameliorates the course of the myocarditis.

3. **Meningococcal infection:** Cardiac involvement is common in fatal infections. Congestive heart failure, pericardial effusion, tamponade, and involvement of the atrioventricular node with resultant heart block may occur.

4. **Mycoplasma pneumonia:** This infection commonly involves the heart, with subclinical findings such as ST and T-wave changes noted on ECG. Pericarditis with an audible friction rub is noted on occasion.

5. **Psittacosis:** Myocarditis is a common finding with this infection. Cardiac involvement usually presents as congestive heart failure and acute (often fibrinous) pericarditis. Immediate treatment with tetracycline is indicated.

6. **Whipple disease:** Intestinal lipodystrophy is associated with rod-like organisms in the intestine and myocardium. The organism and mechanism of damage to the myocardium have not been elucidated. Cardiac involvement includes coronary artery lesions (panarteritis) and valvular fibrosis. Antibiotic therapy is reported to be effective in the treatment of the underlying disease.

7. **Spirochete infections:** Leptospirosis (Weil's disease), Lyme carditis, syphilis, and, in Ethiopia, relapsing fever have myocardial involvement.

8. What are the cardiac findings in Lyme disease?

Lyme disease is caused by the tick-borne spirochete, *Borrelia burgdorferi*. The initial infection is often marked by a rash, followed in weeks to months by involvement of other organ systems, including the heart, neurologic system, and joints. About 1 in 10 patients manifest cardiac involvement, usually with severe atrioventricular (AV) node block which is often associated with syncope, since there is concomitant depression of ventricular escape rhythms. Temporary pacing is indicated (the AV block usually resolves), as is antibiotic treatment with high-dose intravenous penicillin or oral tetracycline.

9. How long after the initial infection with *Trypanosoma cruzi* (Chagas' disease) do the cardiac manifestations occur?

The initial infection with *Trypanosoma* occurs when young adults are bit, usually around the eye, by a reduviid bug. A few individuals (about 1%) develop an acute myocarditis and pericarditis, which usually resolves over time. The major cardiac manifestation of Chagas' disease occurs about 20 years after the initial infection and is evident in 30% of the infected subjects. It involves cardiomegaly, congestive heart failure, arrhythmias, thromboembolism, right bundle branch block, and sudden death.

10. What are some unusual features of the cardiac involvement in Chagas' disease?

The pathologic appearance shows infiltration followed by fibrotic changes. There is a characteristic involvement of the right ventricle early in the process, which explains the early manifestations of right heart failure and tricuspid insufficiency. There is a predilection for involvement of the right bundle branch with subsequent right bundle branch block and an associated left anterior hemiblock. The fibrosis often extends into the apex of the left ventricle, resulting in a thin-walled, thrombus-filled ventricular aneurysm.

Laboratory and noninvasive testing yields in some characteristic findings. The ECG shows characteristic right bundle branch block and left anterior hemiblock. ST and T-wave changes may be present. Ventricular arrhythmia's are common, especially following exercise. Electrophysiologic testing often demonstrates inducible ventricular tachycardia. Echocardiography may demonstrate apical akinesia or a frank apical aneurysm, often with a ventricular thrombus. This pathophysiology explains the high incidence of sudden death and thromboembolic phenomena (seen in 50% of patients).

11. Describe the cardiac manifestations of a pheochromocytoma.

Patients may present with a reversible dilated cardiomyopathy. The cause is assumed to be the high level of circulating catecholamines resulting from the tumor, which may result in cell damage via a variety of pathways. The protective effect of aspirin suggests a role for platelet aggregation.

BIBLIOGRAPHY

1. Adair OV, Randive MD, Krashaw N: Isolated toxoplasm myocarditis in acquired immunodeficiency syndrome. Am Heart J 118:856–857, 1989.
2. Anderson DW, Virmani R: Emerging patterns of heart disease in human immunodeficiency virus infection. Hum Pathol 21:253, 1990.
3. Coplan NL, Bruno MS: Acquired immunodeficiency syndrome and heart disease: The present and the future. Am Heart J 175:1175–1177, 1988.
4. Maguire JH, Hoff R, Sherlock I, et al: Cardiac morbidity and mortality due to Chagas' disease: Prospective electrocardiographic study of a Brazilian community. Circulation 75:1140–1145, 1987.
5. McAlister HF, Klementowicz PT, Andrews C, et al: Lyme carditis: An important cause of reversible heart block. Ann Intern Med 110:339–345, 1989.
6. Midei MG, DeMent SH, Feldman AM, et al: Peripartum myocarditis and cardiomyopathy. Circulation 81:992–928, 1990.
7. Morris SA, Tanowitz HB, Wittner M, Bilezikian JP: Pathophysiological insights into the cardiomyopathy of Chagas' disease. Circulation 82:1900–1909, 1990.
8. Roberts WC, Berard CW: Gas gangrene of the heart in clostridial septicemia. Am Heart J 74:482–488, 1967.
9. Weinstein L, Shelokov A: Cardiovascular manifestations in acute poliomyelitis. N Engl J Med 244:281–285, 1951.

28. DILATED CARDIOMYOPATHY

Robert A. Vaccarino, M.D.

1. What is cardiomyopathy?

Cardiomyopathies comprise a group of diseases in which the dominant characteristic is primary involvement of heart muscle (myocardium only).

2. Describe the classification of cardiomyopathy.

Cardiomyopathy can be classified as primary, which is heart muscle disease of unknown etiology, or secondary, which is heart muscle disease in response to specific or preexisting disease (coronary artery disease, hypertension, valvular heart disease, infection, or coexisting disease). However, the World Health Organization has recommended that cardiomyopathy be classified into three major groups according to pathophysiology regardless of etiology:

1. Dilated
2. Hypertrophic
3. Restrictive

3. What is the incidence of idiopathic dilated cardiomyopathy?

0.7–7.5/100,000 population, with higher incidence rates seen in blacks than whites and males than females.

4. What factors predict increased mortality in patients with dilated cardiomyopathy?

Age > 55 yrs
Left ventricular ejection fraction < 35%
New York Heart Association functional class II or greater
Intraventricular conduction delay on electrocardiography
Left ventricular end-diastolic pressure > 20 mm Hg
Cardiac index < 3.0
Increased serum norepinephrine level
Increased serum level of atrial natriuretic peptide
Increased cardiothoracic ratio of ≥ 0.55 on chest x-ray
Hyponatremia

5. What are the definite indications for endomyocardial biopsy?

Monitoring cardiac allograft rejection
Detecting myocarditis
Monitoring anthracycline cardiotoxins
Diagnosing secondary cardiomyopathy

6. What is the major pathophysiological characteristic of dilated cardiomyopathy?

Dilated cardiomyopathy is characterized by biventricular enlargement with reduced ventricular systolic function.

7. How frequently does cardiomyopathy develop with anthracycline chemotherapeutic agents?

The incidence is 1.7–4.4% depending on which anthracycline agent is used. A clear cumulative dose-related incidence has been found. Patients receiving a cumulative dose of 500–550 mg/m^2 of doxorubicin have a 7% incidence of developing cardiomyopathy. Patients receiving a cumulative dose of > 550 mg/m^2 have a 20–40% incidence of developing cardiomyopathy. If other chemotherapeutic agents, such as mitomycin or cyclophosphamide, and radiation therapy are combined with doxorubicin, cardiomyopathy may develop at a lower cumulative dose (450–500 mg/m^2).

8. Which chemotherapeutic agents most frequently cause cardiomyopathy?
Doxorubicin, cyclophosphamide, amsacrine, and interferon.

9. Does therapy for dilated idiopathic cardiomyopathy differ from that for congestive heart failure secondary to coronary artery disease?
The approach in treating patients with dilated cardiomyopathy and congestive heart failure are similar. Treatment consists of salt restriction, limitation of physical exertion, diuretics, angiotensin-converting enzyme inhibitors, combination of hydralazine and isosorbide nitrates, digitalis, oral anticoagulants, and β-blockade.

10. Name the neuromuscular disorders that are most commonly associated with dilated cardiomyopathy.
Friedreich's ataxia, myotomic muscular dystrophy, Duchenne muscular dystrophy.

11. What is peripartum cardiomyopathy?
Peripartum cardiomyopathy is a form of dilated cardiomyopathy that occurs during the last 3 months of pregnancy and up to 6 months postpartum, in the absence of a previous history of myocardial disorder. Endomyocardial biopsy reveals myocarditis in 30–50% of these cases.

The reported incidence of peripartum cardiomyopathy ranges from 1/3,000 to 1/15,000. The incidence is increased in women who are >30 years of age, hypertensive, toxemic, multiparous, and with twin pregnancies.

12. A 50-year-old woman presents with worsening exertional dyspnea and lower-extremity edema. The physical examination demonstrates elevated jugular venous pressure, bilateral rales, an S$_3$ gallop, and pitting edema of the lower extremities. She is obviously intoxicated. The chest x-ray shows an enlarged cardiac silhouette and a prominent interstitial pattern. What diagnostic possibilities should be considered?
The patient has congestive heart failure. Given that she is acutely intoxicated, further history should be obtained to assess for chronic alcoholism. If the patient is indeed alcoholic, the heart failure may be the result of alcoholic cardiomyopathy. Alcoholic cardiomyopathy is one of the most common secondary causes of dilated cardiomyopathy in the United States. Many patients improve markedly if they stop drinking.

Diagnostic thought should not end there though. Many chronic alcoholics eat poorly and develop multiple nutritional deficiencies. One of these, thiamine deficiency, can cause heart failure, so-called "wet beriberi." Most alcoholic patients with cardiomyopathy should be given a therapeutic trial of thiamine. In addition, ethanol does not provide protection against other diseases that cause cardiomyopathy, such as coronary artery disease.

13. A 47-year-old man, who is tanned and appears healthy, presents with symptoms and signs of heart failure. On questioning, he reveals that he was diagnosed as "borderline diabetic" at a screening examination several years ago, and that his father died suddenly in his late 40s. If you could order only one blood test for diagnostic purposes, what would it be?
Either a serum iron or ferritin, since it may give a clue to the presence of hemochromatosis. Hemochromatosis can cause heart failure, diabetes, and chronic liver disease. It is an important diagnosis to consider in patients with heart failure, because it is one of the few cardiomyopathies that may resolve with treatment. It is more common in men, is frequently familial, and typically presents in the fifth or sixth decade of life. A more aggressive form of the disease, primarily limited to the heart, may present at younger ages.

14. Describe the pathogenesis of restrictive cardiomyopathy.
Restrictive cardiomyopathy is the least common of the cardiomyopathies and is characterized by abnormal diastolic function in the presence of normal ventricular systolic function.

15. What is the most common form of cardiac amyloidosis?
Primary amyloidosis. The amyloid pattern is the terminal component of a light chain immuno-globulin referred to as AL protein. These AL proteins are produced by plasma cells. Secondary amyloidosis usually occurs in chronic inflammatory disease, producing a protein referred to as AA protein. This protein is of unknown origin and is not produced by plasma cells. Senile amyloidosis and familial amyloidosis are rarely associated with cardiomyopathy.

16. What are the most common forms of restrictive cardiomyopathy?
The restrictive cardiomyopathies can be classified into myocardial and endocardial forms. The most common myocardial forms are:

Infiltrative:	amyloid or sarcoid
Noninfiltrative:	idiopathic or scleroderma
Storage disease:	hemochromatosis, Fabry's disease, or glucogen storage disease

The most common endocardial forms are carcinoid, endomyocardial fibrosis, and metastatic malignancy.

17. Describe the characteristic findings in patients with restrictive cardiomyopathy.
The hemodynamic findings in restrictive cardiomyopathy are very similar to those of constrictive pericarditis, and the differential diagnosis by hemodynamic parameters alone may be very difficult. The hemodynamic findings are:

1. An early diastolic dip in ventricular pressure at the onset of diastole, followed by an early diastolic plateau. This early diastolic dip and diastolic plateau is referred to as the "square-root sign."

2. Near-equalization of right and left ventricular filling pressure with left ventricular filling pressure being 2–5 mmHg greater than the right ventricular filling pressure.

3. High pulmonary artery systolic pressure.

4. Deep X descent and prominent A wave. The A wave is the same height and amplitude as the V wave, making the typical M or W waveform in the central venous pressure tracing.

BIBLIOGRAPHY

1. Anderson KP, et al: Sudden death in idiopathic dilated cardiomyopathy. Ann Intern Med 107:104, 1987.
2. Cohn JN, Johnson G, Ziesche S, et al: A comparison of enalapril with hydralazine-isosorbide dinitrate in the treatment of chronic congestive heart failure. N Engl J Med 325:303–310, 1991.
3. Keren A, et al: Mildly dilated congestive cardiomyopathy. Circulation 81:506, 1990.
4. Manolio TA, et al. Prevalence and etiology of idiopathic dilated cardiomyopathy (summary of a National Heart, Lung, and Blood Institutes Workshop). Am J Cardiol 69:1458, 1992.
5. Packer M, Carver JR, Rodeheffer RJ, et al: Effect of oral milrinone on mortality in severe chronic heart failure: The PROMISE study research group. N Engl J Med 325:1509–1510, 1991.
6. Perloff JK: The cardiomyopathies. Cardiol Clin 6:185–320, 1988.
7. SOLVD Investigators: Effect of enalapril on survival in patients with reduced left ventricular ejection fractions and congestive heart failure. N Engl J Med 325:293–302, 1991.
8. Sugrue DD, Rodeheffer RJ, Codd MB, et al: The clinical course of idiopathic dilated cardiomyopathy: A population-based study. Ann Intern Med 117:117–123, 1992.
9. Vaitkus PT, Kussmaul WG: Constrictive pericarditis versus restrictive cardiomyopathy: A reappraisal and update of diagnostic criteria. Am Heart J 122:1431–1441, 1991.

29. HYPERTROPHIC CARDIOMYOPATHY

Ashraf ElSakr, M.D., and Luther T. Clark, M.D.

1. What is hypertrophic cardiomyopathy?

Hypertrophic cardiomyopathy (HCM) is a primary disorder of the heart muscle characterized by inappropriate myocardial hypertrophy of a nondilated left ventricle (LV) and not secondary to a cardiovascular or systemic disease (i.e., hypertension or aortic stenosis). It most often involves the interventricular septum (**asymmetric septal hypertrophy**) and may be associated with dynamic LV outflow tract obstruction (**hypertrophic obstructive cardiomyopathy**). Another term that has been used to describe HCM is **idiopathic subaortic stenosis.**

2. Is HCM genetic or acquired?

In more than half of the patients, the disease appears to be genetically transmitted as a single-gene autosomal-dominant trait with variable expression and penetrance. In the remaining patients, HCM occurs sporadically.

3. What are the most common variants of HCM?

The pattern and extent of LV hypertrophy in patients with HCM vary greatly, and different patterns may occur in the same family pedigree. Asymmetric septal hypertrophy, the most common variant, accounts for 90% of patients. The septal hypertrophy may affect the basal one-third of the septum (subaortic area) only, the basal two-thirds (down to papillary muscles), or the entire septum from base to apex. The other two common variants are apical (involving the apical one-third of the ventricle) and midventricle hypertrophy (maximal thickening at the level of the papillary muscles).

4. Is the histology of HCM unique?

The histologic picture of HCM is characterized by myocardial hypertrophy and myocardial fiber disarray. There is disorganization of the muscle bundles, abnormalities in the cell-to-cell arrangements, and disorganization of the myofibrillar architecture, but these findings also may occur in other acquired and congenital cardiac conditions. The disarray of HCM is unique only in its ubiquity and frequency, with virtually all patients with HCM having some degree of disarray and most having at least 5% of the myocardium affected, whereas in non-HCM patients it usually involves only about 1% of the myocardium.

5. What are the most frequent symptoms in patients with HCM?

Most patients with HCM are asymptomatic and are identified during screening of relatives with known disease. In patients who are symptomatic, the most common symptoms are:
1. **Dyspnea**
   - Present in up to 90% of symptomatic patients
   - Secondary to LV diastolic dysfunction, impaired ventricular filling, and elevation of left atrial and pulmonary venous pressures
2. **Angina pectoris**
   - Occurs in up to 75% of symptomatic patients
   - Secondary to imbalance between oxygen supply and demand with greatly increased myocardial mass, impaired vasodilatory coronary reserve (due to thickened and narrowed small intramural coronary arteries), and subendocardial ischemia (due to increased oxygen demand in the presence of an outflow gradient and increased filling pressure)
3. **Syncope and presyncope**
   - Due to inadequate cardiac output with exertion or to cardiac arrhythmias
   - Identify patients at increased risk for sudden death (especially in children and young adults, the first clinical presentation may be sudden death)

6. Describe the classic murmur of obstructive HCM and bedside maneuvers that help distinguish it from other common etiologies.

The classic murmur of obstructive HCM is a **crescendo-decrescendo systolic murmur,** typically harsh, that usually begins well after the first heart sound (since ejection is not impeded early in systole). Bedside maneuvers that help differentiate this murmur from others are listed in the accompanying table.

Effect of Bedside Maneuvers on Systolic Murmurs

	VALSALVA	HANDGRIP	SQUATTING	AMYL NITRITE	LEG RAISING
Obstructive HCM	↑	↓	↓	↑	↓
Aortic stenosis	↓	↓	↑↓	↑	↑
Ventricular septal defect	↓	↑	No change	↓	↑
Mitral regurgitation	↓ (slight)	↑	No change	↓	↑

7. How does the carotid pulse in obstructive HCM differ from that in valvular aortic stenosis?

In patients with HCM, the carotid pulse has an initial brisk rise, followed by a decline, then a second rise. In aortic stenosis, the carotid upstroke is slowed and the amplitude low (*pulsus parvus et tardus*).

8. Which noninvasive laboratory evaluations are helpful in evaluating patients with suspected HCM?

Useful noninvasive laboratory tests include electrocardiography (ECG), chest x-ray, and echocardiography. The **ECG** may be normal but is usually abnormal in symptomatic patients, showing nonspecific ST and T-wave changes, LV hypertrophy, deep broad Q waves in the inferolateral leads, left axis deviation, and left atrial enlargement. Arrhythmias (supraventricular and ventricular) may be present on ambulatory monitoring.

The **chest x-ray** may be normal but usually shows mild to moderate increase in the cardiac silhouette.

Echocardiography is the cornerstone of the diagnosis of HCM. Ventricular hypertrophy is the cardinal feature seen on the echocardiogram. The septum is usually > 15 mm thick with a septal-to-posterior wall ratio of > 1.3–1.5. Other features include narrowing of the LV outflow tract formed by the interventricular septum anteriorly and the anterior mitral valve leaflet posteriorly (accentuated further with the Valsalva maneuver or amyl nitrite), a small LV cavity, and partial systolic closure or fluttering of the aortic valve. Color flow Doppler imaging may reveal mitral regurgitation.

9. What is SAM? What causes it?

SAM refers to the abnormal **systolic anterior motion** of the anterior (and occasionally posterior) mitral valve leaflet during mid-systole. The role of SAM in producing the outflow gradient is controversial, although the degree of SAM and size of the outflow gradient are related. Three explanations have been offered for SAM:

1. A Venturi effect that draws the mitral valve toward the septum because of the early high-velocity jet of ejected blood and the decreased pressure at the outflow tract;

2. Pulling of the mitral valve against the septum by the contraction of the papillary muscles, which are abnormally located and orientated;

3. Pushing of the mitral valve against the septum, perhaps by the posterior wall because of its abnormal position in the LV outflow tract (*see* figures on next page).

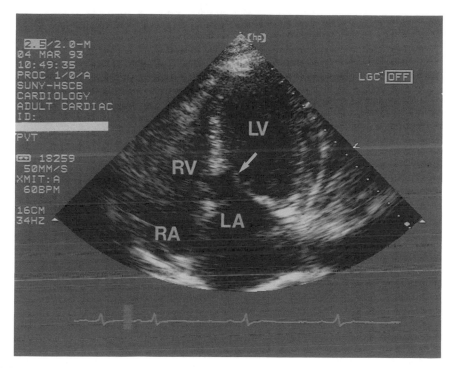

Apical four-chamber view showing SAM (*arrow*) of the anterior mitral leaflet during midsystole. (RV − right ventricle, LV = left ventricle, RA = right atrium, LA = left atrium).

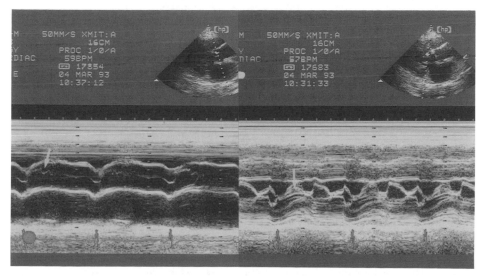

This figure shows two M-mode echocardiographic views in a patient with HCM. *Left,* The M-mode of the aortic root and left atrium. There is late systolic notching (arrow) of the aortic valve leaflets due to partial closure and reopening of the aortic valve. *Right,* SAM of the mitral valve during midsystole (arrow).

10. Which patients with HCM are at greatest risk for sudden death?
Sudden death in patients with HCM is presumed (but not proven) to be due to a ventricular arrhythmia. It may occur in patients who are asymptomatic or whose clinical course has been otherwise stable. Markers of increased risk for sudden death include:
- Age < 30 years at diagnosis
- Family history of HCM and sudden death
- History of syncope (in children)
- Nonsustained ventricular tachycardia on ambulatory ECG monitoring (in adults)

Symptoms, degree of functional limitation, and severity of the outflow tract gradient do not correlate with risk of death. In young competitive athletes who die suddenly, unsuspected HCM is the most common diagnosis at autopsy.

11. Which clinical manifestations of HCM are amenable to medical or surgical therapy?
The goals of management in patients with HCM are to improve symptoms, prevent complications, and reduce the risk of sudden death. The three manifestations of HCM that are amenable to specific medical or surgical therapy are: (1) ventricular outflow obstruction (2) impaired ventricular relaxation during diastole, and (3) atrial and ventricular arrhythmias.

12. In patients with HCM, what are the optimal therapies for relieving outflow obstruction and improving LV relaxation?
Optimal therapy for the various manifestations of HCM has been debated for years. **Outflow obstruction** may be improved with beta-adrenergic blocking agents, calcium antagonists, and disopyramide. Pacemaker implant and, rarely, ventriculomyectomy or mitral valve replacement may be indicated. Patients who do not respond to maximum medical and surgical therapy may be candidates for cardiac transplantation.

Calcium antagonists (i.e., verapamil) and beta-adrenergic blocking agents may improve **ventricular relaxation.** Resting obstruction may be lessened or abolished with disopyramide, thereby improving relaxation. Calcium antagonists should be used with caution because they may worsen or provoke outflow obstruction in some patients.

13. Name three ways to enhance the outflow gradient in HCM.
1. Increase contractility (with inotropic drugs such as digitalis)
2. Decrease preload (hypovolemia, diuretics, nitrates)
3. Decrease afterload (nitrates, vasodilators)

14. What is the natural history of HCM?
The clinical course of patients with HCM is variable. Many patients remain asymptomatic or only mildly symptomatic for years. In those with resting obstruction, approximately two-thirds progress to New York Heart Association Class III–IV over a 4-year period. The degree of ventricular hypertrophy usually remains stable over time but may increase. In about 10% of patients, HCM progresses to LV dilatation and a dilated cardiomyopathy. The onset of atrial fibrillation usually results in worsening of symptoms. Mortality tends to be higher in those with outflow obstruction, who also tend to have the most extensive hypertrophy and the highest incidence of atrial and ventricular arrhythmias. The annual mortality of patients with HCM is about 3% in adults and 6% in children.

BIBLIOGRAPHY

1. Frank S, Braunwald E: Idiopathic hypertrophic subaortic stenosis: Clinical analysis of 126 patients with emphasis on the natural history. Circulation 37:759–788, 1968.
2. Lawson JWR: Hypertrophic cardiomyopathy: Current views and etiology, pathophysiology and management. Am J Med Sci 294:191–210, 1987.
3. Lembo NJ, Dell-Italia LJ, Crawford MH, O'Rourke RA: Bedside diagnosis of systolic murmurs. N Engl J Med 318:1572–1578, 1988.

4. Maron BJ, Bonow RQ, Cannon RO, et al: Hypertrophic cardiomyopathy: Interrelations of clinical manifestations, pathophysiology and therapy. N Engl J Med 316:780–787, 844–851, 1987.
5. Maron BJ, Fananapazir L: Sudden cardiac death in hypertrophic cardiomyopathy. Circulation 85 [Suppl I]: I-57–I-63, 1992.
6. Moro E, Ten Cate FJ, Lenoard JJ, et al: Genesis of systolic anterior motion of the mitral valve in hypertrophic cardiomyopathy: An anatomic or dynamic event? Eur Heart J 8:1312–1321, 1987.
7. Romeo F, Pelliccia F, Cristofan R, et al: Hypertrophic cardiomyopathy: Is a left ventricular outflow tract gradient a major prognostic determinant? Eur Heart J 11:233–240, 1990.
8. Rosing DR, Idänpään-Heikkilä U, Maron BJ, et al: Use of calcium channel blocking drugs in hypertrophic cardiomyopathy. Am J Cardiol 55:185B–195B, 1985.
9. Sasson Z, Rakowski H, Wigle ED, et al: Echocardiographic and Doppler studies in hypertrophic cardiomyopathy. Cardiol Clin 8:217–232, 1990.
10. Seiler C, Hess OM, Schoenbeck M, et al: Long-term follow-up of medical versus surgical therapy for hypertrophic cardiomyopathy: A retrospective study. J Am Coll Cardiol 17:634–642, 1991.
11. Solomon SD, Jarcho JA, McKenna W, et al: Familial hypertrophic cardiomyopathy is a genetically heterogenous disease. J Clin Invest 86:993–999, 1990.
12. Spirito P, Chiarella F, Carratino L, et al: Clinical course and prognosis of hypertrophic cardiomyopathy in an outpatient population. N Engl J Med 320:749–755, 1989.
13. Wynne J, Braunwald E: Hypertrophic cardiomyopathy. In Braunwald E (ed): Heart Disease: A Textbook of Cardiovascular Medicine, 4th ed. Philadelphia, W. B. Saunders, 1992, pp 1404–1415.

30. SYNCOPE AND DIZZINESS

Olivia V. Adair, M.D.

1. What is syncope? How common is it?
Syncope is a transient loss of consciousness, usually for seconds to minutes, with loss of postural tone and resulting in spontaneous recovery. Syncope may also be associated with near-syncope or presyncope as dizziness, almost blacking out. Syncope is not associated with stupor or coma. The condition is very common, seen in 30–50% of the adult population, and accounts for approximately 1–2% of hospital admissions and 3% of emergency room visits per year.

2. How common is dizziness?
Dizziness is one of the most common complaints in ambulatory care and accounts for nearly 8 million outpatient visits/year in the U.S.; after fatigue, it is the most common complaint in general medical clinics. Dizziness is a very heterogeneous symptom and includes sensations of vertigo, presyncope, disequilibrium, and lightheadedness.

3. What prognosis is associated with syncope or dizziness?
The prognosis depends on the underlying cause. Cardiac syncope carries the worse prognosis. Therefore, syncope usually initiates a thorough diagnostic evaluation to rule out a cardiac etiology. Dizziness, on the other hand, is often self-limiting and only rarely relates to life-threatening events, even in elderly patients.

4. What causes dizziness?
- Vertigo (54%), with benign positional vertigo being the most common specific vestibular diagnosis.
- Psychiatric disorders (40%), usually in younger patients
- Multicausal (13%)

5. Describe the workup for dizziness.
Dizziness is often self-limiting, but when it does persist, a directed history and physical examination can establish a presumptive diagnosis in most patients. The best tests to supplement these are vestibular function testing and psychiatric evaluation.

6. What are the major etiologies of syncope?
Three major categories each account for approximately one-third of the cases of syncope: noncardiac, cardiac, and unknown causes. Because syncope is a symptom and not a disease, its etiologies are diverse and may be multicausal. The 1-year mortality for cardiac syncope is the highest, 30%. Those for noncardiac syncope (12%) and undetermined-etiology syncope (6%) are lower, but they still represent a higher mortality than in a general healthy population. The symptom of syncope should be considered serious, and an etiology should be identified.

7. What is the most important evaluation step or test in identifying the etiology of syncope?
A careful **history and physical examination** form the cornerstone for establishing the proper diagnosis of syncope. One study showed that the history and physical exam were sufficient in establishing the diagnosis in 85% of patients. Also, if the answer is not found in the history and physical exam, it may never be found. The surrounding circumstances are important to establish—e.g., loss of consciousness, chest pain, palpitations, running after a bus, or watching TV. Also, other medical problems and medications should be evaluated for a possible effect. Physical examinations should include postural maneuvers, attention to murmurs, carotid pulse,

carotid sinus massage (unless contradicted), careful neurologic examination, as well as rectal examination (to rule out gastrointestinal bleeding).

Routine laboratory studies, a chest roentgenogram, and an **electrocardiogram** (ECG) are recommended. If heart disease is suspected, an echo-Doppler study should be included in the initial workup. Unfortunately, only about one-half of patients will have a correct diagnosis after the routine clinical evaluation.

8. How helpful is 24-hour Holter monitoring for the diagnosis of syncope?

In a large study of patients with syncope unexplained by history or physical examination, 86 patients (mean age, 61 yrs) underwent three serial 24-hour Holter evaluations. The first Holter showed at least one major abnormality in 14 patients (16%); the second showed a major abnormality in 9 (12%) of the remaining 72 patients; only 3 patients (5%) had major abnormalities on the third Holter. The factors associated with major abnormalities on Holter were age > 65 yrs, male gender, history of heart disease, and initial nonsinus rhythm (highest relative risk, 3.5). Therefore, in the 26 patients identified with major abnormalities, 23 of them were identified with 48-hour Holter evaluation. Thus, extending the monitoring duration from 24 to 48 hours almost doubled the diagnostic benefit.

9. Does syncope every occur as the initial presentation of an acute myocardial infarction?

Yes. Five to 10% of patients with acute myocardial infarction have syncope as their initial presentation. This most commonly occurs in association with Q-wave inferior wall infarction and may be fatal. The mechanism is most likely activation of the Bezold-Jarisch reflex, predominantly a vasovagal reaction.

10. Should syncope in the elderly patient be evaluated differently?

The incidence of syncope is increased in the elderly (6–7% annually and 30% recurrence rate), as cerebral blood flow decreases with aging. Also, syncope in the elderly may be the first manifestation of various serious illnesses and thus of graver prognosis. One study reported that patients over 70 years old who experienced syncope had a mortality in 1 year of 16–27% versus a mortality in a young population of 1–8%. The physical injury that may result from a syncopal episode may be especially devastating in elderly persons.

11. How common is carotid sinus syncope?

Hypersensitivity to carotid sinus stimulation has been shown in recent studies to be more common than previously thought. Carotid sinus stimulation may either cause a vasodepressor reaction or a predominant vasovagal reaction, or both. Drugs known to aggravate carotid sinus syncope are digitalis, beta blockers, and calcium channel blockers. The hypersensitivity may be secondary to an abnormality of the carotid sinus mechanism or to underlying conduction system disease. Diagnosis can be made with carotid massage in a head-up tilt position with blood pressure and ECG monitoring, with hypotension being a positive result.

Therapy includes patient education and evaluation of their medications, with possible carotid sinus denervation and pacemaker implantation if symptoms are refractory or associated with significant bradycardias. Dual-chamber pacing is required since single-chamber pacing commonly produces pacemaker syndrome. Pacer therapy reduces the incidence of syncope even without a direct affect on vasodepressor response.

12. When should arrhythmic syncope be suspected?

Arrhythmia is more likely if the patient has underlying heart disease, symptoms of palpitations, abrupt syncope with injury, and syncope not associated with posture changes. Arrhythmic syncope is usually the result of a heart rate either too fast or slow occurring in a patient with limited cardiac reserve (secondary to valvular or myocardial disease). These patients are also more likely to have conduction abnormalities, predisposing them to low cardiac output with an arrhythmia.

13. What is the best approach for work-up of a suspected arrhythmic syncope?
The work-up of syncope can be costly and timely. Therefore, it should usually start with the less expensive and least invasive studies, unless special circumstances dictate otherwise.

The accompanying table shows the usual tests and how they fit into the evaluation of syncope. Obviously, if a specific exertional etiology is suspected from the history and physical examination, this should help dictate the work-up strategy. Because of the importance of left ventricular function in the prognosis of patients, we do echo-Doppler as part of the evaluation of almost all syncope patients referred to the cardiology service.

Laboratory Evaluation of Arrhythmic Syncope

TEST	PURPOSE
Electrocardiogram (ECG)	Defines conduction system disease, Wolff-Parkinson-White syndrome, myocardial infarction, left ventricular hypertrophy, atrial and ventricular ectopy, and occasionally arrhythmia.
Signal-averaged ECG	Screens for ventricular tachycardia after myocardial infarction.
Ambulatory monitoring	Documents arrhythmia and relates to symptoms; aids in defining therapeutic response.
Echocardiography	Evaluates for valve disease, myocardial disease, left ventricular function.
Patient-activated monitoring devices	Documents paroxysmal arrhythmias in low-risk subsets.
Exertional exercise test	Reproduces external arrhythmia; evaluates role of ischemia.
Invasive electrophysiologic study	Defines conduction system disease, elicits supraventricular and ventricular tachycardia, and measures hemodynamic effect of arrhythmias and response to pharmacologic and pacing interventions.
Head-up tilt	Elicits vasodepressor or hemodynamic response to arrhythmia.

Modified from Weissler AM, Boudoulas HB, Lewis RP, et al: Syncope: Pathophysiology, recognition, and treatment. In Hurst JW (ed): The Heart, 7th ed. New York, McGraw-Hill, 1990, p 581.

14. How helpful is signal-averaged ECG in evaluating recurrent syncope?
Signal-averaged ECG is especially helpful in identifying patients with ventricular tachycardia with late potentials. The presence of a late potential predicts ventricular tachycardia as the etiology of syncope with a sensitivity of 73% and specificity of 89%. The combination of heart disease and late potentials is highly predictive of the eventual clinical diagnosis of ventricular tachycardia. Also, combining results of other noninvasive test, such as Holter monitoring, and echocardiogram, greatly increases the usefulness of signal-averaged ECG. The absence of a late potential provides a strong negative predictor of ventricular tachycardia and is therefore a useful screening test in patients with syncope.

15. When should electrophysiology studies (EPS) be considered for arrhythmia detection?
Patients who are best served by EPS are those strongly suspected of having arrhythmic syncope as indicated by the noninvasive test and underlying heart disease. In these patients, EPS reveals a mechanism in two-thirds of patients who undergo the procedure. Also, patients with a negative study have a very low short-term mortality but may have recurrent nonarrhythmic syncope. The most common arrhythmia detected is ventricular tachycardia, and the most powerful predictor of a positive EPS is an ejection fraction of < 40%. The therapeutic strategies formulated by the diagnostic tests are very effective in preventing syncope in most patients, 96%, during an 18-month follow-up.

16. Should you expect to find the cause of syncope in most patients? What should you do if no cause is identified?
With the more common use of EPS and tilt-table testing, fewer patients are given the diagnosis of syncope of unknown cause. However, still about 20% of patients have no etiology established after extensive work-ups. These may include patients with multiple causes, especially older

patients. Close follow-up is important because about one-third will have recurrence. Also, counseling on avoidance of potentially dangerous activities and predisposing factors is essential.

BIBLIOGRAPHY

1. Bass EB, Curtiss EI, Arena VC, et al. The duration of Holter monitoring in patients with syncope. Arch Intern Med 150:1073–1078, 1990.
2. Kapoor WN, Karpf M, Wieand S, et al: A prospective evaluation and follow-up of patients with syncope. N Engl J Med 309:197–204, 1983.
3. Kapoor W, Snustad D, Peterson J, et al: Syncope in the elderly. Am J Med 80:419–428, 1986.
4. Kroenke K, Lucas CA, Rosenberg ML, et al: Causes of persistent dizziness: A prospective study of 100 patients in ambulatory care. Ann Intern Med 117:898–904, 1992.
5. Krol RB, Morady F, Flaker GC, et al: Electrophysiologic testing in patients with unexplained syncope: Clinical and noninvasive predictors of outcome. J Am Coll Cardiol 10:358–363, 1987.
6. Kuchar DL, Thorburn CW, Sammel NL: Signal-averaged electrocardiogram for evaluation of recurrent syncope. Am J Cardiol 58:949–953, 1986.
7. Manolis AS, Linzer M, Salem D, Estes NA III: Syncope: Current diagnostic evaluation and management. Ann Intern Med 112:850–863, 1990.
8. McIntosh HD: Evaluating elderly patients with syncope. Cardiovasc Rev Rep 9:54–58, 1988
9. Sra JS, Anderson AJ, Sheikh SH, et al: Unexplained syncope evaluated by electrophysiologic studies and head-up tilt testing. Ann Intern Med 114:1013–1019, 1991.
10. Wehrmacher WH: Syncope among the aging population. Am J Geriatr Cardiol 2:50–57, 1993.
11. Winters SL, Stewart D, Gomes JA: Signal averaging of the surface QRS complex predicts inducibility of ventricular tachycardia in patients with syncope of unknown origin: A prospective study. Am Coll Cardiol 10:775–781, 1987.

31. TRAUMATIC HEART DISEASE

Edward P. Havranek, M.D.

1. What are the most common causes of nonpenetrating cardiac injury?
Motor vehicle accidents.

2. What cardiac structures can be injured by blunt chest trauma?
Injury to the myocardium itself is most common and may result in contusion or outright rupture of any chamber with cardiac tamponade. Traumatic tear of the aorta or any of the heart valves is also relatively common. The coronary arteries sustain damage with either thrombosis or laceration. The pericardium may rupture. Finally, contusion or localized edema may result in dysfunction of the sinoatrial or atrioventricular nodes, causing sinus bradycardia or heart block, respectively.

3. What techniques are useful in diagnosing traumatic injury to the heart?
The history and physical examination remain the most important diagnostic tools for evaluating suspected cardiac trauma. The most important aspect of the history is the mechanism of injury. Significant damage to the vehicle's steering wheel, for instance, is an important clue to associated heart injury. The physical examination should focus on evidence for chest wall injury and hemodynamic compromise (i.e., tachycardia, hypotension and shock, and jugular venous distention). Jugular venous distention is a component of Beck's triad, as seen in acute pericardial tamponade (*see* chapter 24).

4. What about other noninvasive diagnostic techniques?
   Electrocardiography: The ECG is frequently normal in cases of myocardial contusion and may show nonspecific ST or T-wave changes unrelated to cardiac injury. In some cases, it may show arrhythmia or changes diagnostic of myocardial injury.
   Chest x-ray: Significant cardiac injury may be present when the x-ray is normal. A finding of rib fracture or pulmonary contusion should increase the level of suspicion of cardiac injury.
   Cardiac enzymes: These are usually elevated from associated skeletal muscle injury and cannot be relied on for the diagnosis of myocardial contusion; however, cardiac enzymes (MB) are quite specific and useful.
   Radionuclide ventriculography: A wall motion abnormality generally indicates the presence of myocardial contusion. A normal study does not rule out such injury, since many injuries occur to the right ventricle, which is less well visualized by this technique.
   Echocardiography: In general, this is the most useful technique, because it can show wall motion abnormalities, intracardiac shunts, and valvular regurgitation.

5. How is the diagnosis of myocardial contusion made?
Echocardiography is the procedure of choice. Because many patients with chest trauma have bandages, chest tubes, or subcutaneous emphysema that makes transthoracic echocardiography difficult, transesophageal echocardiograms are assuming a larger role in the evaluation of trauma patients.

6. What is the most common site of injury to the aorta?
The ligamentum arteriosum, where the aorta is tethered to other mediastinal structures. During deceleration injury, shear forces are greatest in this region.

7. Are there any late sequelae of nonpenetrating cardiac trauma?
Yes. Myocardial contusion may be extensive enough to result in significant left ventricular dysfunction of aneurysm formation, although this is distinctly uncommon. Contusion also may lead to ventricular septal defect or mural thrombus formation (these clots may embolize). Any of the cardiac valves may be rendered insufficient. Pericardial damage may result in constrictive pericarditis.

8. A patient is admitted to the emergency department following a motor vehicle accident, and the ECG shows ST-segment elevation in leads II, III, and aVF. What has happened?

The ECG shows evidence of an acute inferior myocardial infarction, but the sequencing of events is ambiguous. Two scenarios are possible.

1. The myocardial infarction occurred spontaneously, and preceded the accident. Inferior myocardial infarction may cause syncope either through acute heart block or sinus bradycardia, with or without right ventricular infarction (*see* chapter 18). Such an event may have caused the accident.

2. Blunt chest trauma during the accident may have resulted in coronary thrombosis, causing an infarction.

9. How should this situation be handled?

Thrombolytic therapy and anticoagulants are inappropriate. If facilities are available, emergent coronary angiography and angioplasty should be considered.

10. An unconscious patient is brought to the hospital following a major motor vehicle accident and is found to have deep T-wave inversion in leads V_1, V_2, and V_3. What has happened?

Again, two scenarios are possible: (1) the ECG changes are the result of myocardial contusion, or (2) more likely, the T wave inversions are those seen in association with an intracranial process. These ECG changes should prompt an evaluation for head trauma.

11. What was the first cardiac surgery, and when was it performed?

This subject of this chapter is cardiac trauma, so if you guessed it was repair of a ventricular laceration, you are correct! The procedure was reported by Rehn in 1897.

12. If stab wounds to the heart can be survived, what about gunshot wounds?

Yes, such injuries are survivable, but the mortality rate following penetrating cardiac injury from a gunshot is much higher than with stab wounds.

13. Is there a role for conservative management of suspected penetrating cardiac wounds?

Not at present. Virtually all patients with suspected penetrating cardiac trauma should undergo emergent thoracotomy.

14. Are there any late sequelae of penetrating cardiac injuries?

An amazing variety of fistulae between contiguous cardiac chambers and great vessels following stab or gunshot wounds have been described. Valvular regurgitation from laceration is possible. Myocardial infarction from coronary artery damage may result in left ventricular dysfunction, aneurysms, and mural thrombi. Post-pericardiotomy syndrome may result in pericardial effusion with or without tamponade. Constrictive pericarditis is also possible. Embolization of retained bullets and the like, either to or from the heart, has been described.

15. How can these complications be diagnosed?

As with nonpenetrating trauma, **echocardiography** is the most useful tool. Many authors recommend that all patients have an echocardiogram during the initial hospital stay, because many cardiac lesions may go undetected at initial thoracotomy. A follow-up echocardiogram three to six months later should be done.

BIBLIOGRAPHY

1. Harman PK, Trinkle JK: Injury to the heart. In Moore EE, Mattox KL, Feliciano DV (eds): Trauma. Norwalk, CT, Appleton & Lange 1991, pp 373–391.
2. Liedtke AJ, DeMuth WE: Nonpenetrating cardiac injuries: A collective review. Am Heart J 86:687–697, 1973.
3. Mattox KL, Limacher MC, Feliciano DV, et al: Cardiac evaluation following heart injury. J Trauma 25:758–764, 1985.
4. Tenzer ML: The spectrum of myocardial contusion: A review. J Trauma 25:620–627, 1985.

32. CARDIAC TUMORS

Karen Cooper, M.D.

1. A 45-year-old woman with a history of metastatic breast cancer develops shortness of breath, cardiomegaly, and elevated neck veins. What findings are consistent with pericardial involvement by tumor?

Generally, signs of pericardial tamponade include equalization of pressures in the pericardial space, right atrium, pulmonary artery wedge, right ventricle, and pulmonary artery during diastole. In tamponade, there is a prominent x descent with a small y descent on the jugular venous pressure contour. The echocardiogram characteristically shows right ventricular free-wall diastolic collapse.

2. What is the most common type of primary cardiac tumor?

Benign myxoma. Most frequently, these arise in the left atrium, where auscultation may reveal a "tumor plop" in diastole as the tumor hits the ventricular wall. Myxomas usually are sporadic but can be familial with autosomal-dominant inheritance. Features of familial syndromes include pigmented nevi, nodular disease of the adrenal cortex, mammary fibroadenomas, and testicular or pituitary tumors.

3. What primary malignant cardiac tumor is seen most frequently in adults?

Sarcoma occurring most frequently in the right atrium. The most common morphologic subtypes include angiosarcoma, rhabdomyosarcoma, and fibrosarcoma. In general, these tumors are fatal, and the interval between diagnosis and death is very short. These sarcomas infiltrate the heart extensively so that resection is not possible, and they tend to extend locally into the pericardium, lung, and other surrounding structures. Eighty percent of these tumors have distant metastases at the time of discovery. Symptoms can range from nonspecific, such as anemia and weight loss, to frank congestive heart failure. On occasion, the first sign can be from a symptomatic metastasis.

4. Name the most common benign cardiac tumor seen in children.

Rhabdomyoma. These tumors arise from the ventricular surfaces and affect the right and left sides equally. They vary in size and cause symptoms either by obstructing intracardiac blood flow or by interfering with normal cardiac conduction. A high percentage (30%) of these tumors are associated with tuberous sclerosis, which ultimately determines their prognosis. They are congenital. Resection has been performed successfully.

5. Which tumor has the greatest propensity for cardiac metastases?

Malignant melanoma, with 50–65% of patients having cardiac metastases.

6. What four tumors are commonly associated with most cardiac metastases?

1. Leukemias
2. Bronchogenic carcinoma
3. Carcinoma of the breast
4. Lymphomas (Hodgkin's and non-Hodgkin's)

The tumors spread to the heart by direct extension from surrounding intrathoracic structures or by hematogenous or lymphatic spread. Direct extension is seen most often with bronchogenic carcinoma that has extended through the pericardium into the left atrium. Malignant pericardial effusions from noncardiac neoplasms can lead to the implantation of viable cells on the epicardial surface.

7. How are cardiac metastases detected?

Most myocardial metastases are symptomatic. Although the metastases can interfere with conduction, valve function, or intracardiac blood flow, most commonly they are relatively small and do not affect global cardiac function. As the tumors become larger, symptoms can occur. Atrial arrhythmias, fibrillation or flutter, occur most often, and these findings in a patient with known carcinoma should arouse suspicion of cardiac metastasis. Diagnosis can be made by two-dimensional echocardiography or cytologic examination of pericardial fluid.

8. What class of cancer drugs is most often associated with electrocardiographic (ECG) abnormalities and arrhythmias?
Anthracycline antibiotics. ECG changes can occur over a wide range of doses and develop as a cumulative effect. The most frequent abnormalities are nonspecific ST-T wave changes, decreased QRS voltage, sinus tachycardia, supraventricular tachyarrhythmias, premature ventricular and atrial contractions, T-wave abnormalities, and QT-interval prolongation. The changes occur during or within a few days of drug administration but are reversible within a few hours after discontinuation of treatment. Most ECG abnormalities commonly encountered with doxorubicin or daunorubicin therapy are benign, and usually it is not necessary to stop therapy, although sudden death and life-threatening ventricular tachyarrthymias have been reported.

9. Describe the pericarditis seen after treatment of Hodgkin's disease.
Radiation-induced pericarditis occurs following radiotherapy, and its effects are related to the dose of radiation administered. The acute pericarditis usually occurs within 12 months of the initiation of radiation therapy but may manifest years later. The clinical course may be mild, but in 50% of patients, a mild to severe tamponade may develop, requiring pericardiocentesis or a pericardial window. Chronic pericarditis is generally benign, with many patients having an asymptomatic enlarged pericardial silhouette on chest x-ray. An effusion may develop 2–5 years after treatment and clears spontaneously. A constrictive pericarditis may occur with an acute pericarditis or chronic effusion, appearing 6–30 months after radiation therapy. Other clinical radiation-induced heart diseases include myocardial fibrosis, accelerated coronary heart disease, and valvular dysfunction.

10. Which cancer drugs have been associated with myocardial ischemia and infarction?
Although rare findings, drug-induced ischemia and infarction are most commonly associated with **5-fluorouracil, doxorubicin,** and the **vinca alkaloids** (vinblastine and vincristine). Rarely do patients who experience 5-fluorouracil-induced myocardial infarction have preexisting coronary artery disease. Chest pain occurs after 3–4 days of consecutive administration. With daunorubicin and doxorubicin, few cases of myocardial ischemia and infarction have been reported, with episodes occurring within hours of drug administration. The vinca alkaloids have been associated with coronary artery-related toxicities that include accelerated atherosclerosis, coronary vasospasm, angina, and myocardial infarction. Prophylactic treatment with nitrates and calcium channel blockers may be useful in abolishing pain and allowing continuation of treatment when necessary.

11. What is the most important factor in the development of cardiomyopathy secondary to anthracycline chemotherapy?
Total dose of drug received. The overall incidence of clinical doxorubicin cardiomyopathy is low, at 1–2%, but is dose-dependent. It is rare at doses <450 mg/m^2 body surface area, but increases along a continuum with an average incidence of 7% at 550 mg/m^2, 15% at 600 mg/m^2, and 30% to 40% at 700 mg/m^2. Congestive heart failure occurs generally 30–60 days after the last dose, but can occur during treatment or years later.

12. How should a patient's cardiac status be followed during treatment with anthracycline drugs?
Recommended guidelines for monitoring patients are based on the patient's cardiac function as measured by the left ventricular ejection fraction (LVEF): **normal baseline** LVEF ($\geq 50\%$):
   1. A second LVEF should be determined after administration of 250–300 mg/ml of anthracycline.

2. In patients with risk factors (heart disease, radiation, abnormal echocardiogram, cyclophosphamide), LVEF should be measured again at 400 mg/ml; in those with no risk factors, at 450 mg/ml.

3. Sequential studies should then be performed prior to each dose.

4. Treatment should be discontinued if the LVEF shows an absolute decrease of 10% or more or a decline to 50% or less.

Abnormal baseline LVEF (< 50% but > 30%)

1. Sequential studies should be performed prior to each dose.

2. Treatment should be discontinued if the LVEF shows an absolute decrease of 10% or more and/or a final LVEF of 30% or less.

13. What is the most accurate method for detecting anthracycline-induced cardiac damage?

The most accurate method is endomyocardial biopsy. The main disadvantages of the biopsy are its invasive nature, limited availability, and expense.

14. How is anthracycline-induced cardiopathy treated?

Treatment of congestive heart failure or cardiomyopathy secondary to anthracyclines is with digoxin, diuretics, vasodilators, and/or captopril. Cardiac dysfunction can improve with standard therapy in some cases, as evidenced by improved long-term assessment.

BIBLIOGRAPHY

1. Haq MM, Legha SS, Choksi J, et al: Doxorubicin-induced heart failure in adults. Cancer 56:1361–1365, 1985.
2. Labianca R, Beretta G, Clerici M, et al: Cardiac toxicity of 5FU: A study on 1083 patients. Tumori 68:505–510, 1982.
3. McAllister HA: Primary tumors and cysts of the heart and pericardium. Curr Probl Cardiol 4(May):1–51, 1979.
4. Piehler JM, Lie JT, Giuliani ER: Tumors of the heart. In Brandenbury RO, et al (eds): Cardiology: Fundamentals and Practices. Chicago, Year Book Medical Publ. 1987, pp 1671–1689.
5. Prichard RW: Tumors of the heart: Review of the subject and report of one hundred and fifty cases. Arch Pathol 51:98–128, 1951.
6. Ritchie JL, Singer JW, Thorning D, et al: Anthracycline cardiotoxicity: Clinical and pathologic outcomes assessed by radionuclide ejection fraction. Cancer 46:1109–1116, 1980.
7. Schwartz RG, McKenzie WB, Alexander J, et al: Congestive heart failure and left ventricular dysfunction-complicated doxorubicin therapy: Seven years' experience using radionuclide angiocardiopathy. Am J Med 82:1109–1118, 1987.
8. Stewart JR, Fajardo LF: Radiation-induced heart diseases: Clinical and experimental aspects. Radiol Clin North Am 9:511–531, 1971.
9. Tori FM, Lum BL: Cardiac toxicity. In DeVita VT Jr, Hellman S, Rosenberg SA (eds): Cancer: Principles and Practice of Oncology, 3rd ed. Philadelphia, J. B. Lippincott, 1989, pp 2153–2161.
10. Van Hoff DD, Layard MW, Basa P, et al: Risk factors for doxorubicin-induced congestive heart failure. Ann Intern Med 91:710–717, 1979.

33. ADULT CONGENITAL HEART DISEASE

Ira M. Dauber, M.D.

1. What are the most common congenital heart diseases of adults?

The spectrum of congenital heart disease in adults is considerably different from that in infants and children. **Bicuspid aortic valve** and **atrial septal defect** are the most common congenital heart lesions found in adults. **Coarctation of the aorta** and **pulmonary stenosis** are considerably less frequent. In children, ventricular septal defects are the most common malformations, but most children who survive to adulthood without surgical correction will have spontaneous closure of the defect. Adults are much less likely than children to have complex congential lesions; the lesions are either corrected in childhood or cause death before adulthood. Adults with *corrected* congenital heart disease are increasingly more common.

2. Can cyanotic congenital heart disease occur in adults?

Yes! In adults, as in children, cyanotic heart disease is caused by right-to-left shunting of blood. In adults, shunting is most often due to increased pulmonary vascular resistance, but obstructive lesions causing reduced pulmonary blood flow (which are more common in children) are also seen. **Atrial** and **ventricular septal defects** and **patent ductus arteriosus** involve acyanotic left-to-right shunting. Increased pulmonary blood flow from these lesions can increase pulmonary vascular resistance with subsequent right-to-left shunting of cyanotic blood (Eisenmenger syndrome). Some patients with obstruction to pulmonary blood flow and an associated right-to-left shunt survive to adulthood. The most common anomalies with pulmonary obstruction are tetralogy of Fallot, pulmonic atresia with ventricular septal defect, and pulmonic stenosis with atrial septal defect or patent foramen ovale.

3. Do bicuspid aortic valves cause symptoms?

Bicuspid aortic valves can be functionally normal at birth and therefore go undetected. Some bicuspid valves remain functionally normal and therefore asymptomatic. Most bicuspid valves eventually develop **aortic stenosis, aortic regurgitation,** or both. Progressive fibrocalcific thickening of a bicuspid valve is a common cause of aortic stenosis, accounting for nearly one-half of adult cases requiring valve surgery. Bicuspid valves are the most common cause of isolated valvular aortic regurgitation. The development of both aortic stenosis and aortic regurgitation is usually gradual. Sudden aortic regurgitation can occur due to **infective endocarditis,** as bicuspid valves are at increased risk for endocarditis.

4. Describe the signs and symptoms of atrial septal defects.

Many atrial septal defects are detected only at autopsy because the physical signs may be subtle and symptoms absent. Life expectancy is shortened, but there is usually a long asymptomatic phase and most patients do not develop symptoms until after age 40. Increased left-to-right shunting associated with age-related reduced left ventricular compliance can lead to **dyspnea on exertion** and **failure.** New-onset **atrial arrhythmias,** especially atrial fibrillation, occur and many precipitate congestive heart failure. Patients with **pulmonary hypertension** from long-standing left-to-right shunting may also have symptoms of effort-related cyanosis, hemoptysis, and chest pain.

5. What are the "classic" features of atrial septal defects?

- Widened and fixed splitting of the second heart sound (due to increased pulmonic blood flow)
- Pulmonic systolic heart murmur (due to increased flow across the pulmonic valve)
- Electrocardiographic (ECG) findings of left axis deviation with evidence of increased right-sided forces (especially in lead V_1).

Pulmonary hypertension secondary to the atrial septal defect can cause cyanosis, clubbing, accentuated pulmonary component of S_2, and right-sided regurgitant murmurs. Because there is an association between ostium secundum atrial septal defect and mitral valve prolapse, findings of a mitral valve click or murmur of mitral regurgitation may occur. An ectopic atrial rhythm may be present in patients with sinus venosum atrial septal defect.

6. Is echocardiography useful for the assessment of atrial septal defects?
Echocardiography can suggest the presence of an atrial septal defect by identifying an attenuated or absent atrial septum, associated atrial and/or right ventricular enlargement, or pulmonary hypertension from right-to-left shunting. Doppler studies may localize a high-velocity flow pattern across the atrial septum. **Contrast echocardiography** may be diagnostic of an atrial septal defect, especially with right-to-left shunting. Injections of saline microbubbles into a peripheral vein can demonstrate transit of the contrast from right to left at the atrial level. In patients with left-to-right shunting, a negative image of contrast-free blood may be seen in the right atrium due to washout from contrast-free left atrial blood.

7. Should atrial septal defects be surgically repaired?
Symptomatic atrial septal defects should be fixed whether symptoms are due to left-to-right or to right-to-left shunting. In asymptomatic patients, recommendations for closure of the defect are intended to prevent the development of pulmonary hypertension, which can develop from persistently increased pulmonary blood flow from left-to-right shunting. Closure is recommended for patients with pulmonary-to-systemic blood flow ratios of 1.5:1.0 or greater. In patients < 45 years of age, surgical risk is < 1%.

8. What is a coarctation of the aorta?
Coarctation of the aorta is a congenital narrowing of the descending thoracic or abdominal aorta. It usually occurs just distal to the origin of the left subclavian artery. Coarctation occurs 5 times more commonly in males. There is a significant association with bicuspid aortic valve and Turner's syndrome (gonadal dysgenesis).

9. Does aortic coarctation have any "classic" findings?
The physical clue to coarctation is **differential pulses** in the arms (strong) versus the legs (weak and delayed). There is often a systolic murmur from the coarctation best heard in the *posterior* left thorax. Chest x-ray may show notching of the ribs due to enlargement of the intercostal arteries. Coarctation is one of the causes of surgically correctable hypertension in the adult. Later symptoms include heart failure and endocarditis.

10. Which congenital heart lesions are at increased risk of endocarditis?
   Bicuspid aortic valve
   Aortic coarctation
   Ventricular septal defect
   Tetralogy of Fallot
   Pulmonic stenosis (moderate or severe)
   Severe mitral or tricuspid regurgitation
   Patients with surgically corrected congenital heart disease involving placement of a prosthetic valve or prosthetic conduit are at even higher risk. Antibiotic prophylaxis is recommended for these patients. Unfortunately, <20% of endocarditis cases in patients with congenital heart disease are associated with identifiable events or medical procedures.

11. How important are congenital anomalies of the coronary arteries?
Congenital coronary artery anomalies have been described with increased frequency due to the increased utilization of coronary angiography, but most are asymptomatic. **Myocardial bridging** due to an intramuscular course of a portion of the coronary artery (usually the left anterior descending) is the most common anomaly. In some patients, sufficient systolic compression of

the artery occurs to produce symptoms of ischemic heart disease (angina, myocardial infarction, sudden death). **Ectopic aortic origin** of either the right or left coronary artery is asymptomatic unless its course is altered to pass between the aorta and right ventricular outflow tract, which causes proximal obstruction of the artery and resultant ischemic symptoms. Anomalous origins from the pulmonary artery and congenital coronary arteriovenous fistulae usually become symptomatic during infancy and childhood.

12. Are arrhythmias a problem in congenital heart disease?
Approximately one-quarter of patients with congenital heart disease have arrhythmias, especially patients who have undergone corrective intracardiac surgery. More than 50% of patients with corrected transposition, 30% with tetralogy of Fallot, 25% with Fontan repair, and 10% with ventricular or atrial septal defect have postoperative arrhythmias. Supraventricular arrhythmias are most common, but sudden death due to ventricular arrhythmias is believed to occur in 5–10% of these patients.

13. Ventricular arrhythmias are most common after repair of tetralogy of Fallot. What are the risk factors for sudden death in these patients?
1. Older age at the time of repair
2. Prolonged postoperative recovery
3. Right ventricular end-systolic pressure > 60 mmHg
4. Right ventricular end-diastolic pressure > 10 mmHg
5. Depressed right ventricular systolic function
6. Significant tricuspid or pulmonic regurgitation

Fifteen percent of postoperative patients have inducible ventricular tachycardia during electrophysiologic testing.

14. Describe the features of Eisenmenger's syndrome. What is Eisenmenger's complex?
Eisenmenger's syndrome is a broad term applied to any anomaly in which the pathophysiologic process (e.g., increased pulmonary blood flow) leads to obliterative pulmonary vascular disease with resultant pulmonary hypertension whether or not there is an associated right-to-left shunt and cyanosis. **Eisenmenger's complex** refers to patients with congenital heart disease involving shunts with pulmonary hypertension severe enough to cause reversal of a left-to-right shunt with resultant right-to-left shunting through the defect. Eisenmenger originally described patients with ventricular septal defects. Pulmonary hypertension due to Eisenmenger-type pathophysiology is usually irreversible but may improve after corrective surgery if the associated pulmonary vascular anatomic changes are not too severe.

15. Who were Blalock and Taussig?
Helen B. Taussig and Alfred Blalock collaborated in establishing the Blalock-Taussig procedure in 1945. This subclavian-to-pulmonary artery anastomosis created a systemic-to-pulmonic shunt. This procedure established the first surgical treatment for "blue babies" suffering from pulmonic stenosis or atresia, a previously fatal condition.

16. Name the four features of tetralogy of Fallot.
1. Ventricular septal defect
2. Obstruction to right ventricular outflow.
3. Overriding of the aorta
4. Right ventricular hypertrophy.

Tetralogy of Fallot accounts for approximately 10% of all congenital heart lesions (including pediatric) and is the commonest cause of cyanotic disease presenting after 1 year of age. The degree of obstruction to pulmonary blood flow is the major factor in the clinical presentation.

17. Is mitral valve prolapse a congenital heart disease?
Although some cases of mitral valve prolapse are associated with congenital heart diseases, mitral

valve prolapse itself is not due to a congenital malformation of the valve. Mitral valve prolapse results from various pathogenetic mechanisms affecting the mitral valve apparatus, of which myxomatous degeneration is the most frequent cause.

18. Are there alternatives to surgery for adults with congenital heart disease?
Catheter-based therapy is increasingly important in the treatment of congenital heart disease in adults. Balloon dilatation of congenital aortic stenosis, umbrella closure of atrial and ventricular septal defects, umbrella closure of patent foramen ovale, and occluder implantation for patent ductus arteriosus are all technically feasible.

CONTROVERSIES

19. Can patients with congenital heart disease participate in athletics?
In general, yes. However, as no formal guidelines are available, recommendations are based on the judgments of individual physicians. The risks of athletic activity vary with the type of disease, functional cardiac status of the patient, and type of activities. The intensity and duration of excrcise, risk of body collision or trauma, conditioning required, and the risk of injury (to both the athlete and spectators) if the athlete develops syncope are also factors in assessing risk.

Recommendations for Athletic Participation in Persons with Congenital Heart Disease

CONGENITAL DISEASE	EXERCISE-INDUCED EFFECTS	RECOMMENDATIONS*
Congenital aortic stenosis	Angina	
Mild (gradient < 20 mmHg)	Syncope	No restrictions if ECG, exercise stress test,
	Sudden death	LV function, and Holter monitoring normal.
Moderate or severe		Avoid strenuous activity until after surgical correction.
Pulmonic stenosis		
Mild (gradient < 25 mmHg)		No restrictions
Moderate or severe		Avoid strenuous activity until after surgical correction.
Tetralogy of Fallot	Breathlessness	Requires careful assessment before athletic
	Cyanosis	participation.
	Arrhythmias	
Anomalous origin of left coronary	Angina	Avoid strenuous activity until after surgical
artery	Myocardial infarction	correction.
	Sudden death	
Pulmonic vascular disease	Syncope	Avoid strenuous activity
(pulmonary hypertension)	Sudden death	
Atrial septal defects	Dyspnea	Exercise recommendations depend on
	Cyanosis	severity of illness.
Small (minimal shunt, no pulmonary hypertension)		No restrictions
Moderate or large (significant shunt, pulmonary hypertension)		Avoid strenuous activity; reevaluate after surgical correction

*Patients on anticoagulation therapy should consider risk for trauma-induced bleeding.

20. Is congenital heart disease a contraindication to pregnancy?
The most common congenital malformation in women surviving to childbearing age are atrial septal defect (secundum), patent ductus arteriosus, pulmonary valvular stenosis, aortic coarctation, aortic valve disease, and tetralogy of Fallot. Few congenital heart lesions interfere with the initiation of pregnancy. Maternal mortality is related to functional class and varies from 0.4% for New York Heart Association Classes I and II to 6.8% for Classes III and IV. Fetal mortality varies from essentially 0% in Class I to 30% for Class IV.

The effects of pregnancy on common congenital defects also relate to clinical status. Asymptomatic atrial septal defects, bicuspid aortic valves, and aortic coarctation require special attention to risks of embolism and endocarditis but have little effect on mortality. In contrast, elevations of pulmonary vascular resistance significantly increase the risks of pregnancy, and Eisenmenger's complex is associated with cumulative maternal death rates of 30–70% during and after pregnancy. Risks of pregnancy are lower in patients with surgically corrected disease but are still determined by the degree of cardiac and vascular reserve and the residual defects after surgery. The major risks to the fetus stem from functional class of the mother, presence of maternal cyanosis, and use of anticoagulants (especially with prosthetic heart valves).

BIBLIOGRAPHY

1. Blalock A, Taussig HB: Surgical treatment of malformation of the heart in which there is pulmonary stenosis or pulmonary atresia. JAMA 128:189–202, 1945.
2. Borow KM, Alpert JS, Braunwald E: Congenital heart disease in the adult. In Braunwald E (ed): Heart Disease, 4th ed. Philadelphia, W. B. Saunders, 1992.
3. Brannell HL, Vogel JH, Pryor R, et al: The Eisenmenger syndrome. Am J Cardiol 28:679, 1971.
4. Fisher J, Platia EV, Weiss JL, Brinker JA: Atrial septal defect in the adult: Clinical findings before and after surgery. Cardiovasc Rev Rep 4:396, 1983.
5. Fraker TD, Harris PJ, Behar VS, Kisslo JA: Detection and exlusion of interatrial shunts by two dimensional echocardiography and peripheral venous injection. Circulation 59:379, 1979.
6. Graham TP, Bricker JT, James FW, Strong WB: Twenty-sixth Bethesda Conference: Recommendations for Determining Eligibility for Competition in Athletes with Cardiovascular Abnormalities. Task Force 1: Congenital Heart Disease. J Am Coll Cardiol 24:867–873, 1994.
7. Jeresaty RM: Mitral valve prolapse: Definition and implications in athletes. J Am Coll Cardiol 7:231–236, 1986.
8. Liberthson RR: Congential Heart Disease: Diagnosis and Management in Children and Adults. Boston, Little, Brown, 1989.
9. Linde LM: Psychiatric aspects of congenital heart disease. Psychiatr Clin North Am 5:399–406, 1982.
10. Lock JE: The Adult with Congenital Heart Disease: Cardiac Catheterization as a Therapeutic Intervention. J Am Coll Cardiol 18:330–331, 1991.
11. Perloff JK, Child JS: Congenital Heart Disease in Adults. Philadelphia, W.B. Saunders, 1991.
12. Perloff JK. Congenital heart disease in adults. Circulation 84:1881–1890, 1991.
13. Pitkin RM, Perloff JK, Koos BJ, Beall MH: Pregnancy and congenital heart disease, Ann Intern Med 112:445–454, 1990.
14. Rashkind WJ: Historical aspects of surgery for congenital heart disease. J Thorac Cardiovasc Surg 84:619, 1982.
15. Serfas D, Borow KM: Coarctation of the aorta: Anatomy, pathophysiology and natural history. J Cardiovasc Med 8:575, 1983.
16. Vetter VL, Horowitz LN: Electrophysiologic residua and sequelae of surgery for congenital heart defects. Am J Cardiol 50:588–604, 1982.

34. HEART DISEASE IN WOMEN

Olivia V. Adair, M.D.

1. Is ischemic heart disease a problem in women?
Yes. Ischemic heart disease causes 250,000 deaths/year in women in the U.S. This represents 23% of all deaths in women, making ischemic heart disease the leading cause of death in women over age 50.

2. What are the risk factors for coronary artery disease (CAD) in women?
The effects of risk factors are not well studied, but age, smoking, hypertension, lipoprotein profile, obesity, diabetes, and family history do predict CAD in women. Also, oral contraceptives and menopause increase the risk, while postmenopausal hormonal replacement decreases the risk.

3. Does the natural history of atherosclerotic CAD differ in females and males?
Yes. The Framingham Study has shown that 23% of all female mortality and 52% of all cardiovascular female deaths are due to atherosclerotic CAD, whereas figures for males are 34% and 64%, respectively. Sudden cardiac death is less common in women, and women manifest symptoms approximately 10 years later than men.

4. Do women and men present with the same symptoms when they have CAD?

Common Presenting Manifestations of CAD

	MALES	FEMALES
Angina	33%	50%
Myocardial infarction	33%	33%
Sudden death	33%	17%

5. What tests are used for diagnosing CAD in women?
The **exercise treadmill test** is of limited value in the diagnosis of CAD in women, having a sensitivity and specificity of 70%; however, the addition of thallium increases the specificity to 90%. **Radionuclear ventriculography** with exercise has also been disappointing in diagnosing CAD in females. The diagnostic accuracy for the presence of CAD is increased with stress testing in women if two or more cardiac risk factors are present; mitral valve prolapse is excluded; the ST segments normalize after > 6 minutes into recovery; target heart rate is achieved; or exercise duration is < 5 minutes on a full Bruce protocol.

6. Why is thallium perfusing imaging less sensitive in diagnosing CAD in women?
Though studies predominantly in men show exercise thallium perfusion imaging to improve the sensitivity of the stress test for CAD diagnosis, in women with single-vessel and multivessel disease the sensitivity is lower. This may be influenced by women's inability to attain target heart rate, low exercise levels, or imaging artifact from breast attenuation.

7. Is there another test to diagnose CAD in women before going to angiography?
Exercise echocardiography has been shown to have excellent accuracy, independent of chest pain being typical or atypical and the prevalence of CAD in women. Also, exercise echocardiography can detect noncoronary causes of chest pain, such as mitral valve prolapse, pericardial effusion, pulmonary hypertension, hypertrophic cardiomyopathy, and valvular disease. **Coronary angiography** should be used when noninvasive risk stratification and testing suggest a high probability of significant CAD. Women who despite medical therapy are symptomatic during

low-level exercise in their daily routine or who have had frequent noninvasive testing for multiple bouts of chest pain (even with minimal risk factors) should be considered for coronary angiography.

8. Is there a difference in the extent of CAD in females compared to males?

Yes. As a subset study in CASS, Chaitman et al. showed less extensive left main and triple-vessel CAD in women as compared to men in coronary angiography studies. Women also retained angiographic systolic function to a greater extent, suggesting a resistance to developing chronic left ventricular dysfunction and heart failure.

9. Do women fare as well as men post heart transplantation?

Although this issue has not been studied well, the Italian Multicenter Study Group followed 65 women and 238 men with documented idiopathic cardiomyopathy. Though the women presented with a more advanced phase of the disease—i.e., more dilated left ventricles, thicker left ventricular walls, shorter exercise duration, and worse symptoms—the 18-month follow-up transplant-free survival was not significantly different by gender, and there was no difference in prognosis. Therefore although women presented with more symptomatic disease after transplant, they did equally well as men.

10. Should women be treated differently than men for CAD?

There is little information available comparing the efficacy of medical management for CAD by gender. In two studies, the protective effects of β-blockers and aspirin as secondary prevention of CAD were shown not to extend to women, whereas one study showed a regimen of 1–6 aspirin/week decreased the risk of the first myocardial infarction in women. Recent studies show success of percutaneous transluminal coronary angioplasty is no longer adversely influenced by female gender. Coronary artery bypass surgery in women is associated with an increased operative mortality, perhaps related to smaller vessels, and vein graft (including the internal mammary artery) patency is less at 5 years (87–97% survival in women vs. 90–94% in men). These differences post-bypass, however, disappear at 10-year follow-up studies.

11. Diabetes is an important risk factor for CAD. Are there gender differences in risk when diabetes and CAD coexist?

In a study of 585 men and 389 women with CAD assessed by angiography, diabetic women had greater than two times the relative risk of death over a 4–6-year follow-up for all causes of death as well as cardiac death; whereas in nondiabetic patients, death was significantly lower in women. Therefore, diabetes confers a substantially higher risk of mortality in women when it coexists with CAD than in men, and the favorable cardiac risk profile premenopausal women have compared to men is lost in the presence of diabetes. Hypertriglyceridemia may also be of greater risk for women than men.

12. How does estrogen replacement affect the risk of atherosclerosis and myocardial infarction in postmenopausal women?

Estrogen reduces the risk of atherosclerosis and myocardial infarction in postmenopausal women. There is a reduction of up to 50% in myocardial infarction and stroke and a reduction in the incidence of hypertension.

13. Do cardiac rehabilitation program show similar results for women and men?

A recent study showed older women were less likely to enter cardiac rehabilitation than older men, due primarily to the stronger recommendations to men by their physicians. Although before entrance to programs, women were less fit than men (peak oxygen consumption 18% lower in women), both groups improved aerobic capacity similarly in response to a 12-week aerobic conditioning program.

14. Are there other gender-specific characteristics of myocardial infarction in women with CAD?

Non–Q-wave myocardial infarction, supraventricular arrhythmias, and infarct expansion are all more common in women, whereas pericarditis and ventricular arrhythmias are more common in men.

BIBLIOGRAPHY

1. Becker RC, Alpert JS: Cardiovascular disease in women. Cardiology 77(suppl 2):1–39, 1990.
2. De Maria R, Gavazzi A, Recalcati F, et al: Comparison of clinical findings in idiopathic dilated cardiomyopathy in women versus men: The Italian Multicenter Cardiomyopathy Study Group (SPIC). Am J Cardiol 72:580–585, 1993.
3. Liao Y, Cooper RS, Ghali JK, et al: Sex differences in the impact of coexistence of diabetes on survival in patients with coronary heart disease. Diabetic Care 16:708–713, 1993.
4. Rehnquist N, Hartford M, Schenck-Gustafsson K, et al: Coronary artery disease in women. J Myocard Ischemia 5:29–35, 1993.
5. Salvage MP, et al: Clinical and angiographic determinants of primary coronary angioplasty success. J Am Coll Cardiol 17:22–28, 1991.
6. Sawada SG, Ryan T, Fineberg NS, et al: Exercise echocardiographic detection of coronary artery disease in women. J Am Coll Cardiol 14:1440–1447, 1989.
7. Wren BG: The effect of estrogen on the female cardiovascular system. Med J Aust 157:204–208, 1992.

35. HEART DISEASE IN THE ELDERLY

Evelyn Hutt, M.D.

1. What cardiovascular changes are part of normal aging?

This question is a difficult one to answer because coronary artery disease is so prevalent among the elderly, affecting 50% of Americans aged 65–74 years and 60% of those > 75 years. There are virtually no studies that address this question in the oldest old, those over 80. Studies which were careful to screen out underlying atherosclerotic disease indicate the following:

1. **The heart ages well.**
   - Normal morphology changes little except for a mild increase in left ventricular wall thickness.
   - Contractile function is well preserved.
   - Decrease in early diastolic filling results from diminished myocardial compliance, increased isovolumic relaxation time, and sclerosis of the mitral valve.
2. **Resting heart rate does not change.**
   - Maximum heart rate declines (about 1 beat/year due to diminished β-adrenergic responsiveness).
   - Cardiac output in both rest and exercise is preserved.
   - End-diastolic volume and stroke volume increase.
3. **Arteries and veins do not fare so well.**
   - Arterial media thickens and becomes less elastic.
   - Vascular resistance increases.
   - Autonomic nervous system becomes less efficient.
   - Blood pressure falls significantly on standing (baroreceptor reflex attenuated).

2. What is diastolic dysfunction?

Diastolic dysfunction is increased resistance to filling of one or both cardiac ventricles and is particularly prevalent in older patients, especially in association with hypertension and senile amyloidosis and in women and blacks. The cellular mechanism is thought to be a decline in the cells' ability to sequester calcium after contraction, mediated by cyclic AMP. A decrease in cyclic AMP may be related to the decreased β-adrenergic responsiveness of normal aging.

Diastolic dysfunction should be suspected when a patient presents with dyspnea and fatigue without the classic x-ray findings of congestive heart failure or obvious pulmonary disease. The diagnosis is important because it is treated differently than systolic failure, responding best to agents that increase the diastolic filling time, such as beta blockers and calcium channel blockers.

3. Are myocardial infarctions more difficult to recognize clinically in older people?

Yes. The older a patient is, the more likely he or she is to present with dyspnea, syncope, delirium, or stroke and the less likely to have chest pain. This change again may be related to diminished adrenergic responsiveness. Given the prevalence of atherosclerotic disease in older men *and* women, the clinician should consider infarction high in the differential diagnosis of any acutely ill older patient.

4. Do people over 70 benefit from bypass grafting and angioplasty as much as younger people do?

Limited data suggest that in well-selected patients, a low operative mortality and good symptom relief can be achieved for patients 75 and older by **coronary artery bypass grafting.** Preoperative factors that predict mortality include emergency operation, cachexia, New York Heart Association functional class IV disease, and previous myocardial infarction. The major perioperative risk factor for death is prolonged pump and cross-clamp time. Postoperative problems include atrial fibrillation, delirium, depression, anorexia, and delays in starting ambulation.

Several case series have looked at success rates and complications from **percutaneous transluminal angioplasty** in elders. Clinical and arteriographic success rates are similar for middle-aged, young-old (60–69 years) middle-old (70–79 years), and old-old (> 80 years), but complication rates are higher for old-old patients (who had more extensive atherosclerotic disease and a higher prevalence of preoperative heart failure).

5. Is age over 75 a strong contraindication to thrombolytic therapy in acute myocardial infarction?

This is a controversial question. On one hand, the risk of major hemorrhagic complications during thrombolysis clearly rises with age. However, the mortality associated with myocardial infarction also rises with age. Subgroup analyses of larger trials (ISIS-2 in particular) show a reduction in mortality from 37–20% in patients over 80 who were given thrombolytic therapy.

The decision to use thrombolysis in the elderly must be individualized. Vigorous patients with classic signs, symptoms, and a large area of involved myocardium who present early in the course of their event should probably not be denied thrombolytic therapy solely because of their age.

6. What is the most common valvular heart disease in older people?

Aortic stenosis. Autopsy studies show that it occurs in 4–6% of people over 65. In the absence of symptoms, it is very difficult to distinguish true stenosis from the much more common murmur of aortic sclerosis, which occurs in about one-third of patients over 65. Concern over this murmur should prompt echocardiography with Doppler flow studies.

7. How does orthostatic hypotension affect the elderly?

Orthostatic hypotension, a drop in blood pressure from lying to standing of ≥ 20 mmHg due to decreased β-adrenergic responsiveness, is a common cause of syncope. It may be worse in the morning on first arising and after meals, and especially affects patients with systolic hypertension, whose treatment may exacerbate it. Blood pressure should be checked with the patient lying down for a minute, immediately upon standing, and after 1 and 5 minutes of standing.

8. How should orthostatic hypotension be managed in the elderly?

In patients without hypertension, control of symptoms can be achieved without medication. Patients should arise more slowly, increase salt and caffeine intake, and elevate the head of the bed at night (lessens diurnal fluid shifts). More refractory cases which cause the patient to fall can be treated with a very low dose of mineralocorticoid, watching carefully for signs of volume overload.

Patients with hypertension and orthostatic hypotension need careful selection of antihypertensive drugs to minimize symptoms. Avoid diuretics and selective α-antagonists; calcium channel blockers may be the "first line."

9. At what age can you stop checking cholesterol?

It is known that approximately 10 years' treatment of elevated cholesterol levels is required to effect a change in risk for myocardial infarction. Given the average life expectancy of 80 for men and 85 for women, it is probably reasonable to stop screening the general population at about age 70. This does *not* pertain to cholesterol management in patients with symptomatic atherosclerotic heart disease, in whom lowering cholesterol achieves much more rapid benefits.

10. Does estrogen replacement therapy affect the incidence of heart disease in older women?

The answer to this question is not known. Both epidemiologic and biochemical evidence suggests that it should decrease risk for myocardial infarction. Epidemiologically, the incidence of atherosclerotic disease rises dramatically after menopause and is the leading cause of death of older women. Biochemically, estrogen raises high-density lipoprotein (HDL) and lowers low-density lipoprotein (LDL) cholesterol, which should improve cardiac risk.

11. What are appropriate goals and treatment regimens for controlling cholesterol in the elderly?

In attempting cholesterol lowering, a reasonable goal is to get the LDL cholesterol below 100 plus the patient's age. As in younger people, the first step is an adequate trial of diet, exercise, and, for women, estrogen replacement. Because constipation is common in the elderly, psyllium can be added early and is generally well tolerated *if* the patient drinks sufficient water.

Choosing a medical regimen involves balancing side effects and cost. The bile acid-binding residues and niacin are generally poorly tolerated. Gemfibrozil is less expensive than the HMG-CoA reductase inhibitors, is the only cholesterol-lowering agent that raises HDL, and is generally effective and well-tolerated. The HMG-CoA reductase inhibitors have the advantages of once-daily dosing and greatest efficacy.

12. What common side effects of cardiac medications are the elderly most vulnerable to?

Side effects of cardiac medications that present a real danger to the elderly can be divided into four broad categories:

1. Mental status changes
   Antihypertensives
   Antianginals
   Antiarrhythmics
   Drugs with anticholinergic effects (e.g., atropine)
   Centrally acting alpha agonists (e.g., clonidine)
   Lipophyllic beta blockers (e.g., propranolol)

2. Orthostatic hypotension
   Antihypertensives
   Antianginals (e.g., isosorbide, nitroglycerin)

3. Cardiac conduction delays
   Drugs with anticholinergic effects
   Tricyclic antidepressants and major tranquilizers
   Antiarrhythmics
   Calcium channel blockers (e.g., verapamil)
   Beta blockers

4. Gastrointestinal problems
   Nausea and anorexia
      Digoxin (even below toxic levels)
      Angiotensin-converting enzyme inhibitors
      Peripherally acting calcium channel blockers (e.g., nifedipine)
   Constipation
      Centrally acting calcium channel blockers (e.g., verapamil)
      Drugs with anticholinergic effects

13. How common is atrial fibrillation in the elderly?

Atrial fibrillation affects 5–10% of ambulatory elderly. The incidence among hospitalized elderly is probably twice that. Unlike in younger people, atrial fibrillation is a harbinger of underlying cardiac disease in the elderly. The rate of stroke is 10 times higher in older than younger patients with atrial fibrillation.

14. Is anticoagulation therapy more risky in an elderly patient with atrial fibrillation than in younger patients?

Solid evidence demonstrates that the risk of bleeding from appropriately dosed and monitored warfarin does not rise with age alone. Instead, increased risk of bleeding is associated with frailty, a tendency to fall, history of peptic ulcer disease, or underlying malignancy.

15. Who is too old for a pacemaker?

No one. Sinus and atrioventricular nodal dysfunction are more common in the elderly and are a common cause of syncope and falls. Both quality and length of life can be improved by appropriate use of pacemakers.

BIBLIOGRAPHY

1. Bayer AJ, Chadha JS, Farag RR, Pathy MSJ: Changing presentation of myocardial infarction with increasing old age. J Am Geriatr Soc 34:263–266, 1986.
2. Denke MA, Grundy SM: Hypercholesterolemia in elderly persons: Resolving the treatment dilemma. Ann Intern Med 112:780–792, 1990.
3. Edmunds LH, Stephenson LW, Edie RN, Ratcliffe MB: Open heart surgery in octogenarians. N Engl J Med 319:131–136, 1988.
4. Ezekowitz MD, et al: Warfarin in the prevention of stroke associated with nonrheumatic atrial fibrillation. N Engl J Med 327:1406–1412, 1992.
5. Forman DE, Berman AD, McCabe CH, et al: PTCA in the elderly: The 'young-old' versus the 'old-old.' J Am Geriatr Soc 40:19–22, 1992.
6. Grossman W: Diastolic dysfunction in congestive heart failure. N Engl J Med 325:1557–1564, 1991.
7. Krumholz HM, Pasternak RC, Weinstein MC, et al: Cost effectiveness of thrombolytic therapy with streptokinase in elderly patients with suspected acute myocardial infarction. N Engl J Med 327:7–13, 1992.
8. Muller DWM, Topol EJ: Selection of patients with acute myocardial infarction for thrombolytic therapy. Ann Intern Med 113:949–960, 1990.
9. Pritchett ELC: Management of atrial fibrillation. N Engl J Med 326:1264–1271, 1992.
10. Topol EJ, Traill TA, Fortiun NJ: Hypertensive hypertrophic cardiomyopathy of the elderly. N Engl J Med 312:277–283, 1985.

36. HEART TRANSPLANTATION

Brian D. Lowes, M.D., and JoAnn Lindenfeld, M.D.

1. Who should be considered for heart transplantation?

Approximately 40,000 people/year under age 65 die of heart failure. In most of these patients, heart transplantation could be life-saving, but unfortunately only about 2,100 heart transplants are being done per year, predominantly due to a shortage of donor organs.

Adult patients are generally considered to be candidates for transplantation when medical therapy has been maximized and the patient's prognosis or quality of life can still be significantly improved by transplantation. This is generally the case if a patient's maximal oxygen consumption is < 14 mL/kg/min and the left ventricular ejection fraction is < 25%. Occasionally, transplantation is considered for patients with better left ventricular function but with severe ischemia not amenable to revascularization by angioplasty or surgery or those with recurrent symptomatic ventricular arrhythmias unresponsive to therapy.

2. Are there patients who cannot be considered for a heart transplant?

Contraindications to transplantation include coexisting systemic illness that limits a patient's survival:

    Severe irreversible pulmonary, renal, or hepatic disease
    Irreversible pulmonary hypertension (pulmonary vascular resistance >6 Wood units)
    Active infection
    Insulin-dependent diabetes mellitus with end-organ damage
    Acute pulmonary embolism
    History of recent malignancy
    Psychosocial instability.

3. What quality of life can patients reasonably expect post transplantation?

About 30–50% of patients return to work after transplantation, and 80–85% consider themselves to be physically active. One-year survival post-transplantation is about 90% at better centers and the 5-year survival is about 75%. Overall, 90% of patients consider themselves to be normal or have minimal symptoms of disease.

The function of a transplanted heart, however, is not completely normal. Several factors, such as cardiac denervation, altered neurohormonal activity with exercise, organ preservation injury, and differences in the donor and recipient body size, contribute to decreased cardiac function. Thus, while transplant recipients have a better functional capacity than pretransplantation, they are frequently impaired in comparison to normal controls.

4. What medicines are commonly used for immunosuppression in heart transplant patients?

The combination of cyclosporine, azathioprine, and prednisone has become standard immunosuppressive maintenance therapy in most transplant centers. This combination has been extremely effective in preventing rejection while minimizing the side effects that were associated with dual therapy with high-dose steroids and azathioprine, which had greater side effects. The dose of azathioprine is usually adjusted to maintain a white blood cell count of 4000–6000/mL, while the cyclosporine dose is adjusted by plasma levels depending on the time post-transplantation as well as manifestations of toxicity (e.g., worsening renal function, neurologic symptoms, or biliary stasis). Immediately after transplantation, patients receive methylprednisolone and then are switched to prednisone within 24 hours at a dose of approximately 1 mg/kg/day, which is gradually weaned to a maintenance dose of 0.1 mg/kg/day over the next 6 months. Some centers have discontinued steroids completely in about half of patients, whereas other centers maintain patients on a low dose of prednisone indefinitely.

5. What are the side effects of the commonly used immunosuppressive medicines?

Cyclosporine's most common side effect is nephrotoxicity, which is believed to be predominantly due to renal arterial vasoconstriction from cyclosporine's effect on endothelin and prostaglandin production as well as a direct vasoconstrictor effect. Hyperkalemia of hyperuricemia may also develop, but tends to be dose related and reversible with discontinuation or lower doses. Cyclosporine also results in hypertension (in up to 90% of patients). Cholelithiasis is also a common problem among transplant recipients secondary to cyclosporine's effects on bile metabolism. Hirsutism, often a welcome side effect in men, is quite distressing to women. Many of cyclosporine's side effects can be avoided by close monitoring of trough cyclosporine levels and adjusting the dose as needed to maintain safe levels.

Bone marrow suppression is the commonest problem with **azathioprine** but is usually dose-related and responsive to decreasing dosing. A drug-induced hepatitis or cholestasis can also occur with azathioprine.

Steroids at high doses are associated with numerous side effects including osteoporosis, glucose intolerance, and hyperlipidemia.

All these drugs result in an increased susceptibility to infection.

6. What infections are common in heart transplant patients and when do they usually occur?

Infection remains a major cause of death in the transplant population. In a recent multicenter review, 21% of patients had one or more serious infections within their first year posttransplantation.

Within the first month post transplant, nosocomial bacterial infections with staphylococci or gram-negative organisms tend to predominate. Herpes simplex mucocutaneous infections tend to occur as well within the first several weeks post transplant. After the first month and through the next several months, patients are at higher risk for other viruses such as CMV or opportunistic infections such as fungi, *Pneumocystis carinii,* or toxoplasmosis.

The lung tends to be the most frequent site of infection in heart transplant patients, and CMV remains the most common single infection. Prophylactic therapy with trimethoprim-sulfamethoxazole appears to be effective in preventing *Pneumocystis* infection in heart transplant recipients.

7. What malignancies are common in heart transplant patients and what predisposes patients to them?

Skin and lip cancers are fairly common post-transplantation and are believed to be secondary to a metabolite of azathioprine which causes increased photosensitivity. Unlike non-transplant patients, in transplant patients **squamous cell tumors** are more frequent than basal cell tumors by a ratio of 2:1. These tumors tend to be more aggressive and metastasize more quickly in transplant patients. Other tumors which are substantially more common are non-Hodgkin's lymphomas, Kaposi's sarcoma, and uterine, cervical, vulvar, and perineal tumors. Common tumors such as those of the lung, breast, and colon fortunately do not seem to be markedly increased in the transplant population.

A special form of lymphoma known as **post-transplant lymphoproliferative disease** is a common tumor that has been associated with cyclosporine-based immunosuppression. This tumor is usually of B-cell origin and is believed to be induced by the Epstein-Barr virus. Patients with this disease will often respond to decreased levels of immunosuppression and possibly antiviral therapy, suggesting a relationship to intensity of immunosuppression. Use of OKT3 and other antilymphocyte antibodies has also been implicated in increasing the risk of this disease.

8. What is the leading cause of death in heart transplantation after the first year?

Coronary artery disease (graft atherosclerosis) remains the leading cause of death in patients after their first transplant year. Graft atherosclerosis can develop within months of transplantation but usually appears gradually, so that 5 years post transplantation 30–50% of patients have angiographic evidence of disease. Detection of graft atherosclerosis is a difficult clinical problem since cardiac transplant patients do not usually have angina due to cardiac denervation from the surgical procedure. In addition, noninvasive tests such as exercise testing and radionuclide scans are less reliable in the cardiac transplant patient. Thus yearly coronary angiography is still routinely employed in these patients. Patients with severe disease usually present with sudden death or congestive heart failure secondary to a myocardial infarction. The etiology of this accelerated graft atherosclerosis is unknown but it is believed to be secondary to immune mediated endothelial injury.

Histopathologically, arteries with graft atherosclerosis usually have diffuse concentric lesions that involve the length of the vessel in comparison to typical coronary artery disease, where lesions tend to be more focal and nonconcentric. This usually makes heart transplant patients poor candidates for revascularization by angioplasty or surgery and leaves retransplantation as the only definitive therapy for this life-threatening process.

9. What predisposes heart transplant patients to coronary artery disease?

Although the exact mechanism of graft atherosclerosis remains unclear, certain variables strongly correlate with its development. Humoral rejection, circulating HLA antibodies, HLA mismatch at the DR locus, hyperlipidemia, and CMV infection all have been variably associated with its development. Medical attempts to prevent or slow this process, such as exercise, lipid-lowering agents, and blood pressure control, have not met with success. The calcium channel blocker diltiazem may result in modest slowing of this disease process.

10. What noninvasive tests are useful for the diagnosis of coronary artery disease in heart transplant patients?

Unfortunately, routine exercise testing, nuclear myocardial blood flow scans with thallium and sestamibi, as well as dobutamine stress echocardiography all lack the sensitivity to be useful tests in screening for graft atherosclerosis. The reason is likely the diffuse nature of graft coronary artery disease, which complicates interpretation of results. Surveillance angiography is the gold standard for screening for graft atherosclerosis, and noninvasive tests are used predominantly to assess functional capacity as well as clarify the significance of certain lesions.

11. What are some of the signs and symptoms of rejection?

The clinical diagnosis of rejection is often difficult. Frequently, patients have rejection on biopsy without symptoms. Less often patients may have nonspecific complaints of fatigue or malaise as the original symptom. Left untreated, a patient may progress to having dyspnea on exertion, orthopnea, and paroxysmal nocturnal dyspnea consistent with overt heart failure. Signs on physical exam often alert a physician to the presence of rejection before a patient is critically ill. Elevated neck veins, tricuspid regurgitation, and a third heart sound are all very suggestive, although not diagnostic, of rejection. Fevers without a source, arrhythmias of any kind, and hypotension also may be presentations of cardiac rejection.

12. How is the diagnosis of rejection made?

Endomyocardial biopsy remains the gold standard for the diagnosis of rejection. It is extremely sensitive and specific. The International Society of Heart and Lung Transplantation developed a scale for grading the severity of cellular rejection that is now widely used and that is based on the amount of lymphocytic infiltrate and degree of myocyte damage. Humoral (vascular) rejection is much less common than cellular rejection, although it may occur in up to 20% of patients receiving antilymphocyte preparations. This antibody-mediated rejection is characterized by an increased incidence of fatal rejection, development of graft atherosclerosis, and a poorer long-term prognosis. The diagnosis of antibody-mediated rejection is based on endothelial cell swelling on microscopy along with immunofluorescent staining of complement and immunoglobin on the vascular endothelium. Hyperacute rejection is another form of rejection that is mediated by preformed antibodies in the recipient against antigens on the donor heart. This type of rejection is often characterized by immediate graft failure post transplantation and has an extremely poor prognosis.

13. Are noninvasive tests such as cardiac echocardiography useful in the diagnosis of rejection?

In general, cardiac imaging studies lack the sensitivity and specificity to be useful in diagnosing rejection. By the time left ventricular function deteriorates, the level of rejection is usually fairly advanced and more difficult to treat. Echocardiography, however, is not entirely useless in the management of heart transplant recipients. Doppler echocardiographic evaluation of patients to assess diastolic function is a fairly sensitive technique for following the changes that occur with rejection. Other echocardiographic findings such as increased wall thickness or edema may provide clues about humoral rejection that is not routinely detected by standard biopsy staining techniques. Echocardiography can also provide evidence of wall motion abnormalities, suggesting ischemic disease, and can assist in the evaluation of valvular dysfunction, which may explain worsening cardiac function.

14. What are the different kinds of rejection?

Rejection currently accounts for 17% of deaths in transplanted patients. Hyperacute, cellular, and humoral rejection are the major forms of rejection as we currently understand them.

Hyperacute rejection usually presents immediately after transplantation as severe graft dysfunction. It occurs when the recipient has preformed antibodies to HLA antigens on the donor heart. These antibodies can be formed when there is previous exposure to HLA antigens common to the donor, as may occur with blood transfusions, pregnancy, or previous organ transplantation. Most instances of hyperacute rejection can be prevented by screening recipients for anti-HLA antibodies prior to transplantation. Patients who have a broad spectrum of anti-HLA antibodies are usually required to undergo crossmatching prior to transplantation.

Cellular rejection is the commonest form of rejection. T-lymphocytes mediate this process, which involves perivascular and perimyocytic lymphocytic infiltrates. This form of rejection is diagnosed by H&E staining of biopsy specimens and usually responds very well to increased levels of immunosuppression. Cellular rejection occurs most frequently and most aggressively in the first few months following transplantation. It is uncommon after the first 6 months unless the recipient has a concurrent infection, a recent reduction in immunosuppression, or has had frequent previous episodes of rejection.

Humoral (vascular) rejection is much less common than cellular rejection but carries a much worse prognosis. Patients with this type of rejection characteristically have deposition of immunoglobin and complement in a vascular pattern by immunofluorescent staining. They also have generalized endothelial cell swelling by light microscopy. Vascular rejection is seen more commonly in patients with sensitization to OKT3.

15. How is rejection treated?

Treatment of rejection depends on the type and severity of the pathologic grade as well as clinical symptoms and the presence of hemodynamic changes (*see* table).

Patients with grade 1 rejection without hemodynamic changes are often not treated but followed closely for progression. Rejection often resolves spontaneously, avoiding the risks of additional immunosuppression. Grade 3 and 4 rejection, in comparison, requires significant changes in therapy. These episodes of rejection are usually treated with high doses of intravenous or oral steroids for 3 days, followed by a rapid steroid taper. Steroid-resistant episodes are treated with OKT3, a mouse monoclonal antibody to the CD3 molecule, which is part of a multi-molecular complex found on mature C cells.

International Society of Heart and Lung Transplantation Scale for Cardiac Rejection

GRADE	PATHOLOGIC FINDINGS ON BIOPSY
0	No rejection
1	Perivascular or interstitial infiltrate without necrosis
2	One focus of aggressive infiltrate or focal myocyte damage
3	Multifocal aggressive infiltrates or myocyte damage
4	Diffuse infiltrate with necrosis, edema, vasculitis, or hemorrhage

16. Who should be considered as potential donor candidates?

Due to the shortage of donor organs and the poor prognosis of patients awaiting cardiac transplantation, the initial screening of donors should be very liberal. The initial step involves the recognition and declaration of brain death in the donor. After consent has been obtained, the donor is screened for suitability by the designated organ recovery system. The relative contraindications could potentially complicate a transplantation, but this must be weighed against the recipient's clinical situation and short-term survival.

Contraindications to Organ Donation

ABSOLUTE CONTRAINDICATIONS	RELATIVE CONTRAINDICATIONS
HIV-positive status	Sepsis
Death due to CO poisoning	Prolonged inotropic support or CPR
Structural heart disease	Prolonged hypotension
Previous myocardial infarction	Noncritical coronary artery disease
Intractable ventricular arrhythmias	Hepatitis B or C positivity
Severe hypokinesis	History of metastatic cancer
Severe occlusive coronary artery disease	Evidence of cardiac contusion
	History of intravenous drug abuse

BIBLIOGRAPHY

1. Baldwin J, Anderson JL, Boucek M, et al: Donor guidelines. J Am Coll Cardiol 22:15–20, 1993.
2. Bolman RM, Saffitz J: Early postoperative care of the cardiac transplantation patient: Routine considerations and immunosuppressive therapy. Cardiovasc Dis 33:137–148, 1990.
3. Desruennes M, Corcos T, Cabrol A, et al: Doppler echocardiography fo the diagnosis of acute cardiac allograft rejection. J Am Coll Cardiol 12:63–70, 1988.
4. Edwards BS, Rodeheffer RJ: Prognostic features in patients with congestive heart failure and selection criteria for cardiac transplantation. Mayo Clin Proc 67:485–492, 1992.
5. Hammond EH, Yowell RL, Nunoda S, et al: Vascular (humoral) rejection in heart transplantation: Pathologic observations and clinical implications. J Heart Transplant 8:430–443, 1989.
6. Levine AB, Levine TB: Patient evaluation for cardiac transplantation. Prog Cardiovasc Dis 33:219–228, 1991.
7. Miller L, Schlant R, Kobashigawa J, et al: Task force 5: Complications. J Am Coll Cardiol 22:41–51, 1993.
8. Mudge G, Goldstein S, Addonizio LJ, et al: Recipient guidelines/prioritization. J Am Coll Cardiol 22:21–30, 1993.
9. Smart FW, Grinstead WC, Cocanougher B, et al: Detection of transplant arteriopathy: Does exercise thallium scintigraphy improve noninvasive diagnostic capabilities? Transplant Pro 23:1189–1192, 1991.
10. Young JB, Winters WL, Bourge R, et al: Function of the heart transplant recipient. J Am Coll Cardiol 22:31–40, 1993.

37. PERIPHERAL VASCULAR DISEASE

David Tanaka, M.D.

1. What is peripheral vascular disease (PVD)?

This term peripheral vascular disease is usually used to describe atherosclerotic peripheral arterial disease. Other names for this condition are peripheral arterial disease and arteriosclerosis obliterans.

2. How is claudication different from other types of leg pain?

Claudication is the characteristic symptom of PVD. It is an intermittent pain which results from inadequate tissue perfusion during exercise. It consists of three essential features:

1. The pain is always experienced in a functional muscle unit (calf, buttock, thigh, etc.).
2. It is reproducibly precipitated by exercise.
3. It is promptly relieved by rest.

Claudication does not necessarily have to be pain; it can be cramping, weakness, or numbness.

3. An elderly woman complains of calf pain that occurs when she walks more than two blocks. She has a normal pulse in the dorsalis pedis and posterior tibial arteries. Does she have claudication?

Possibly. Several conditions share the characteristic onset of leg pain with exercise, including arterial embolism, muscle phosphorylase deficiency, drug toxicity (vasospasm), as well as nonvascular causes such as arthritis and lumbar disc disorders. They can be differentiated from PVD by the reproducibility of pain (recurs consistently after the same amount and type of activity in PVD), means of pain relief, and presence of distal pulses (reduced in PVD).

The patient should be asked what she does to relieve the pain—sit down, stand up, slow down? Does the pain develop in other activities? In this case, the patient can relieve the pain only by sitting down, and the pain sometimes develops after she stands too long. These differences suggest pseudoclaudification, which is from spinal stenosis. Spinal stenosis causes a pain very similar to claudication that is relieved by sitting or bending over, but not by standing up straight (as it is in PVD). The presence of normal distal pulses also makes PVD less likely.

4. What can cause claudication-like symptoms is young, athletic people with normal pulses?

Chronic compartment syndrome. This overuse injury, usually of well-conditioned athletes, is not responsive to anti-inflammatory medication or physical therapy. Rest improves the pain, but it usually returns with resumption of exercise. The diagnosis is made by measuring the compartment pressures (normal pressure is < 15 mmHg and in chronic compartment syndrome it is > 20 mmHg). Treatment is surgical, either open fasciectomy or subcutaneous fasciotomy.

5. Which arteries are affected in PVD?

The most commonly affected artery is the **superficial femoral artery.** The aortoiliac and tibioperoneal arteries are affected less commonly. One-third of patients will have more than one area involved.

6. Can the history help in localizing the area of disease?

Aortoiliac disease may cause claudication of the buttock or thigh or impotence in men. Disease at this level may cause isolated calf claudication. Femoropopliteal disease also causes calf claudication.

7. What is the best physical finding for diagnosing PVD?
An abnormal posterior tibial pulse has a sensitivity of 70% and a specificity of 91% in diagnosing PVD.

8. Will PVD gradually worsen in a patient and cause loss of the leg?
Only 2–4% of all patients with claudication will require amputations. Smoking and diabetes increase the rate of amputations by four and seven times, respectively. Unfortunately, the overall mortality for patients is increased two to three times over that of aged- and sex-matched controls, mainly due to coronary artery and cerebrovascular disease.

9. Are the risk factors for coronary artery disease and PVD the same?
Yes and no. The general risk factors are the same, but there are some differences:
    1. **Smoking** is more pervasive in patients with PVD (80%). Smoking status influences limb prognosis, patency of vessels after surgery or angioplasty, and mortality.
    2. **Diabetes** increases the risk of progression of disease. Diabetics also have a higher incidence of vascular disease distal to the popliteal artery.
    3. **Hyperlipemia** is a risk factor for PVD, but the risk profile is different than for coronary artery disease. Low levels of high-density lipoprotein (HDL) cholesterol and elevated triglycerides are independent risk factors for PVD, but elevated low-density lipoprotein (LDL) cholesterol is not.
    4. **Hypertension** is a risk factor for PVD, but there is no evidence that treatment of hypertension influences the prognosis of PVD. Most patients with claudication can be treated for hypertension without worsening their claudication, although in some patients with severe disease, worse symptoms might develop. In general, beta blockers can be safely used to treat hypertension or angina in the presence of claudication.

10. What noninvasive vascular studies are useful in PVD?
    1. **Ankle:brachial index** (ABI) is the ankle systolic pressure as determined by Doppler divided by the brachial systolic pressure. An abnormal index is < 0.90. The sensitivity is approximately 90% for diagnosis of PVD.
    2. **Plethysmography** measures changes in volume of toes, fingers, or parts of limbs that occur with each pulse beat as blood flows into or out of the extremity. This method may be used to determine toe pressures and pulse volume recordings, which are helpful when ankle pressures are falsely elevated because of calcified lower-extremity vessels. A toe:brachial index of < 0.6 is abnormal, and values of < 0.15 are seen in patients with rest pain (toe pressures of < 20 mmHg).
    3. **Ultrasound:Doppler velocity, duplex, and color-flow Doppler** are methods of evaluating artery stenosis and blood flow. These methods can localize and quantify the degree of stenosis. They are dependent on operator skill and are not as sensitive as the ankle:brachial index for screening purposes.
    4. **Transcutaneous oxygen tension measurements** are useful in assessing tissue viability for wound healing. Measurements over 55 mmHg are considered normal and those below 20 mmHg are associated with nonhealing ulcers.
    5. **Exercise testing** measures treadmill walking time and pre-exercise and post-exercise ankle:brachial indices. In those without significant PVD, the ABI is unchanged after exercise. In patients with PVD, the ABI falls after exercise. This testing is more sensitive for detecting disease than a resting ABI alone.

11. What is claudication at rest and what is its significance?
Claudication at rest occurs when blood flow is reduced below a level sufficient for supplying the metabolic needs of the tissue at rest. The pain is typically in the forefoot, often occurs at night when the feet are elevated, and is often relieved by placing the feet in a dependent position. Ulcers and gangrene often accompany claudication at rest.

12. What is the general approach to outpatient management of PVD?

First, treat other conditions that might adversely affect tissue oxygen delivery, such as congestive heart failure, anemia, and hypoxia. Modify risk factors. Smoking cessation has been shown to improve the morbidity and mortality in patients with PVD. Despite the lack of firm evidence, it is prudent to treat hypertension, control hyperglycemia, and lower cholesterol. In severe cases, especially in diabetics, meticulous local care of skin, feet, and nails is necessary if infection and limb loss are to be prevented. Have your patients take off their shoes and socks during the examination.

13. Can claudication be improved?

Exercise has been shown to improve pain-free walking time. The magnitude of the improvement has been up to 290% with an average of approximately 134%. Patients should be encouraged to walk to the point of claudication and then to rest until pain-free and then resume walking.

Pentoxifylline is presently the only medication for claudication. It is believed to improve erythrocyte deformability, platelet reactivity, and blood viscosity. The magnitude of improvement is less than with exercise (25–100%), and should be used when the response to exercise is inadequate.

14. What about anticoagulation, aspirin, and vasodilators?

None of these medications has been proved to reduce claudication or prevent progression of atherosclerosis in PVD patients. Aspirin should be prescribed routinely because it reduces the incidence of myocardial infarctions and strokes in patients with PVD.

15. When is surgery or angioplasty indicated?

- Symptoms interfere with lifestyle
- Failure to respond to medical interventions
- Development of claudication at rest
- Skin ulceration or gangrene

16. Is angioplasty preferable over surgery?

If feasible, angioplasty is recommended because it has a lower complication rate, is less expensive, and does not preclude future surgery.

17. What are the appropriate lesions for angioplasty?

Angioplasty is most effective for localized disease, especially of the iliac and femoral arteries. Extensive disease (lesion > 10 cm in length) or disease at multiple sites is often best treated surgically. These decisions are best made in consultation with a vascular surgeon and interventional radiologist.

18. How do you evaluate operative risk in a patient scheduled for vascular surgery?

The major concern for PVD patients is evaluating risk of a perioperative cardiac complication. This is the most common cause of mortality with vascular surgery because approximately one-half of such patients have significant coronary artery disease. Many of these patients do not have angina and cannot exercise because of their PVD.

The proper preoperative evaluation of the patient for vascular surgery has been extensively studied but remains controversial. One approach is based on the clinical evaluation and begins with the assessment of the patient for the following risk factors: age > 70, diabetes, previous myocardial infarction, angina, or history of ventricular ectopy.

If the patient has no risk factors and can walk approximately two blocks, then he or she is at **low risk** and can proceed to surgery.

If the patient has three or more risk factors, then he or she is at **high risk** for surgery. Consideration should be given to performing a lower risk procedure, such as axillofemoral bypass or angioplasty, or foregoing surgery. Coronary angiography should also be considered, but the risk of any intervention based on coronary angiography must be considered in addition to the risk of the vascular surgery. Invasive monitoring with Swan-Ganz and arterial catheters, perioperative use of beta blockers and nitrates, and careful monitoring for ST depression perioperatively (up to 48 hours postoperatively) may decrease the risk of cardiac complications.

If the patient has one or two risk factors or is unable to walk two blocks, then he or she is at **intermediate risk.** Dipyridamole-thallium imaging should be done. If the study is negative, the patient is at low risk and can proceed to surgery. If the study is positive, then the patient is at high risk and is approached as above.

BIBLIOGRAPHY

1. Consensus Document: Chronic critical leg ischemia. Eur J Vasc Surg 6(suppl A):1–32, 1992.
2. Criqui MH, Fronek A, Klauber MR, et al: The sensitivity, specificity and predictive value of traditional clinical evaluation of peripheral arterial disease: Results from noninvasive testing in a defined population. Circulation 71:516–522, 1985.
3. DeWeese JA, Leather R, Porter J: Practice guidelines: Lower extremity revascularization. J Vasc Surg 18:280–294, 1993.
4. Eagle KA, Coley CM, Newell JB, et al: Combining clinical and thallium data optimizes preoperative assessment of cardiac risk before major vascular surgery. Ann Intern Med 110:859–866, 1989.
5. Hertzer NR, et al: Coronary artery disease in peripheral vascular patients. Ann Surg 199:223–233, 1984.
6. Hiatt WR, Regensteiner JG: The value of exercise programs and risk factors modifications in claudicators. Semin Vasc Surg 4:188–194, 1991.
7. Mannick JA: Evaluation of chronic lower extremity ischemia. N Engl J Med 309:841–843, 1983.
8. Turnipseed W, Metmer DE, Girdley F: Chronic compartment syndrome: An unusual cause for claudication. Ann Surg 210:557–563, 1989.
9. Wilt TJ: Current strategies in the diagnosis and management of lower extremity peripheral vascular disease. J Gen Intern Med 7:87–101, 1992.

38. PULMONARY EMBOLISM

Michael E. Hanley, M.D.

1. What three primary factors promote thromboembolic disease?

Development of venous thrombosis is promoted by (1) venous blood stasis, (2) injury to the intimal layer of the venous vasculature, and (3) abnormalities in coagulation and/or fibrinolysis.

2. What are risk factors for thromboembolic disease?

Previous history of thromboembolic disease
Obesity
Pregnancy
Prolonged immobilization
Lower-extremity or pelvic trauma or surgery
Surgery with greater than 30 minutes of general anesthesia
Congestive heart failure
Nephrotic syndrome
Cancer
Estrogen-containing compounds
Advanced age

3. What is the natural history of venous thrombosis?

Resolution of fresh thrombi occurs by fibrinolysis and organization. Fibrinolysis results in actual clot dissolution. Organization reestablishes venous blood flow by reendothelializing and incorporating into the venous wall residual clot not dissolved by fibrinolysis. In the absence of new clot formation, the two processes generally are complete in 7–10 days.

4. Can patients with deep venous thrombosis be accurately diagnosed clinically?

No. The clinical diagnosis of deep venous thrombosis is neither sensitive nor specific. Less than 50% of patients with confirmed deep venous thrombosis present with classic symptoms of pain, erythema, and edema. Similarly, radiologic tests confirm the diagnosis in only 50% of patients who present with a high clinical suspicion of deep venous thrombosis.

5. How is the diagnosis of lower extremity deep venous thrombosis confirmed?

The test of choice depends on the likely location of the deep venous thrombosis. Contrast venography remains the gold standard but is associated with a higher incidence of adverse effects, primarily phlebitis. Radiolabelled fibrinogen scanning is highly sensitive for deep venous thromboses in the calf and lower thigh but loses sensitivity above midthigh, because accumulated radiofibrinogen in the large pelvic blood pool interferes with scanning. In contrast, impedance plethysmography is sensitive above but not below the knee. Similarly, Doppler/ultrasound has a sensitivity and specificity of 90–95% for proximal clots located cephalad of the popliteal vein. Its accuracy for vein thromboses in the calf is not well defined.

6. When should prophylaxis of deep venous thromboses be considered?

Two factors must be weighed in deciding to initiate prophylaxis of deep venous thrombosis: the degree of risk for thrombosis (see question 1 and 2) and the risk of prophylaxis. The risk factors for deep venous thrombosis are cumulative. The primary risk of pharmacologic prophylaxis is hemorrhage, which is generally uncommon if no coagulation defects or lesions with bleeding potential exist.

7. What prophylactic measures are available?

Approaches to prophylaxis of deep venous thrombosis include **antithrombotic drugs** and **pneumatic-compressive devices.** Both heparin and warfarin are effective in preventing deep venous thrombosis. Subcutaneous heparin offers a low risk of bleeding and rapid onset of prophylaxis but is ineffective in patients undergoing prostate or hip surgery. Low-dose warfarin (with prolongation of the prothrombin time to 1.2–1.3 times normal) also has a low risk of bleeding and is effective in patients with trauma, burns, and hip surgery. It takes several days, however, to develop a full antithrombotic effect. Antiplatelet drugs such as aspirin and dipyridamole are not effective in prophylaxis.

Intermittent pneumatic-compressive devices effect prophylaxis by maintaining venous flow in the lower extremities and are especially efficacious in patients who cannot receive anticoagulant medications. Modalities available include compressive devices applied to the feet alone, covering the calves, or extending to the thighs. No version has been shown to provide superior prophylaxis.

8. Should all deep venous thromboses be treated with anticoagulation?

No. Deep venous thromboses are treated primarily to prevent fatal pulmonary embolism. Because the risk of fatal embolism is low for deep venous thromboses limited to calf veins, many authorities do not recommend anticoagulation in this setting. Lack of extension into the popliteal system must be confirmed and followed (for 14 days) by impedance plethysmography. If this or other reliable tests for popliteal extension are not available, deep venous thromboses in the calf should be treated.

9. Where do most pulmonary emboli originate?

Thromboses in the deep veins of the lower extremities account for 90–95% of pulmonary emboli. Less common sites of origin include thromboses in the right ventricle; in upper-extremity, prostatic, uterine, and renal veins; and, rarely, in superficial veins.

10. Are pulmonary embolism and pulmonary infarction synonymous terms?

No. The pulmonary parenchyma is supplied by both the pulmonary and bronchial (systemic) circulations. Pulmonary infarction results when embolized lung parenchyma is inadequately perfused by the bronchial circulation. Infarction complicates only 10% of pulmonary emboli. The two conditions are treated in the same fashion.

11. What are the most common findings on chest roentgenogram and electrocardiogram (ECG) in patients with pulmonary emboli?

Most patients with pulmonary embolism have a normal chest roentgenogram. When the chest roentgenogram is abnormal, the findings are nonspecific and include an elevated hemidiaphragm, focal or multifocal infiltrates, pleural effusion, platelike atelectasis, enlarged pulmonary arteries, focal oligemia (Westermark's sign), and right ventricular enlargement. Most patients with pulmonary embolism present with sinus tachycardia. Other EKG findings include arrythmias (premature atrial and ventricular beats, first-degree atrioventricular (AV) block, supraventricular arrhythmia); right ventricular strain (right axis deviation, right ventricular hypertrophy); p-pulmonale; right bundle-branch block; $S_1S_2S_3$ and $S_1Q_3T_3$ pattern; and depression, elevation, or inversion of S-T and T waves.

12. What is the differential diagnosis of the patient suspected of having pulmonary emboli?

Other diagnoses that should be entertained in patients suspected of pulmonary embolism include infectious pneumonitis, viral pleuritis, atelectasis, cardiovascular collapse secondary to sepsis or hemorrhage, pulmonary edema, bronchial asthma, and hyperventilation syndrome.

13. How is the diagnosis of pulmonary embolism confirmed?

The diagnosis of pulmonary embolism requires laboratory confirmation, because clinical diagnosis is quite unreliable. Helpful diagnostic tests include tests for lower-extremity deep vein thrombosis (see question 5), ventilation/perfusion lung scans, and pulmonary angiography. Pulmonary angiography remains the gold standard. Although angiography is safe when performed by experienced angiographers, morbidity and mortality are increased in patients with pulmonary hypertension, cor pulmonale, or acute right ventricular strain. Ventilation/perfusion lung scanning is safer and less invasive than angiography but also less specific. Specificity is improved when only segmental or larger perfusion defects are considered significant. When ventilation/perfusion lung scans are nondiagnostic, some authorities advocate evaluation for evidence of lower-extremity deep vein thromboses before proceeding to angiography. Although definitive proof of deep vein thromboses does not prove pulmonary embolism, it renders the issue inconsequential, because anticoagulation is generally indicated for both conditions.

14. What is the treatment of pulmonary embolism?

Treatment of pulmonary embolism includes cardiopulmonary supportive measures (fluids and vasopressors for hemodynamic support, oxygen) and specific measures for thromboembolism, such as anticoagulation, placement of an intracaval filter, or thrombolytic therapy. Anticoagulation remains the treatment of choice for most patients. The primary debate regards length of therapy. The goal of therapy is to prevent new clot formation and/or thrombus growth while existing clots become organized or resolve. Because organization and resolution require 7–10 days, all patients must be anticoagulated during this period. Controversy surrounds the need for more chronic anticoagulation. Although most authorities recommend anticoagulation for 3 months for deep vein thromboses and 6 months for proved pulmonary embolism, some advocate anticoagulation beyond 7–10 days only in patients at high risk for recurrence {continued thromboembolic risk factors [see questions 1 and 2] and/or persistent venous obstruction, as assessed by impedance plethysmography}. Either oral warfarin or subcutaneous heparin is effective if chronic anticoagulation is indicated.

15. What are the indications for intracaval filters?

Absolute indications for interruption of the inferior vena cava through insertion of a filter include failure of anticoagulation and/or a contraindication to anticoagulation. In addition, some experts advocate placement of an intracaval filter for massive pulmonary embolism, because failure of anticoagulation in this setting frequently has a fatal outcome.

16. When is thrombolytic therapy indicated for pulmonary embolism?

Although thrombolytic therapy for pulmonary embolism in general is associated with more rapid clot dissolution than anticoagulation (heparin) alone, no well-controlled studies have demonstrated a difference in morbidity or mortality between the two therapeutic modalities. Thrombolytic therapy is therefore indicated only for massive pulmonary embolism characterized by refractory hypotension and/or refractory hypoxemia.

CONTROVERSIES

17. Is surgery indicated in massive pulmonary embolism?

Massive pulmonary embolism is a life-threatening occurrence with significant morbidity and mortality. Surgical embolectomy (via thoracotomy, suction catheter, or balloon catheter) is a potentially life-saving procedure. Attempts at medical therapy may waste precious time and, if unsuccessful, almost certainly result in a fatal outcome. On the other hand, many patients with massive pulmonary embolism die within the first hour of presentation (before surgical services can be mobilized); medical therapy is highly effective if instituted quickly; and results of surgical embolectomy are not impressive. Surgical embolectomy therefore should be reserved for rare cases when the diagnosis is irrefutable, medical therapy has failed or is contraindicated, and surgical intervention can be performed immediately.

BIBLIOGRAPHY

1. Cameron J, Pohlner PG, Stafford EG, et al: Right heart thrombus: Recognition, diagnosis and management. J Am Coll Cardiol 5:1239, 1985.
2. Dalen JE, Haffajee CI, Alpert JS III, et al. Pulmonary embolism, pulmonary hemorrhage, and pulmonary infarction. N Engl J Med 296:1431–1435, 1977.
3. Huisman MV, Buller HR, Ten Cate JW: Utility of impedance plethysmography in the diagnosis of recurrent deep-vein thrombosis. Arch Intern Med 148:681–683, 1988.
4. Hull R, Delmore T, Carter C, et al: Adjusted subcutaneous heparin versus warfarin sodium in the long-term treatment of venous thrombosis. N Engl J Med 306:189–194, 1982.
5. Hull R, Hirsh J, Carter CJ, et al: Pulmonary angiography, ventilation lung scanning and venography for clinically suspected pulmonary embolism in the abnormal perfusion scan. Ann Intern Med 98:891–899, 1983.
6. Hull R, Raskob GE, Hirsh J: Prophylaxis of venous thromboembolism: An overview. Chest 89:374S–383S, 1986.
7. Kelley MA, Carson JL, Palevsky HI, Schwartz JS: Diagnosing pulmonary embolism: New facts and strategies. Ann Intern Med 114:300–306, 1991.
8. Kipper MS, Moser KM, Kortman KE, Ashburn WL: Long-term follow-up of patients with suspected pulmonary embolism and normal lung scan. Chest 82:411–415, 1982.
9. Marder VJ, Sherry S: Thrombolytic therapy: Current status. N Engl J Med 318:1585–1595, 1988
10. Novelline RA, Baltarowich OH, Athanasoulis CA, et al: The clinical course of patients with suspected pulmonary embolism and a negative pulmonary arteriogram. Radiology 126:561–567, 1978.
11. PIOPED Investigators: Value of the ventilation/perfusion scan in acute pulmonary embolism: Results of the Prospective Investigation of Pulmonary Embolism Diagnosis (PIOPED). JAMA 263:2753–2795, 1990.
12. Stein PD, Willis PW, DeMets DL: History and physical examination in acute pulmonary embolism in patients without preexisting cardiac or pulmonary disease. Am J Cardiol 47:218–223, 1981.
13. White RH, McGahan JP, Daschbach MM, Hartling RR: Diagnosis of deep-vein thrombosis using duplex ultrasound. Ann Intern Med 111:297–304, 1989.

39. PULMONARY HYPERTENSION

David B. Badesch, M.D.

1. What are the typical presenting symptoms in patients with pulmonary hypertension?
Dyspnea on exertion is most common. Because this symptom is nonspecific, patients are often thought to have some other respiratory or cardiac disorder. Other symptoms include chest pain, presyncope or syncope, and edema.

2. What are the usual physical findings in patients with pulmonary hypertension?
By the time most patients present, pulmonary hypertension is already severe. Findings on physical examination might include:
Loud pulmonic valve closure sound (P_2)
Right ventricular heave
Murmur of tricuspid regurgitation (a systolic murmur over the left lower sternal border)
Murmur of pulmonic insufficiency (a diastolic murmur over the left sternal border)
Jugular venous distention (indicating elevated central venous pressures)
Peripheral edema
Hepatomegaly
Hepatojugular reflux
Ascites
Cyanosis
Clubbing

3. How is pulmonary hypertension classified?
1. **Etiology: primary vs. secondary.** Primary pulmonary hypertension is not associated with any of the known causes of pulmonary hypertension. Secondary pulmonary hypertension is due to an underlying disease.
2. **Location: precapillary vs. post-capillary.** Precapillary pulmonary hypertension is caused by increased resistance to flow in the pulmonary arteries and arterioles. Post-pulmonary hypertension is caused by back pressure from the left heart and/or increased resistance to flow in the pulmonary veins.
3. **Duration: acute vs. chronic.** Acute pulmonary hypertension is caused by such things as thromboembolism or adult respiratory distress syndrome. Most other forms of pulmonary hypertension are chronic.
4. **Histopathology: plexiform vs. thrombotic.** The plexiform lesion is characterized by focal medial disruption and aneurysmal dilatation, with formation of a complex proliferative tuft of intimal cells and channels. Thrombotic histopathology is characterized by intravascular thrombus.

4. What should the clinical evaluation for possible pulmonary hypertension include?
As always, the evaluation begins with a thorough history and physical examination. Possible causes of secondary pulmonary hypertension, as listed in the accompanying figure, should be addressed in the history. In addition, travel to or residence in an area endemic for shistosomiasis should be considered. All patients should receive a basic initial screening evaluation, consisting of chest x-ray, electrocardiogram, and echocardiogram.

Patients with no clues to the etiology on history or physical examination are given a broad "detailed" evaluation; patients with a suspected secondary cause receive a "focused" evaluation to verify that etiology, followed by the broad evaluation if necessary. In addition to these tests, arterial blood gases and pulmonary angiography may be indicated. If undertaken, pulmonary angiography should be performed by someone experience in working with pulmonary hypertension patients. See figure.

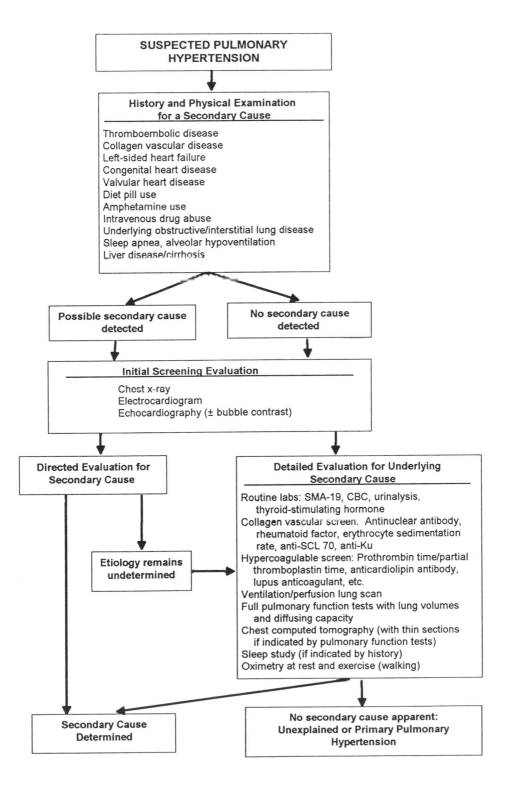

5. List some causes of secondary pulmonary hypertension:
Recurrent pulmonary emboli
Chronic exposure to high altitude
Chronic lung diseases, especially COPD
Sleep apnea
Obesity with hypoventilation
Sickle cell disease
Schistosomiasis
Left heart failure
Mitral valve disease, especially stenosis
Pulmonary veno-occlusive disease
Collagen vascular disease

6. Which connective tissue diseases most commonly cause pulmonary hypertension?
Scleroderma (especially CREST syndrome)
Mixed connective tissue disease
Systemic lupus erythematosus
Rheumatoid arthritis
Dermatomyositis

7. Which occurs more frequently, primary or secondary pulmonary hypertension?
Primary (unexplained) pulmonary hypertension is a rare disorder. Secondary pulmonary hypertension is seen considerably more often in practice.

8. What population group is most frequently affected by primary pulmonary hypertension?
Although primary pulmonary hypertension occurs in both sexes and virtually all age groups, it has a tendency to affect young females. The female-to-male predominance is 1.7:1, and the mean age is 36 years.

9. Is surgical therapy now an option for patients with pulmonary hypertension secondary to chronic recurrent thromboembolism?
Appropriate prevention of recurrent thromboembolism continues to be extremely important. In addition to this prevention, it is now possible to remove organized thrombus surgically from the proximal pulmonary arteries of patients with pulmonary hypertension secondary to chronic recurrent thromboembolism. Operative mortality was 8.7% in a recent study from the most experienced center.

10. What is the average survival for the patient with primary pulmonary hypertension?
According to the National Institutes of Health Registry on Primary Pulmonary Hypertension, the median survival is approximately 2.8 years from the date of diagnosis. It should be noted, however, that there is large interindividual variability. Although some patients progress quickly to death over a period of months, others live for years with little change in symptoms or hemodynamics. Response to therapy with calcium channel antagonists has recently been reported to be associated with an improved prognosis.

11. What is now considered "conventional therapy" for patients with primary pulmonary hypertension?
"Conventional therapy" includes **supplemental oxygen** as needed to maintain an oxygen saturation of at least 91%, **diuretics** if the patient has clinically significant edema or ascites, **oral vasodilators** (usually calcium channel antagonists), **anticoagulation** in the absence of contraindications, and occasionally **digitalis.**

12. How are oral vasodilators used in the treatment of primary pulmonary hypertension?

Many oral vasodilators have been tried in the treatment of primary pulmonary hypertension. Most recently, interest has focused on the calcium channel blockers **nifedipine** and **diltiazem.** A recent study suggests that approximately one-quarter of patients with primary pulmonary hypertension have a favorable response to calcium channel blockers. Patients who respond are thought to have a better prognosis. However, continued follow-up remains important, because patients who demonstrate favorable initial response later deteriorate.

The response to vasodilator therapy in an individual patient is difficult to predict. There is significant risk of adverse reactions, particularly systemic hypotension, since most of the drugs utilized are not selective pulmonary vasodilators. For these reasons, a trial of a short-acting intravenous vasodilator should be done in the cardiac catheterization laboratory or intensive care unit.

13. Why is anticoagulation recommended for patients with primary pulmonary hypertension?

Although no prospective randomized studies have not been done, retrospective data suggest that anticoagulation decreases mortality.

14. Is heart-lung transplantation the transplant procedure of choice in patients with severe pulmonary hypertension?

In most cases, it is no longer thought necessary to transplant the heart in patients with severe pulmonary hypertension. When its afterload is reduced by the transplantation of one or both lungs, the right ventricle is able to recover function. Transplantation of the heart, therefore, is often unnecessary and adds the potential for cardiac rejection and accelerated coronary vascular disease. Occasionally, heart-lung transplantation is still needed in the patient with an underlying congenital heart defect that cannot be repaired at the time of transplantation.

15. Which patients are appropriate candidates for lung transplantation?

Patients with severe pulmonary hypertension unresponsive to other modes of therapy who are otherwise healthy, of reasonable age (generally < 60), and have adequate psychosocial strength and family (or important other) support should be considered for possible lung transplantation. Significant renal, hepatic, or coronary vascular disease is usually considered a significant impediment to lung transplantation. Most experts now consider transplant when signs of right heart failure develop, but some advocate earlier transplantation.

CONTROVERSY

16. Is bilateral lung transplantation better than single lung transplantation in patients with severe pulmonary hypertension?

For: Single lung transplantation in severe pulmonary hypertension is associated with more postoperative and long-term complications. In the postoperative period, the grafted lung is highly susceptible to the development of pulmonary edema due to ischemia and reperfusion. The majority of blood flow is directed toward the graft by the high resistance to flow in the remaining native lung, increasing the likelihood of pulmonary edema. Ventilation is directed to the remaining native lung, however, causing ventilation-perfusion mismatch. In addition, the long-term risks associated with rejection and infection are also greater. As with reperfusion edema, rejection or pneumonia in the single lung transplant can lead to mismatching of ventilation and perfusion. For all these reasons, it is likely, though not proven, that bilateral lung transplantation leads to better long-term survival than single lung transplantation.

Against: Bilateral lung transplantation is thought to be associated with a higher intraoperative risk than single lung transplantation, due to the longer and more complicated operation. Bilateral lung transplantation also uses up more donor organs and may lengthen waiting times for the patient as well as others on the list, thereby increasing their risk of dying while awaiting transplantation. If the overall goal is to help as many patients as possible, bilateral lung transplantation, in the absence of convincing evidence of improved long-term survival, is difficult to justify.

Current Practice: We currently lean toward single lung transplantation in older candidates and bilateral lung transplantation in younger candidates. However, there are no studies to support this, and a randomized multicenter trial is needed.

BIBLIOGRAPHY

1. Alpert M, Goldberg S, Singsen B, et al: Cardiovascular manifestations of mixed connective tissue diseases in adults. Circulation 68:1182–1193, 1983.
2. Alpert MA, Pressly TA, Mukerji V, et al: Short- and long-term hemodynamic effects of captopril in patients with pulmonary hypertension and selected connective tissue disease. Chest 102:1407–1412, 1992.
3. D'Alonzo GE, Barst RJ, Ayres SM, et al: Survival in patients with primary pulmonary hypertension: Results from a national prospective registry. Ann Intern Med 115:343–349, 1991.
4. Fuster V, et al: Primary pulmonary hypertension: Natural history and importance of thrombosis. Circulation 70:580–587, 1984.
5. Groves BM, Badesch DB, Turkevich D, et al: Correlation of acute prostacyclin response in primary (unexplained) pulmonary hypertension with efficacy of treatment with calcium channel blockers and survival. In Weir K (ed): The Role of Ion Flux in Pulmonary Vascular Control. New York Plenum Publishing Corp., in press.
6. Jamieson SW, Auger WR, Fidulo PF, et al: Experience and results with 150 pulmonary thromboendarterectomy operations over a 29 month period. J Thoracic Cardiovasc Surg 106:116–127, 1993.
7. Kasukawa R, Nishimaki T, Takagi T, et al: Pulmonary hypertension in connective tissue disease: Clinical analysis of sixty patients in a multi-institutional study. Clin Rheum 9:56–62, 1990.
8. Palevsky HI, Fishman AP: The management of primary pulmonary hypertension. JAMA 265:1014–1020, 1991.
9. Pietra GG, Edwards WD, Kay JM, et al: Histopathology of primary pulmonary hypertension: A qualitative and quantitative study of pulmonary blood vessels from 58 patients in the National Heart, Lung, and Blood Institute, Primary Pulmonary Hypertension Registry. Circulation 80:1198–1206, 1989.
10. Rich S, Dantzker DR, Ayres SM, et al: Primary pulmonary hypertension: A national prospective study. Ann Intern Med 107:216–223, 1987.
11. Rich S, Kaufman E, Levy PS: The effect of high doses of calcium-channel blockers on survival in primary pulmonary hypertension. N Engl J Med 327:76–81, 1992.
12. Rubin LJ: Primary pulmonary hypertension: Practical therapeutic recommendations. Drugs 43:37–43, 1992.
13. Salerni R, Rodnan GP, Leon DF, Shaver JA: Pulmonary hypertension in the CREST syndrome variant of progressive systemic sclerosis (scleroderma). Ann Intern Med 86:394–399, 1977.
14. Sfikakis P, Kyriakidis M, Vergos C, et al: Cardiopulmonary hemodynamics in systemic sclerosis and response to nifedipine and captopril. Am J Med 90:541–546, 1991.
15. Weir EK: Acute vasodilator testing and pharmacological treatment of primary pulmonary hypertension. In Fishman AP (ed): The Pulmonary Circulation: Normal and Abnormal. Mechanisms, Management, and the National Registry. Philadelphia, University of Pennsylvania Press, 1990.

40. PULMONARY DISEASE AND THE HEART

David A. Kaminsky, M.D., and Thomas A. Neff, M.D.

1. How can diseases of the left heart affect the lungs?

The heart and lungs are intimately linked by the pulmonary vasculature; thus, it is not surprising that the pulmonary vasculature is most commonly affected by left-heart disease. Any process that raises left ventricular (LV) end-diastolic pressure or left atrial pressure will result in elevated pulmonary venous pressure (PVP). Such processes include diseases that reduce LV contractility, such as ischemic heart disease, mitral regurgitation, or cardiomyopathy, as well as processes that decrease LV compliance, such as ischemic heart disease, aortic stenosis, and hypertension. Mitral stenosis results in elevated left atrial pressures. In all of these circumstances, PVP is increased and leads to elevations of pulmonary capillary and pulmonary arterial pressures.

2. What are the mechanical effects of the heart on the lungs?

The heart and lungs both occupy an enclosed space within the thoracic cavity. Any process that results in changes in the size or position of the heart may alter pulmonary function. Cardiomegaly may produce pulmonary symptoms such as cough, dyspnea, and wheezing by compressing mediastinal structures such as the trachea or bronchi. A dilated main pulmonary artery or enlarged left atrium may cause gas trapping and hyperinflation by occluding bronchi. Massive cardiomegaly or pericardial effusion may cause left lower lobe atelectasis.

3. Describe the pulmonary vascular consequences of elevations in PVP.

Pulmonary capillary pressures are elevated in the setting of increased PVP. Normal Starling forces in the alveolar interstitium yield a net filtration force of 4 mmHg outward from the pulmonary capillaries to the interstitium. However, net fluid accumulation does not occur due to the absorbtive capacity of the pulmonary lymphatics, which may increase fluid transport 5- to 10-fold in response to increased fluid formation. Eventually, the lymphatics reach their limit, and net fluid formation in the form of interstitial edema occurs, usually at capillary pressures > 20 mmHg. Alveolar flooding, or pulmonary edema, may be seen with elevations in pressure > 25 mmHg. While these pressure limits apply to acute pulmonary edema, situations in which PVP is chronically elevated, such as mitral stenosis, may require much higher pressures before alveolar edema occurs.

4. What are the two primary diagnoses to consider when Kerly B lines are seen on chest x-ray?

Left-heart disease (congestive heart failure or mitral stenosis) and lymphangitic carcinomatosis. Radiographically, pulmonary congestion, with redistribution of flow to the upper zones of the lung, is typically seen with pulmonary capillary pressures of 18–20 mmHg. As pressure increases further, interstitial edema occurs with the appearance of perihilar haze, peribronchial cuffing, and Kerly B lines. So-called periacinar rosettes, or radiolucent grapelike clusters surrounded by radiodense fluid, may appear as fluid encroaches upon the alveolar space. At 25–30 mmHg pressure, frank pulmonary edema occurs, with fluffy alveolar infiltrates typically in a perihilar distribution. Fairly accurate assessments of true pulmonary capillary pressures, as measured by Swan-Ganz catheter readings, can be made if one looks closely at the chest radiograph.

5. Describe the pulmonary function abnormalities associated with elevations in PVP due to cardiac disease.

Patients with elevated PVP, such as seen in chronic congestive heat failure, may show a combined restrictive and obstructive ventilatory defect on pulmonary function testing. Restriction occurs as a result of loss of lung volume due to increased blood and fluid within the interstitial and alveolar spaces; compliance is reduced.

Airflow limitation is evident as a fall in **forced expiratory volume** in the first second (FEV_1) and **forced vital capacity** (FVC). Since both FEV_1 and FVC fall, the ratio of FEV_1/FVC may be normal. A very low ratio usually implies the concurrence of additional airways disease, such as chronic obstructive pulmonary disease (COPD). Increased airway resistance due to elevations of PVP occurs predominantly in the lung periphery.

Diffusing capacity for carbon monoxide (DLCO) may be *increased* early on due to increased pulmonary blood volume, but with worsening interstitial edema and ultimate injury to the pulmonary vessels, DLCO normalizes and is then reduced.

6. What is "cardiac asthma"?

Patients with elevations in PVP, such as in congestive heart failure or mitral stenosis, have airflow limitation due to increased airways resistance. On physical examination, this may be manifested as wheezing. Although blood vessel engorgement and edema are thought to be responsible for this process, smooth muscle constriction may also be involved. Bronchial hyperresponsiveness to methacholine and acetylcholine has been demonstrated in cardiac asthma. Obviously, it is important to distinguish wheezing due to heart failure from wheezing due to intrinsic airway disease, as the treatment is substantially different. A careful history and physical examination, followed by a therapeutic trial of diuretics or bronchodilators, will answer the question.

7. Besides wheezing, patients with congestive heart failure often have coarse crackles. What other pulmonary diseases can cause crackles?

1. Bronchiectasis
2. Chronic obstructive pulmonary disease (COPD, especially chronic bronchitis)
3. Pneumonia
4. Interstitial lung disease.

As with cardiac asthma, a careful history is the best initial approach to diagnosis. Sophisticated analysis of crackles in different disease states has shown that cardiac crackles are typically more coarse and prolonged than the fine, late-inspiratory, short-duration crackles of interstitial lung disease. COPD crackles also tend to be of short duration, but are early in inspiration and are relatively infrequent and scant. Differentiating crackles of congestive heart failure from those of pneumonia and bronchiectasis is more difficult.

8. What "new" respiratory care modality can be used to treat cardiogenic pulmonary edema and congestive heart failure?

Continuous positive airway pressure (CPAP). CPAP is applied via a tight-fitting mask over the mouth and nose or nose alone. It is usually used to treat respiratory insufficiency due to obstructive sleep apnea or severe COPD. However, CPAP has also been shown to be effective in improving symptoms of acute pulmonary edema and may buy time when one is trying to avoid intubation while waiting for pharmacologic therapy to take effect.

9. What are the long-term consequences of elevations in PVP?

Pulmonary hypertension. The typical pathologic change associated with left-heart-related pulmonary hypertension is medial thickening due to vascular smooth muscle hypertrophy and/or hyperplasia. Pulmonary parenchymal abnormalities may also be seen, especially in advanced mitral stenosis. These include alveolar wall thickening, fibrosis, hemosiderosis, and even parenchymal calcification.

10. Can other classes of cardiac disease alter the pulmonary vasculature?

Congenital heart disease with left-to-right shunting will affect the pulmonary vasculature by causing large increases in pulmonary blood volume and flow. These diseases include atrial septal defects, ventricular septal defects, patent ductus arteriosus, and anomalous pulmonary venous return. The increased flow seen with these lesions may ultimately cause pulmonary hypertension. Ultimately, patients may develop pulmonary vascular resistance sufficiently high that shunt flow equalizes or reverses to right-to-left (Eisenmenger's syndrome).

11. What are the pleural manifestations of cardiac disease?

Normally, a thin layer of fluid exists between the visceral and parietal pleura. Net filtration is favored by Starling forces into the pleural space from the parietal pleura, but the visceral pleura absorbs the fluid to prevent its accumulation. However, increased hydrostatic pressure as in heart failure results in a transudative pleural effusion. The parietal pleura is supplied by the systemic circulation, so any increase in systemic venous pressure, as occurs in right-heart failure, promotes increased fluid formation. The visceral pleural is supplied by the pulmonary circulation, so any increase in pulmonary pressure, as in left heart failure, impedes fluid resorption.

Effusions from heart failure are usually bilateral, but when unilateral, they occur more frequently on the right side.

12. How can heart disease cause an *exudative* pleural effusion?

Following many forms of cardiac injury, including myocardial infarction, surgery, or trauma, a syndrome of pericarditis, pleuritis, and rarely pneumonitis may develop over the ensuing 1–12 weeks. This process is called **Dressler's syndrome** and may be seen in 1–3% of patients following myocardial infarction and up to 30% of cardiac surgery patients. Symptoms include pericardial and pleuritic chest pain, and signs of fever, pericardial or pleural friction rub, and elevated white blood cell count and sedimentation rate are typically seen. Pleural effusions occur in 60–80% of cases, and 50% have an enlarged cardiac silhouette due to pericardial effusion. The pleural effusion is exudative with high protein (usually >3 g/100 ml), pH (>7.40), lactate dehydrogenase, and red blood cell count. The etiology of Dressler's syndrome is unknown but is thought to be due to an antibody-mediated response to myocardial antigens exposed upon injury. Treatment is supportive with nonsteroidals or corticosteroids.

13. A patient presents with fevers, hemoptysis, and multiple pulmonary infiltrates with central radiolucencies on chest x-ray. What is the diagnosis?

Right-sided endocarditis with septic pulmonary emboli. Cardiac disease may lead to pulmonary embolism in the setting of right-sided endocarditis affecting the tricuspid valve. Rarely, septic emboli may arise from indwelling catheters in the superior vena cava. Right-sided endocarditis accounts for 5–10% of all cases of endocarditis and is most often seen in intravenous drug abusers. The most common infecting organism is *Staphylococcus aureus,* although *Streptococcus,* gram-negative, and *Candida* species also may be involved. The radiographic appearance is very characteristic and includes multiple, patchy, ill-defined densities scattered throughout the lung fields, especially in the periphery. They may appear to change in number and size on serial x-rays, reflecting the ongoing shower of emboli to the lungs. Cavitation is seen in 25% of patients.

14. What are the pulmonary effects of various cardiovascular drugs?

Angiotensin-converting enzyme inhibitors cause cough in approximately 15% of all patients but twice as frequently in women than men. The mechanism is not known. β-**blockers** are well-known in their ability to precipitate bronchospasm in patients with asthma and occasionally bronchitis. The drugs **procainamide** and **hydralazine** may cause a lupus-like syndrome in susceptible individuals. With procainamide, the reaction is much more common and involves a positive antineutrophil antibody test in 50–80% of patients, with 30–40% developing pulmonary infiltrates and 40–50% having pleuropericardial disease. The latter manifestations are rare with hydralazine. **Amiodarone** causes pulmonary toxicity, with 5–15% of treated patients developing a severe pneumonitis, which is fatal in 5–10%. This side effect is dose-dependent, usually occurring only in patients who have been treated with > 400 mg/day for > 4 months.

15. What are the main pulmonary complications of cardiac surgery?

Atelectasis, pneumonia, and exacerbation of COPD. Atelectasis and pneumonia are usually due to the inability of the patient to cough adequately or deep breathe following surgery, often because of the pain of the thoracotomy and the heavy use of analgesics and sedatives. These complication are less common following median sternotomy than after lateral thoracotomy. Left lower lobe atelectasis may also be due to concomitant phrenic nerve dysfunction, which may result from mechanical injury or from the cooling associated with cardioplegia. Phrenic nerve function usually recovers within the first 30 days to 1 year but may take as long as 2 years. Bronchospasm may be worsened. Pleural effusions are also common. Some special pulmonary concerns in cardiac transplant surgery, in addition to those above, include postoperative elevations in pulmonary vascular resistance and the numerous infectious complications associated with immunosuppression.

16. Differentiate dyspnea due to cardiac disease from that due to pulmonary disease.

This is a common clinical problem, as many patients have concomitant cardiac and pulmonary disease, often in association with cigarette smoking. The most important feature in distinguishing these two etiologies is clues of underlying disease. Thus, a history of angina, hypertension, or previous myocardial infarction, together with signs of heart failure on examination, make cardiac disease more likely; whereas a history of bronchitis and heavy smoking, with *diminished breath sounds* on examination, and a normal cardiac silhouette with hyperinflated lungs on chest x-ray suggest primary pulmonary disease. In many cases, however, further testing including pulmonary function, arterial blood gases, and a cardiac function assessment with echocardiography or radioisotope scanning, are necessary. Exercise testing with measurement of expired gases can be helpful in difficult cases.

17. Can the pattern of dyspnea help distinguish between cardiac and pulmonary causes?

Yes and no. **Paroxysmal nocturnal dyspnea** (PND) is thought to be specific for heart failure, but patients with COPD may also complain of PND due to the development of increased secretions upon lying down. Asthmatics may also have PND due to nocturnal worsening of bronchospasm. **Orthopnea** is likewise not specific for congestive heart failure because COPD patients sometimes complain of orthopnea due to partial loss of diaphragmatic and accessory muscle function when supine. **Sleep apnea** is often associated with hypertension or left-heart failure, but secondary pulmonary hypertension may result from years of hypoxia. **Cheyne-Stokes respirations,** or periodic breathing, is characteristic of left ventricular dysfunction and rarely associated with pulmonary disease per se. A recent study of patients with congestive heart failure and Cheyne-Stokes respirations found that such patients were more likely to have awake hypocapnia due to hyperventilation. Such patients may complain of PND during periods of hyperpnea.

18. Can pulmonary function predict cardiovascular morbidity and mortality?

Yes. Recent studies have shown an inverse relationship between pulmonary function, as measured by FEV_1 or FVC, and the incidence of coronary artery disease and congestive heart failure, independent of cigarette smoking. One explanation for these findings is that decreased pulmonary function is a marker of centripetal obesity and decreased physical activity, which are themselves related to increased insulin resistance, lower high-density lipoproteins, and higher triglycerides. Hyperinsulinemia is associated with increased sympathetic nervous activity and therefore may result in increased risk of hypertension and myocardial infarction.

BIBLIOGRAPHY

1. Badgett RG, Tanaka DJ, Hunt DK, et al: Can moderate chronic obstructive pulmonary disease be diagnosed by historical and physical findings alone? Am J Med 94:188–196, 1993.
2. Baratz DM, Westbrook PR, Shah PK, Mohsenifar Z: Effect of nasal continuous positive airway pressure on cardiac output and oxygen delivery in patients with congestive heart failure. Chest 102:1397–1401, 1992.
3. Brunnee T, Graf K, Kastens B, et al: Bronchial hyperreactivity in patients with moderate pulmonary circulation overload. Chest 103:1477–1481, 1993.
4. Cabanes LR, Weber SN, Matran R, et al: Bronchial hyperresponsiveness to methacholine in patients with impaired left ventricular function. N Engl J Med 320:1317–1322, 1989.
5. Ettinger NA, Trulock EP: Pulmonary considerations of organ transplantation: State of the art. Am Rev Respir Dis 144:433–451, 1991.
6. Gibson GJ: Lung function in mitral-valve disease. Pract Cardiol 11:88, 91–92, 95–96, 98–100, 1985.

7. Hanly P, Zuberi N, Gray R: Pathogenesis of Cheyne-Stokes respiration in patients with congestive heart failure. Chest 104:1079–1084, 1993.
8. Higgins M, Keller JB, Wagenknecht LE, et al: Pulmonary function and cardiovascular risk factor relationships in black and in white young men and women: The CARDIA Study. Chest 99:315–322, 1991.
9. McFadden ER Jr, Ingram RH: Relationship between diseases of the heart and lungs. In Braunwald E (ed): Heart Disease, 3rd ed. Philadelphia, W. B. Saunders 1988, pp 1870–1882.
10. McParland C, Krishnan B, Wang Y, Gallagher CG: Inspiratory muscle weakness and dyspnea in chronic heart failure. Am Rev Respir Dis 146:467–472, 1992.
11. Messner-Pellenc P, Ximenes C, Brasileiro CF, et al: Cardiopulmonary exercise testing: Determinants of dyspnea due to cardiac or pulmonary limitation. Chest 106:354–360, 1994.
12. Piirila P, Sovijarvi ARA, Kaisla T, et al: Crackles in patients with fibrosing alveolitis, bronchiectasis, COPD and heart failure. Chest 99:1076–1083, 1991.
13. Remetz MS, Cleman MW, Cabin HS: Pulmonary and pleural complications of cardiac disease. Clin Chest Med 10:545–592, 1989.
14. Rosenow EC III, Myers JL, Swenson SJ, Pisani RJ: Drug-induced pulmonary disease: An update. Chest 102:239–250, 1992.
15. Stelzner TJ, King TE, Antony VB, Sahn SA: The pleuropulmonary manifestations of the postcardiac injury syndrome. Chest 84:383–387, 1983.
16. Turino GM: The lungs and heart disease. In Murray JF, Nadel JA (eds): Textbook of Respiratory Medicine. Philadelphia, W. B. Saunders, 1988, pp 1883–1893.

41. PREOPERATIVE EVALUATION FOR CARDIAC RISK

Jeffrey Pickard, M.D.

1. What type of anesthesia is the safest?

It is a common misconception that spinal anesthesia is safer and better tolerated than general anesthesia. Both confer equal risks of postoperative fatal and nonfatal myocardial infarctions. Regional or local anesthesia may be less risky than the same procedure done under general or spinal anesthesia. The type of anesthesia is best determined by the anesthesiologist.

2. How does a history of a myocardial infarction affect a patient's perioperative risk?

Most investigators and clinicians believe that within the first 3–6 months after a myocardial infarction, perioperative cardiac morbidity and mortality are significantly increased. Therefore, nonemergent surgery should be delayed, if possible, until after this time. After 6 months, perioperative risk remains relatively stable, assuming there are no sequelae (e.g., congestive heart failure, rhythm disturbances). Some believe the level of risk returns to what it was before the infarct (< 1% in the general population), whereas others believe the risk remains somewhat elevated (2–8%).

3. What is meant by a patient's preoperative cardiac risk index?

This refers to a quantitative assessment of a patient's risk of an adverse cardiac outcome based on various preoperative clinical, historical, and laboratory variables. The first and probably most widely used of these indices was published by Goldman et al. in 1977.

Computation of the Cardiac Risk Index

CRITERIA	MULTIVARIATE DISCRIMINANT-FUNCTION COEFFICIENT	"POINTS"
1 History:		
(a) Age > 70 yr	0.191	5
(b) MI in previous 6 mo	0.384	10
2 Physical examination:		
(a) S, gallop or JVD	0.451	11
(b) Important VAS	0.119	3
3 Electrocardiogram:		
(a) Rhythm other than sinus or PACs on last preoperative ECG	0.283	7
(b) >5 PVCs/min documented at any time before operation	0.278	7
4 General status: PO$_2$<60 or PCO$_2$>50 mmHg, K<3.0 or HCO,<20 mEq/L,BUN>50 or Cr>3.0 mg/dl, abnormal SGOT, signs of chronic liver disease or patient bedridden from noncardiac causes	0.132	3
5 Operation:		
(a) Intraperitoneal, intrathoracic or aortic operation	0.123	3
(b) Emergency operation	0.167	4
Total possible		53 points

*MI denotes myocardial infarction, JVD jugular-vein distention, VAS valvular aortic stenosis, PACs premature atrial contractions, ECG electrocardiogram, PVCs premature ventricular contractions, PO$_2$ partial pressure of oxygen, PCO$_2$ partial pressure of carbon dioxide, K potassium, HCO, bicarbonate, BUN blood urea nitrogen, Cr creatinine, and SGOT serum glutamic oxaloacetic transaminase.
From Goldman L, et al: Cardiac risk in noncardiac surgery. N Engl J Med 297 (Suppl 16):845–850, 1977, with permission.

Cardiac Risk Index

CLASS	POINT TOTAL	NO OR ONLY MINOR COMPLICATION (N=943)	LIFE-THREATENING COMPLICATIONS (N=39)	CARDIAC DEATHS (N=19)
I (N = 537)	0–5	532 (99)†	4 (0.7)	1 (0.2)
II (N = 316)	6–12	295 (93)	16 (5)	5 (2)
III (N = 130)	13–25	112 (86)	15 (11)	3 (2)
IV (N = 18)	>26	4 (22)	4 (22)	10 (56)

From Goldman L, et al: Cardiac risk in noncardiac surgery. N Engl J Med 297 (Suppl 16):845–850, 1977, with permission.

4. How accurate are these indices?
In general, these indices appear to have a fairly high positive predictive value in assessing preoperative cardiac risk, but their low negative predictive value may make them less helpful, especially when dealing with patients who are undergoing vascular surgery. Patients who appear to be at high risk for perioperative complications, based on their risk scores, have a higher percentage of adverse outcomes than those with low risk scores. However, some patients who have low risk assessment scores may still be at substantial risk and may benefit from further study.

5. Which types of surgery carry higher risks of cardiac complications?
Vascular surgery appears to carry the greatest risk. Intrathoracic, intraperitoneal, and emergency procedures also carry higher risk.

6. Why is the risk of cardiac complications higher in vascular surgery than in other types of surgery?
The incidence of significant coronary artery disease (CAD) in patients undergoing vascular surgery is about 30%. Many vascular surgery patients have asymptomatic myocardial ischemia; because they are made sedentary by claudication, they are not active enough to induce angina and thus their CAD is undiagnosed. Some vascular procedures require significant manipulation of tissue and clamping and unclamping of vessels, which can cause marked increases in afterload and myocardial oxygen demand. Vascular surgery patients are often relatively old (mean age, 59–71 years), and older patients are at higher risk for perioperative complications.

7. Which patients should be evaluated for CAD prior to surgery?
Patients who are undergoing high-risk procedures (especially vascular procedures which require cross-clamping of the aorta) may require additional evaluation for CAD, such as exercise treadmill testing. Patients with unstable angina, new electrocardiographic (ECG) changes (especially ischemic), or high cardiac risk indices should also be considered for further cardiac evaluation. Patients who are unable to exercise (e.g., those with peripheral vascular disease) or who have baseline ECG abnormalities may require a dipyridamole-thallium scan to detect ischemia.

Patients with evidence of ischemic disease on noninvasive testing may require coronary angiography with an eye toward coronary artery bypass grafting (CABG) prior to high-risk surgery. CABG, of course, carries its own operative risks, but patients who have had successful CABG reduce their perioperative cardiac risk to approximately that of the normal population.

8. What techniques can be used to identify patients at risk for perioperative cardiac complications?
The history, physical examination, and ECG are important. Coronary angiography is costly and invasive, carries its own risk, and does not assess function. Radionuclide ventriculography, arm ergometry, and Holter monitoring have been advocated, but their predictive values are inade-

quate. The exercise treadmill test estimates cardiac risk and functional status but often cannot be done, especially in patients with peripheral vascular disease. Stress echocardiography (often done with dobutamine or dipyridamole) may become a valuable way of predicting perioperative complications in patients who cannot exercise but so far has been studied in only a limited number of patients. Vasodilator myocardial imaging remains the most popular technique overall for assessing perioperative cardiac risk. (*See* Chapter 37 for an algorithm on using these techniques.)

9. How is vasodilator myocardial imaging done?

The technique involves administration of a vasodilator (usually dipyridamole) and a contrast agent (thallium-201), followed by myocardial perfusion scanning. Intravenous dipyridamole dilates normal coronary arteries by enhancing their sensitivity to adenosine, a potent coronary artery dilator. Stenotic or occluded vessels remain unaffected. After dipyridamole is infused, thallium-201 is injected, and myocardial scanning is done immediately and 4 hours later. Patients with adequate myocardial perfusion have normal scans. Patients with defects on the initial scan and no defects after 4 hours have ischemic myocardium. Perfusion defects which do not change after 4 hours usually indicate old infarction.

Adenosine-thallium scanning appears to be equally accurate in predicting perioperative risk. It may have an advantage over dipyridamole-thallium scanning because adenosine is rapidly metabolized and so side effects are transient. However, adenosine causes a higher incidence of chest pain.

10. How accurate is vasodilator myocardial imaging in assessing perioperative cardiac risk?

Most patients, even those undergoing major vascular surgery who have underlying CAD, have no perioperative cardiac complications. Therefore, preoperative cardiac risk tests will have low specificity and low positive predictive value. Many studies have a high sensitivity (> 90%) in this procedure but lower specificity. Positive predictive value is generally low. Even selective testing does little to improve these percentages.

Dipyridamole-Thallium-201 Scintigraphy (DTS) and Perioperative Myocardial Infarction or Death in Vascular Surgery Patients

REFERENCE*	YEAR	n	OVER CARDIAC EVENT† RATE (PRETEST PROBABILITY)	RATE OF CARDIAC EVENTS†—POSITIVE DTS (PREDICTIVE VALUE +)	RATE OF CARDIAC EVENTS†—NORMAL OR FIXED DTS FINDINGS (PREDICTIVE VALUE−)
Leppo et al.[44]	1987	96	16%	28%	3%
Cutler et al.[43]	1987	107	8%	28%	0%
Sachs et al.[45]	1988	46	4%	21%	0%
Lette et al.[46]	1989	60	15%	40%	0%
Lane et al.[47]	1989	101	9%	14%	3%
Eagle et al.[29]	1989	200	8%	16%	2%
McEnroe et al.[26]	1990	83	6%	32%	4%
Marwick et al.[48]	1990	83	7%	20%	6%
Makaroun et al.[49]	1990	46	13%	25%	4%

*For complete reference citations, see the reference list.
†Myocardial infarction or death.
From Granieri, R, Macpherson DS: Perioperative care of the vascular surgery patient: The perspective of the internist. J Gen Intern Med 7:102–113, 1992, with permission.

11. How is a patient with a prosthetic valve managed perioperatively?

If cardiac function is relatively normal, there are two major risks to which patients with prosthetic valves are exposed: infective endocarditis and thromboembolism. **Infective endocarditis** in patients with prosthetic valves is associated with significant morbidity and mortality. Regardless of the risk of individual procedures for blood contamination, most patients should be given endocarditis prophylaxis perioperatively.

For **thromboembolism** most patients can be safely managed by discontinuing warfarin therapy 3–4 days before the procedure and then restarting it when adequate hemostasis has been achieved postoperatively, usually in the evening after surgery. In high-risk patients (e.g., the patient with a prosthetic mitral valve in atrial fibrillation), this regimen may not afford adequate protection against thromboembolism, and so it may be appropriate to hospitalize the patient and switch to continuous intravenous heparin 3 days before surgery. The infusion can be stopped approximately 6 hours before the procedure. The infusion is started again, along with warfarin, when adequate hemostasis is assured postoperatively and is continued for 3 days, at which time oral anticoagulation alone should be adequate.

AHA Recommendations for the Prevention of Bacterial Endocarditis in At-Risk Patients (including Prosthetic Heart Valves)

For dental, oral, and upper respiratory tract procedures
I. Standard regimen
    Amoxicillin, 3 g orally 1 hr before procedure, then 1.5 g 6 hrs after initial dose
    For amoxicillin/penicillin-allergic patients:
        Erythromycin ethylsuccinate, 800 mg, or erythromycin stearate, 1 g orally 2 hrs before procedure, then
    ¹/₂ dose 6 hrs after initial dose, *or*
        Clindamycin, 300 mg orally 1 hr before procedure, then 150 mg 6 hrs after initial dose
II. Alternate regimen
    For patients unable to take oral medications:
        Ampicillin, 2 mg iv (or im) 30 min before procedure, then 1 g iv (or im) (*or* amoxicillin, 1.5 g orally)
    6 hrs after initial dose
    For ampicillin/amoxicillin/penicillin-allergic patients unable to take oral medications:
        Clindamycin, 300 mg iv 30 min before procedure, then 150 mg iv (or orally) 6 hrs after initial dose
    For high-risk patients who are not candidates for Standard Regimen:
        Ampicillin, 2 g iv (or im), plus gentamicin, 1.5 mg/kg iv (or im) (not to exceed 80 mg) 30 min before
    procedure, then amoxicillin, 1.5 g orally 6 hrs after initial dose (or repeat parenteral regimen 8 hrs after initial
    dose)
        For amoxicillin/ampicillin/penicillin-allergic patients at high risk:
        Vancomycin, 1 g iv given over 1 hr starting 1 hr before procedure (no repeat dose needed)
For genitourinary and gastrointestinal procedures
I. Standard regimen*
    Ampicillin, 2 g iv (or im), plus gentamicin, 1.5 mg/kg iv (or im) (not to exceed 80 mg) 30 min before
    procedure, then amoxicillin, 1.5 g orally 6 hrs after initial dose (or repeat parenteral regimen once 8 hrs after
    initial dose)
    For amoxicillin/ampicillin/penicillin-allergic patients:
        Vancomycin, 1 g iv given over 1 hr, plus gentamicin, 1.5 mg/kg iv (or im) (not to exceed 80 mg), 1 hr
    before procedure (may be repeated once 8 hrs after initial dose)
II. Alternate oral regimen for low-risk patients*
    Amoxicillin, 3 g orally 1 hr before procedure, then 1.5 g 6 hrs after initial dose

*For initial pediatric doses, substitute: ampicillin, 50 mg/kg; gentamicin, 2.0 mg/kg; amoxicillin, 50 mg/kg; vancomycin, 20 mg/kg. Follow-up doses are one-half of initial dose. Total pediatric dose should not exceed total adult dose.
    Adapted from AHA Committee on Rheumatic Fever, Endocarditis, and Kawasaki Disease: Prevention of bacterial endocarditis: Recommendations by the American Heart Association. JAMA 264:2919–2922, 1990; used with permission of the American Heart Association.

12. When during the perioperative period is a patient most likely to suffer an ischemic cardiac complication?

Ischemia and infarction generally occur in the early *post*operative period (up to 4 days after surgery), with a peak incidence at about 48 hours. It is during this period that patients experience the greatest increases in myocardial oxygen demand because of a hyperadrenergic state associated with pain, emotional stress, withdrawal of anesthesia, and other factors. Patients are also more apt to have diminished oxygen delivery to the myocardium because of anemia, hypoxemia, and hypotension. In addition, the clotting system is activated postoperatively, rendering patients relatively hypercoagulable and at risk for coronary thrombosis.

13. Which patients should have coronary revascularization prior to vascular surgery?
Some institutions recommend coronary angiography for all patients with clinical evidence of CAD before vascular surgery. CABG is then done on patients with severe CAD regardless of symptoms. This approach has been justified by studies indicating that patients who have successfully undergone CABG do better than patients who undergo vascular surgery without CABG. However, these patients may have a better prognosis simply because they are able to withstand revascularization (selection basis).

In a more conservative approach, CABG is generally reserved for patients with left main coronary disease or triple-vessel disease with left ventricular dysfunction. However, morbidity and mortality of the workup and of revascularization itself may be significantly higher in patients with diffuse vasculopathy. This, as well as the delay of vascular surgery, must be considered when deciding who should have CABG.

14. Is the risk associated with carotid surgery the same as for other vascular procedures?
No. Carotid endarterectomy is a relatively low-risk procedure, and these patients may proceed to surgery without preoperative coronary assessment. The exceptions are patients with unstable angina or recent myocardial infarction, in whom it is reasonable to assess coronary anatomy with an eye toward doing a combined carotid-coronary procedure.

BIBLIOGRAPHY

1. Cambria RP, Brewster DC, Abbott WM, et al: The impact of selective use of dipyridamole-thallium scans and surgical factors on the current morbidity of aortic surgery. J Vasc Surg 15:43–51, 1992.
2. Detsky AS, Abrams HB, Forbath N, et al: Cardiac assessment for patients undergoing non-cardiac surgery. Arch Intern Med 146:2131–2134, 1986.
3. Fleisher LA, Barash PG: Pre-operative cardiac evaluation for non-cardiac surgery: A functional approach. Anesth Analg 74:586–598, 1992.
4. Goldman L, Caldera DL, Nussbaum SR, et al: Multifactorial index of cardiac risk in non-cardiac surgical procedures. N Engl J Med 296:845–850, 1977.
5. Granieri R, MacPherson DS: Peri-operative care of the vascular surgery patient: The perspective of the internist. J Gen Intern Med 7:102–113, 1992.
6. Krupski WC, Layug EL, Reilly LM, et al (eds): Comparison of cardiac morbidity between aortic and infrainguinal operations. J Vasc Surg 15:354–365, 1992.
7. Lalka SG, Sawada SG, Dalsing MC, et al: Dobutamine stress echocardiography as a predictor of cardiac events associated with aortic surgery. J Vasc Surg 15:831–842, 1992.
8. Lette J, Waters D, Lapointe J, et al: Usefulness of the severity and extent of reversible perfusion defects during thallium-dipyridamole imaging for cardiac risk assessment before non-cardiac surgery. Am J Cardiol 64:276–281, 1989.
9. Mangano DT: Peri-operative cardiac morbidity. Anesthesiology 72:153–184, 1990.
10. Massie BM, Mangano DT: Assessment of peri-operative risk: Have we put the cart before the horse? J Am Coll Cardiol 21:1353–1356, 1993.
11. Massie BM, Mangano DT: Risk stratification for non-cardiac surgery: How and why? Circulation 87:1752–1755, 1993.
12. Weitz HH: Cardiac risk stratification prior to vascular surgery. Med Clin North Am 77:377–396, 1993.

42. RHEUMATIC HEART DISEASE AND MITRAL STENOSIS

Edward A. Gill, M.D.

1. What causes most cases of mitral stenosis?
Rheumatic heart disease.

2. What is rheumatic fever?
Rheumatic fever is an acute, systemic, inflammatory disease that occurs as a reaction to a recent streptococcal soft-tissue infection, most commonly pharyngitis.

3. How long does it take from the onset of rheumatic fever until mitral stenosis develops?
It can be as short as 2 years. Progression seems to be particularly rapid in developing countries, for reasons which are not entirely understood but could relate to the lack of appropriate penicillin treatment of rheumatic fever or nutritional factors.

4. List the Jones criteria.
The Jones criteria are guidelines for making the diagnosis of an initial attack of rheumatic fever. There is a high likelihood that the disease is present if there is supporting evidence of antecedent group A streptococcal infection (positive throat culture, positive rapid streptococcal antigen test, elevated or rising streptococcal antibody titer), as well as either two major or one major plus two minor manifestations.

Major manifestations	Minor manifestations
Carditis	Arthralgia
Polyarthritis	Fever
Chorea	Elevated sedimentation rate
Erythema marginatum	Elevated C-reactive protein
Subcutaneous nodules	Prolonged PR interval

5. Besides mitral stenosis, how does rheumatic disease affect the heart?
Aortic regurgitation is the second most common lesion, followed by mitral regurgitation and aortic stenosis. The tricuspid valve is less commonly involved, either with stenosis or regurgitation. Involvement of the pulmonary valve is rare. Constrictive pericarditis is thought not to be a sequela to rheumatic fever.

6. What are the typical symptoms of mitral stenosis?
Dyspnea on exertion is the classic presenting symptom. However, mitral stenosis can present with an arrhythmia, such as atrial fibrillation, or a systemic embolic event, since atrial thrombi are common in mitral stenosis.

7. What are less typical presentations?
Severe mitral stenosis can present as pulmonary edema or severe right-sided heart failure if pulmonary pressures become severely elevated. Approximately 15% of patients with mitral stenosis experience angina. Although this symptom may arise from right ventricular hypertension, concomitant atherosclerosis, or embolization of a left atrial thrombus to a coronary artery, in many cases the explanation for chest pain in mitral stenosis cannot be determined.

8. What are the physical findings in mitral stenosis?
Most notable are a loud S_1, an opening snap early in diastole, followed by a diastolic murmur which is mostly decrescendo. By phonocardiogram, the murmur actually has two brief crescendo periods, the first just after the opening snap, and the second with atrial contraction. These periods of crescendo murmur correspond to the two periods of the greatest transvalular gradient in diastole.

9. Why is the first heart sound (S_1) accentuated?
The explanation for this is uncertain. McCall and others have suggested that the mitral valve leaflets must be pliable for the S_1 to be accentuated. The accentuated S_1 then is caused in part by the rapidity of the upstroke of the left ventricular pressure at the time of mitral valve closure. In addition, the wide excursion or displacement of the mitral valve leaflets prior to closure is felt to play a role in the accentuated S_1. Marked calcification or thickening of the mitral valve reduces the amplitude of S_1. Finally, the presystolic accentuation of mitral blood flow caused by atrial contraction blends into S_1 and may contribute to the perceived accentuation.

10. What are the hemodynamic findings in mitral stenosis?
The most important finding is the presence of a pressure gradient across the mitral valve. That is, during diastole, the pressure in the left atrium is greater than the pressure in the left ventricle. This gradient is measured by recording the left ventricular diastolic pressure simultaneously with the pulmonary capillary wedge pressure (PAW). The PAW is used as a close approximation of the left atrial pressure. The mean gradient across the mitral valve can then be determined, and with the Gorlin formula, the valve area (in cm^2) can be calculated:

$$\text{Valve area} = \frac{\text{Cardiac output/(heart rate} \times \text{avg. diastolic period)}}{37.7 \times \sqrt{\text{mean gradient}}}$$

(Note 37.7 is constant empirically derived for the mitral valve)

11. Describe the echocardiographic findings in mitral stenosis.
   M-mode echocardiography. The most specific finding by M-mode echocardiography is the posterior mitral valve leaflet moving in an anterior direction with the anterior mitral valve leaflet in diastole. This demonstrates the tethering of the valve leaflets caused by fusion of the commissures (Fig. 1). Other, less specific findings include increased echoes from the mitral valve due to thickening and/or calcification, and decreased E-F slope due to low flow across the mitral valve (Fig. 1). Decreased E-F slope is a frequent finding in severe heart failure and could be confused with mitral stenosis in this setting.
   Two-dimensional echocardiography. The findings of mitral stenosis include diastolic bowing (''hockey stick'' formation) of the anterior mitral leaflet (Fig. 2), thickening and increased echogenicity of the mitral valve leaflets, annulus, and subvalvular apparatus, and narrowed orifice of the valve as measured by short axis. The actual valve area can be measured by 2-dimensional echocardiography in the short-axis view (Fig. 3).
   Doppler echocardiography. Findings in mitral stenosis include an elevated velocity across the mitral valve (>1.3 m/s or 130 cm/s), indicating an abnormally high transvalvular gradient, and prolonged pressure half-time.

12. How is the pressure half-time calculated from Doppler echocardiography?
   The pressure half-time is the time required for the peak transvalvular pressure gradient to be reduced by one-half and is quantitatively related to the degree of mitral stenosis. The pressure gradient is measured by calculating the velocity of flow across the mitral valve and converting the velocity to pressure, using the modified Bernoulli equation: $P = 4V^2$, where P = pressure and V = velocity of flow. The figure below shows a typical velocity envelope across the mitral valve. The maximum velocity is 296 cm/s. A normal pressure half-time is about 70 ms. In severe mitral stenosis, the pressure half-time is greater than >200 ms. The mitral valve area can be calculated

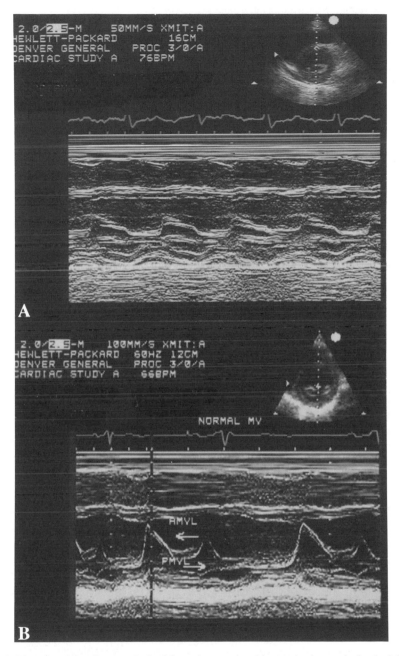

Figure 1. M-mode echocardiogram obtained from the parasternal long-axis view at the level of the mitral valve. *A*, The posterior and anterior mitral leaflets can be seen tracking together. The posterior leaflet moves anterior (toward the top of the figure) during diastole. Ordinarily, the posterior leaflet should move posterior when it opens. Note that the E-F slope is markedly reduced compared to that seen in *B*, an example of a normal mitral valve. This is a semiquantitative measure to show that the mitral valve does not open briskly during diastole.

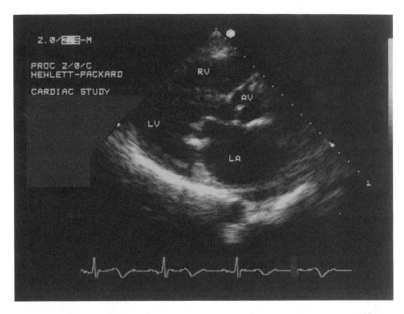

Figure 2. Parasternal long-axis view of the left atrium, left ventricle, and mitral valve. Note the diastolic bowing of the anterior mitral valve leaflet.

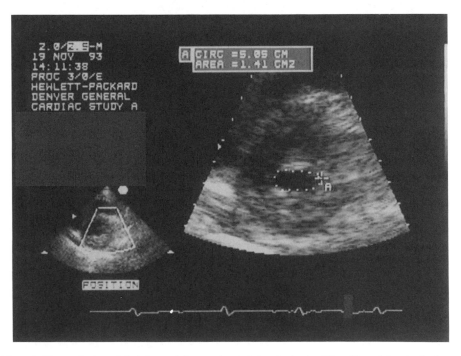

Figure 3. Short-axis view of the left ventricle at the level of the mitral valve. The orifice of the mitral valve can be measured by planimetry.

using the formula MVA = 220/pressure half-time. For example in a patient with severe mitral stenosis, the pressure half-time might be 250 ms and the MVA = 220/250, or 0.7 cm^2.

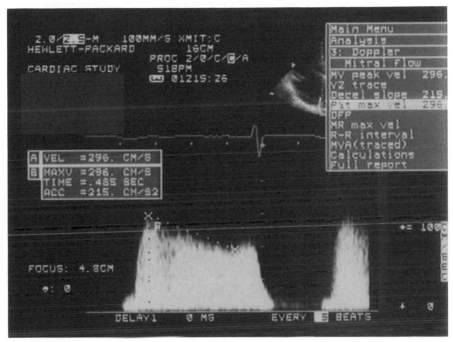

Continuous-wave Doppler measurement of the velocity across the mitral valve.

13. How do regurgitant lesions affect the calculation of valve areas?

The presence of severe aortic regurgitation will cause a slight underestimation of the severity of the mitral stenosis (overestimation of the valve area) determined by Doppler pressure half-time, because the gradient between the left atrium and left ventricle decreases faster due to the aortic regurgitation (hence a shorter pressure half time). On the other hand, the valve area as determined by cardiac catheterization will tend to overestimate the severity of the mitral stenosis (underestimate the valve area), because the cardiac output is in the numerator of the Gorlin equation. The cardiac output used in the formula is the forward cardiac output measured by the Fick equation and therefore does not take into account the regurgitant volume, underestimating the flow across the valve. Mitral regurgitation does not affect the pressure half-time significantly, but it does affect the Gorlin area, as with aortic regurgitation.

14. What treatment options are available?

- Surgical replacement of mitral valve
- Surgical repair (open commissurotomy), where the fused leaflets are separated
- Balloon mitral valvuloplasty (commisurotomy done with a percutaneous balloon technique)

15. What is a normal mitral valve area? When is the mitral valve orifice small enough to warrant surgical or other intervention?

A normal mitral valve orifice is 4–6 cm^2, and intervention is usually considered warranted when the orifice is ≤1.0 cm^2. However, some patients with valve areas of 1.0–1.5 cm^2 may have pulmonary hypertension or exertional dyspnea, warranting intervention.

16. What echocardiographic parameters are used to predict the success of mitral valvuloplasty?
The mitral valve is more amenable to valvuloplasty if the valve is pliable and the valve and subvalvular apparatus are not severely calcified or thickened. An echocardiographic grading system has been developed by Weyman et al. based on valve mobility, thickening or calcification, and subvalvular thickening. Each of these four variables is assigned a score from 1–4 (4 being most severe), with a maximum score being 16. In general, a score of 8 or less suggests that the valve would respond well to valvuloplasty. The presence of more than mild mitral regurgitation precludes valvuloplasty, because in most cases this procedure will increase the degree of mitral regurgitation.

17. What is the role of an exercise evaluation in a patient with mitral stenosis?
One of the most common clinical applications of simultaneous exercise and hemodynamic measurements is in the patient with mitral stenosis and borderline resting measurements. Exercising such a patient to the level of a symptomatic state with simultaneous Doppler measurement of mitral valve gradient and pulmonary artery pressure (or similar measurements made in the catheterization laboratory) may better elucidate the physiologic severity of the mitral valvular disease.

18. What are the other causes of mitral stenosis besides rheumatic heart disease?
Congenital mitral stenosis is the second most common cause of mitral stenosis and is far less frequent than rheumatic fever. Rarely, mitral stenosis can be a complication of malignant carcinoid, systemic lupus erythematosus, rheumatoid arthritis, and the mucopolysaccharidoses of the Hunter-Hurler phenotype. Two obscure causes of mitral stenosis are eosinophilic fibroelastosis and the drug methysergide (a vasodilator used for headaches), which is now rarely, if ever, used. Degenerative mitral annular calcification also can cause stenosis.

19. What myocardial tumor can mimic mitral stenosis?
Atrial myxoma, specifically left atrial myxoma, can present with similar findings on physical examination, including a diastolic rumble and a loud S_1. An opening snap is characteristically absent. The presence of systemic symptoms, such as fever, arthralgia, malaise, cachexia, rash, and Raynaud's phenomenon, can be clues to the presence of myxoma.

20. What is the NAME syndrome?
This syndrome is the association of:
    N = Nevi
    A = Atrial myxoma
    M = Myxoid neurofibromas
    E = Ephelides (freckles)
The syndrome is inherited with an autosomal dominant pattern. Seven percent of all atrial myxomata are inherited.

21. What is Ortner's syndrome?
Hoarseness caused by a dilated left atrium compressing the left recurrent laryngeal nerve.

22. What is Lutembacher's syndrome?
It is the combination of mitral stenosis and atrial septal defect. The significance of this lesion is the presence of a left-to-right shunt that is increased by worsening severity of mitral stenosis. In addition, the mitral valve gradient and pressure half-time will be inaccurate because of rapid deterioration of the pressure gradient due to left atrial-to-right atrial shunting.

The author thanks Doug Voorhees and Sue Rainguet for preparation of the echocardiography figures, and Jo-Anne Orwig for preparation of the manuscript.

BIBLIOGRAPHY

1. Gorlin R, Gorlin G: Hydraulic formula for calculation of area of stenotic mitral valve, other cardiac valves and central circulatory shunts. Am Heart J 41:1, 1951.
2. Grossman W: Cardiac Catheterization and Angiography, 4th ed. Philadelphia, Lea & Febiger.
3. McCall BX, Price JL: Movement of mitral valve cusps in relation to the first heart sound and opening snap in patients with mitral stenosis. Br Heart J 29:417, 1967.
4. Nakatani S, Masuyama T, Kodama K, et al: Valve and limitations of Doppler echocardiography in the quantification of stenotic mitral valve area: Comparison of the pressure half-time and the continuity equation methods. Circulation 77:78–85, 1988.
5. Sharma NGK, Kapoor CP, Mahambre L, Borker MP: Ortner's syndrome. J Indian Med Assoc 60:427, 1973.
6. Wilkins GT, Weyman AE, Abascal VM, et al: Percutaneous balloon dilatation of the mitral valve: An analysis of echocardiographic variables related to outcome and the mechanism of dilatation. Br Heart J 60:299–308, 1988.
7. Wood P: An appreciation of mitral stenosis. BMJ 1(Pt 2):1051 and 1113, 1954.
8. Wranne B, Ask P, Lloyd D: Analysis of different methods of assessing the stenotic mitral valve area with emphasis on the passage gradient half-time concept. Am J Cardiol 66:614–620, 1990.

V. Valvular Heart Disease

43. AORTIC STENOSIS AND REGURGITATION

Edward P. Havranek, M.D.

1. What is the classic triad of symptoms in significant aortic stenosis?
Dyspnea, syncope, and angina.

2. What are the usual physical findings in aortic stenosis?
The hallmark of aortic stenosis is a **crescendo-decrescendo systolic murmur.** This murmur is heard best at the upper right or left sternal border, radiates to the carotids, and is harsh. The murmur of significant aortic stenosis typically is at least III/VI in intensity, in severe stenosis with left ventricular systolic failure, the murmur may be less intense.

The **carotid pulses** offer important clues in the diagnosis of aortic stenosis. As the valvular disease progresses, the carotid upstroke becomes slowed, the contour sustained, and the amplitude small. In elderly patients, however, relatively inelastic arteries many make the pulse seem normal even in severe disease.

Palpation of the precordium may demonstrate the findings of left ventricular hypertrophy—a sustained, forceful apical impulse, and a palpable atrial filling wave.

The **second heart sound** (actually the aortic component of S_2) is diminished in intensity. In aortic stenosis caused by a congenitally bicuspid valve, an ejection sound may be heard

In advanced disease, when systolic dysfunction occurs, the findings of **congestive heart failure** are present: a displaced apical impulse, rales, jugular venous distension, hepatomegaly, and the like.

3. Which noninvasive tests are useful in evaluating suspected significant aortic stenosis?
The single most useful test is **Doppler echocardiography,** which allows measurement of the velocity of blood flow through the stenotic valve: the more severe the stenosis, the higher the velocity. A simple formula relates the velocity to the estimated pressure gradient across the valve:

$$\Delta P = 4V^2$$

where ΔP is the pressure gradient (in mmHg), and V is the maximum outflow tract velocity (in m/s). When ventricular function is normal, a pressure gradient of > 50–60 mmHg is likely to be associated with hemodynamically significant stenosis. The remainder of the echocardiogram should demonstrate a calcified, poorly mobile aortic valve and left ventricular hypertrophy.

An **electrocardiogram** should be examined. The presence of left ventricular hypertrophy and left atrial enlargement suggest significant stenosis. The **chest radiograph** may show evidence of a calcified aortic valve, cardiomegaly, and congestive heart failure.

4. What are the causes of aortic stenosis?
In patients over age 70 years, the most common cause is senile calcific degeneration. In younger patients, the most common cause is calcific degeneration of a congenitally bicuspid valve. Rheumatic heart disease is diminishing in importance as a cause for aortic stenosis. In children and young adults, congenital stenosis is most common. Methysergide, a vasodilator medication used for migraines, is a rare cause of aortic stenosis.

5. Of what value is cardiac catheterization?

The main value of catheterization is to define the degree of stenosis accurately. This is done by estimating the valve orifice area through use of an equation relating area to cardiac output, pressure gradient across the valve, and duration of systole, all of which are measured during catheterization. The procedure is also useful for defining left ventricular function and for assessing coronary artery disease in patients over age 40. Significant coronary stenoses should be bypassed at the time of valve replacement.

6. Describe the natural history of aortic stenosis.

In patients with mild to moderate stenosis (valve area > 1.0 cm^2), the prognosis is excellent. The mean time between diagnosis and surgery is well over a decade. In patients with severe stenosis, the outlook is not as good. In one study of patients who refused surgery, survival rates depended on symptoms. Mean survival was 45 months for those with angina, 27 months for those with syncope, and only 11 months for those after the onset of left-heart failure. Patients with severe stenosis seldom die suddenly prior to the onset of symptoms.

7. When should aortic valve surgery be considered?

Most agree that aortic valve replacement should be performed only when stenosis causes symptoms. Some believe that valve replacement should be performed in asymptomatic patients when the valve reaches a critical degree of narrowing, usually defined as a valve area < 0.8 cm^2 as determined at catheterization. Firm evidence that this latter approach improves outcome is lacking, however.

8. When is balloon valvuloplasty a useful procedure?

This procedure has not replaced surgical valve replacement because of high rates of restenosis and complications. It may be useful in patients with severe symptoms whose lifespans are limited by other diseases such as malignancy. It may also "buy time" in patients with severe heart failure or intercurrent illness, such as pneumonia, in order to improve surgical risk. The procedure may be more useful in children or young adults with congenital stenosis.

9. Can chronic aortic regurgitation cause heart failure?

Yes. Although aortic regurgitation is generally better tolerated than stenosis, it may lead to irreversible left ventricular dysfunction. This may occur *prior to the development of symptoms*. Thus, patients with severe aortic insufficiency must be followed carefully.

10. What symptom is found with aortic regurgitation?

Dyspnea.

11. What are the major physical findings?

Physical findings in aortic regurgitation vary with the severity of disease. The **murmur** is diastolic, decrescendo, and heard along the left sternal border. It is frequently missed because it is very similar to normal breath sounds. Listening during held expiration improves chances of correctly identifying the murmur.

A **third heart sound** is common. An **Austin-Flint murmur** may be present. This murmur sounds exactly like that of mitral stenosis. Its pathogenesis is incompletely understood but results from interaction between the regurgitant jet and mitral valve inflow.

Significant aortic regurgitation is usually accompanied by a **wide pulse pressure.** This pulse pressure is typically at least 60 mmHg, and the diastolic pressure is typically < 70 mmHg.

12. What are the peripheral pulse findings?

The wide pulse pressure can produce many abnormalities in the peripheral pulses:
> Bifid carotid pulse
> Visible carotid pulsations (Corrigan's pulse)
> Head bobbing (de Musset's sign)

Bobbing of the uvula (Müller's sign)
Femoral artery bruit induced by light pressure over the artery (Duroziez's murmur)
"Pistol shot" sound over the femoral artery (Traube's sound)
Visible pulsations in the nail beds (Quincke's pulses).

13. How are the noninvasive tests useful?

In severe regurgitation, the **electrocardiogram** generally shows left ventricular hypertrophy, and the **chest radiograph** shows cardiomegaly.

Doppler echocardiography can confirm the diagnosis and grade the severity of the regurgitation. Because irreversible left ventricular dysfunction can occur prior to the onset of symptoms, noninvasive tests provide clues to early decompensation, such as a progressive increase in left ventricular end-systolic diameter and decrease in measures of contractility. Thus, serial echocardiography is useful in following patients with severe regurgitation. Some cardiologists find serial radionuclide ventriculography to be useful for the same purpose.

14. What are the causes of aortic regurgitation?

Causes of Aortic Regurgitation

Long-standing hypertension (most common)
Inflammatory disease of the valve and aortic root (rheumatic fever, rheumatoid arthritis, ankylosing spondylitis, tertiary syphilis)
Connective tissue disorders (Marfan's syndrome, Ehlers-Danlos syndrome)
Congenital disease (congenitally malformed aortic valve, prolapse from long-standing ventricular septal defect)
Aortic insufficiency
Torn cusp (blunt chest trauma, dissecting aortic aneurysm, infective endocarditis)

15. What about acute aortic regurgitation?

Unlike chronic aortic regurgitation, acute regurgitation is generally poorly tolerated. Because the ventricle does not have sufficient time to dilate, the volume of blood flowing back into the ventricle produces a dramatic rise in end-diastolic pressure, which in turn produces signs and symptoms of heart failure. Acute aortic regurgitation generally requires early surgical treatment.

BIBLIOGRAPHY

1. Horsttkotte D, Loogen F: The natural history of aortic valve stenosis. Eur Heart J (suppl E):57–64, 1988.
2. Lombard TJ, Selzer A: Valvular aortic stenosis: A clinical and hemodynamic profile of patients. Ann Intern Med 106:292–298, 1987.
3. Ross J: Left ventricular function and the timing of surgical treatment in valvular heart disease. Ann Intern Med 94:498–504, 1981.

44. MITRAL VALVE PROLAPSE AND MITRAL REGURGITATION

Mark Keller, M.D.

1. Describe the mitral valve prolapse syndrome.

Mitral valve prolapse syndrome is an overused diagnosis. It applies to patients who present with an abnormal murmur, an abnormally thickened prolapsing mitral valve, and various clinical symptoms often including chest pain. Unfortunately, this diagnoses is often applied inappropriately to people who present with chest pain without the characteristic physical findings or echocardiographic evidence of mitral valve prolapse.

2. What physical findings are associated with mitral valve prolapse?

A mid-systolic click indicative of prolapse of the valve is the hallmark sign of this disorder. The click is followed immediately by a mid- to late-systolic murmur of mitral regurgitation which occurs once the valve leaflet has prolapsed into the atrium.

3. What maneuvers can be used to increase the murmur and click in mitral valve prolapse?

In general, maneuvers that increase left ventricular filling tend to make prolapse occur later in the cardiac cycle and decrease the intensity of the murmur. Maneuvers that decrease left ventricular filling have the opposite effect; they move the click earlier in systole and increase the murmur intensity. Therefore, a simple test is have the patient **squat.** This increases left ventricular filling and therefore moves the click later in the cycle and decreases the murmur. Then, while listening closely with the stethoscope, have the patient **stand up** from the squatting position. This will decrease left ventricular filling and increase of the murmur intensity while moving the click earlier in the cardiac cycle.

4. What are the echocardiographic findings?

The mitral valve should appear thickened. During systole, the valve leaflets prolapse superiorly into the left atrium. It may be associated with at least mild mitral regurgitation.

5. What symptoms are associated with mitral valve prolapse?

Many patients with mitral valve prolapse are entirely asymptomatic. However, this is such a common disease that it is found in association with many other cardiac disorders. Therefore, patients may present with symptoms attributable to other cardiac disorders and have mitral valve prolapse seen as an incidental diagnosis.

Patients with "classic mitral valve prolapse syndrome" often present with chest pain. The chest pain may not be due to cardiac ischemia, because it is not brought on by exertion and occurs at rest. The pain is often fleeting, sharp, or stabbing in nature. Often the chest pain syndrome is due to anxiety, and the patients are found to have mitral valve prolapse when an echocardiogram is performed.

6. Outline the proper management for patients with mitral valve prolapse.

Asymptomatic patients need no definitive therapy performed. They should undergo routine follow-up on a regular basis, every 6 months to 1 year. Physical examination should assess the mitral regurgitation murmur for worsening.

In **older patients,** there is a tendency for chordae tendineae to rupture and mitral regurgitation to become much worse. Since the valve is abnormal, these patients are also at risk for endocarditis. Therefore, they should be given antibiotic prophylaxis for any dental or urinary tract procedure which will result in bacteremia.

In **patients with palpitations,** a beta blocker is often a useful medication, although this should not be instituted until the arrhythmia has been assessed thoroughly with Holter monitoring or other available means, i.e., stress exercise testing.

7. What are the common causes of mitral regurgitation?

The architecture of the mitral valve is complex and includes the mitral leaflets, chordae tendineae which support the leaflets, the papillary muscles which support the chordae, the mitral valve annulus, and the left ventricular chamber itself. Abnormalities of all or any one of these structures can result in significant mitral regurgitation.

Involvement of the leaflets is seen in disorders such as rheumatic heart disease, systemic lupus erythematosus, infective endocarditis, and mitral valve prolapse syndrome. Regurgitation due to the chordae tendineae most often results from spontaneous rupture of the chordae tendineae. Papillary muscles can also rupture secondary to myocardial infarction. Any disease which results in enlargement of the left ventricle can produce abnormal papillary muscle function and dilation of the annulus, both of which can result in mitral regurgitation.

8. What is the most common physical finding of mitral regurgitation?

The most characteristic feature of mitral regurgitation is the **loud systolic murmur** heard over the apex of the heart. This murmur is holosystolic and commences with the first heart sound and ends with a second heart sound. The murmur generally radiates into the axilla but can often be heard along the spine or, in severe cases, on top of the head. Patients with severe regurgitation, chronic mitral regurgitation, or severely decreased left ventricular function may have a soft murmur.

9. Which maneuvers can be used to change the intensity of the murmur?

Sudden standing or the use of amyl nitrate will decrease afterload and result in the decrease of the murmur.

CONTROVERSY

10. When should patients undergo surgery for mitral regurgitation?

There is controversy as to the best timing for surgery. Patients presenting with acute severe mitral regurgitation are generally critically ill and require urgent surgery. However, in patients with chronic mitral regurgitation, the timing is more uncertain.

In the past, cardiologists recommended waiting until severe symptoms developed before proceeding to surgery. However, waiting often was associated with a bad outcome, and left ventricular function did not respond well to the sudden change in afterload imposed by putting an artificial valve in a patient who had severe regurgitation. Now, many recommend operating as soon as significant symptoms develop. Some, in fact, even recommend that these patients *not* be treated with medication so as not to mask symptoms and that surgery be done as soon as *any* symptom presents.

However, replacement of a native valve with a prosthetic one is not a cure for the patient, but rather a shift to a new set of problems associated with the prosthetic valve. Newer forms of therapy include valve repair with an annular ring and valve reconstruction and appear to provide better and more natural results in patients while avoiding the use of anticoagulant medications. Long-term follow-up of this procedure from multiple surgical sites is not yet available.

BIBLIOGRAPHY

1. Anwar A, Kohn SR, Dunn JF, et al: Altered beta adrenergic receptor function in subjects with symptomatic mitral valve prolapse. Am J Med Sci 302:89–97, 1991.
2. Boudoulas H, Kolibash AJ, Baker P, et al: Mitral valve prolapse and the mitral valve prolapse syndrome. Am Heart J 118:796–818, 1989.
3. Braunwald E: Valvular heart disease. In Braunwald E (ed): Heart Disease, 4th ed. Philadelphia, W.B. Saunders, 1992.

4. Devereux RB, Kramer-Fox R, Kligfield P: Mitral valve prolapse: Causes, clinical manifestations, and management. Ann Intern Med 111:305–317, 1989.
5. Farb A, Tang AL, Atkinson JB, et al: Comparison of cardiac findings in patients with mitral valve prolapse who die suddenly to those who have congestive heart failure from mitral regurgitation to those with fatal noncardiac conditions. Am J Cardiol 70:234–239, 1992.
6. Galloway AC, Colvin SB, Bauman G, et al: Long-term results of mitral valve reconstruction with Carpentier techniques in 148 patients with mitral insufficiency. Circulation 78(Suppl I):I-97–I-105, 1988.
7. Wooley CF, Baker PB, Kolibash AJ, et al. The floppy, myxomatous mitral valve, mitral valve prolapse, and mitral regurgitation. Prog Cardiovasc Dis 33:397–433, 1991.

45. PROSTHETIC VALVES

Norman Krasnow, M.D.

1. When is a mechanical prosthesis preferred over a bioprosthetic valve?

Bioprosthetic valves in the aortic position may not require anticoagulation, whereas mechanical valves always require such therapy. **Bioprosthetic valves** are therefore preferred in patients for whom anticoagulation poses additional risks or problems: young vigorous patients whose occupations or sports activities present risks of trauma, patients who have clotting disorders or bleeding problems (e.g., peptic ulcer disease), and patients who are unable to follow instructions or have appropriate monitoring of clotting factors. **Mechanical prostheses** may be preferred in young patients with expected considerable longevity, those for whom anticoagulation is not difficult to manage, those who may calcify tissue excessively (e.g., patients with renal failure), and those who may have already failed a bioprosthetic implant.

2. Which type of valve has a lower incidence of bacterial endocarditis? Which has a lower overall complication rate?

Bacterial endocarditis (or, more broadly, infective endocarditis to include fungal organisms) occurs in about 1% of valve replacement per year of implant. The incidence is approximately the same for bioprosthetic and mechanical valves. When infection occurs on a bioprosthetic valve, cure with antibotics alone is feasible in many cases, especially when the infection is on the leaflet. When infection is present in mechanical prostheses, the valve ring is always involved, and therefore medical cure is extremely difficult (though not impossible). Surgical therapy is usually required, with valve replacement.

The complication rate is somewhat lower with bioprosthetic valves than mechanical valves, but when the decreased long-term survival of the bioprosthetics is considered, the overall patient survival and requirement for reoperation are about the same for both types.

3. When is replacement indicated for aortic regurgitation in a patient without symptoms?

When congestive heart failure occurs in association with aortic regurgitation, it is generally agreed that surgical valve replacement is the treatment of choice. In patients with definite severe aortic regurgitation but who have no symptoms and may be fully functional, one or more parameters of left ventricular (LV) function are measured, usually be echocardiography, and followed serially. An end-systolic diameter of 5.5 cm has been advocated by some as an upper limit beyond which surgery leads to better functional results and survival. Similarly, a decrease in ejection fraction from normal to borderline (e.g., 45–50%) is also used. The absolute end-diastolic diameter of the LV is a less reliable parameter indicating surgery, though markedly enlarged hearts (e.g., diameters of 8–9 cm by echocardiography) are perhaps less likely to return entirely to normal even if surgery is performed; increasing end-diastolic diameters serve to alert the physician to the need for surgery in the near future.

4. Is Doppler echocardiography accurate in diagnosing prosthetic aortic stenosis?

When bioprosthetic leaflets thicken and calcify, they may become stenotic. Doppler echocardiography may accurately define the pressure gradient in these cases, just as in stenosis of native valves. However, mechanical prostheses have a variety of orifices, depending on the type of valve. In these cases, the spectral Doppler recording may be in significant error, particularly in overestimating the gradient. St. Jude Medical valves, for example, have a narrow central orifice between the two leaflets. The velocity of blood flow through this slit may be very high, leading to a false diagnosis of prosthetic stenosis. When there is doubt about the severity of prosthetic obstruction, transesophageal echocardiography or cardiac catheterization with hemodynamic recording of pressure is extremely helpful.

5. When is valve replacement indicated for aortic stenosis?

When congestive heart failure, angina pectoris, and syncope appear. Usually, the aortic valve area associated with such symptoms is about 0.7 cm^2 or less. Because aortic stenosis occurs most often in older patients, knowledge of the coronary artery anatomy and its contribution to the angina and congestive heart failure is required. Patients with significant aortic stenosis but without symptoms may be followed closely without surgery. Occasionally, severe LV hypertrophy may be present causing LV diastolic dysfunction with symptoms of pulmonary congestion but with well-maintained systolic function; in these cases, surgery is often warranted.

6. How may prosthetic mitral valves be evaluated for stenosis?

When a patient with a prosthetic mitral valve begins to develop new or increased symptoms of pulmonary congestion, the possibility of prosthetic stenosis due to thrombus formation, fibrosis with leaflet restriction, or valve dysfunction must be considered. The appearance of the leaflets, both bioprosthetic and mechanical, on the two-dimensional echocardiographic image is of considerable use, especially if the leaflets are well visualized and are seen to move well. Because such visualization is not always achieved, alternative approaches are necessary. Bioprosthetic valves may be evaluated reasonably well with spectral Doppler recordings. The peak inflow velocity and the pressure half-time of the deceleration phase of inflow may be used to compute a mitral valve area. These parameters are not accurate with mechanical prostheses, although abnormal values may be useful clues to dysfunction. In these cases, transesophageal echocardiograph, hemodynamic study by cardiac catheterization may be needed.

7. When is valve replacement indicated for mitral regurgitation?

When mitral regurgitation is severe (or at least moderate), it may be associated with LV failure and symptoms of dyspnea on exertion, orthopnea, and edema. When LV function is well maintained despite the volume overload causing symptoms, surgical correction is indicated. Depending on the cause of the regurgitation—e.g., rheumatic valvular disease, prolapse, or ruptured chordae tendineae—the surgeon may elect to repair the valve without replacement. Such repair is being done increasingly, as it leads to better preservation of ventricular function. When repair is not possible, valve replacement offers a good alternative.

However, when LV function has already deteriorated due to the chronic volume overload and the ejection fraction is about 30% or less, surgical mortality and late results are less favorable. This is because implanting a competent valve where there was previously a low-resistance regurgitant "shunt" to the left atrium in effect imposes a significant afterload on the ventricle; if function is already poor, it may then decrease further.

Patients who are asymptomatic but have evidence of severe mitral regurgitation pose a difficult problem in the timing of surgery. By analogy with aortic regurgitation, some recommend surgery based on deterioration of echocardiographic parameters of LV size and/or function. Also, evidence of deteriorating right ventricular function and development of pulmonary hypertension are used as guides.

8. How is mitral regurgitation across a prosthetic valve diagnosed?

Valve dehiscence, thrombotic obstruction of leaflets, or endocarditis are among common causes for prosthetic valve dysfunction with regurgitation. Ordinarily, mitral regurgitation may be usefully evaluated by color-flow Doppler and semi-quantitative estimation based on various parameters of the visualized jet. However, prosthetic mitral valves, especially mechanical types, cause severe shadowing artifacts on the color-flow image, leading to significant underestimation of the degree of regurgitation. In these cases, imaging by the transesophageal route eliminates the shadowing artifact, allowing more accurate visualization of the regurgitant jet. Thereafter, angiography is used to define somewhat more quantitatively the degree of regurgitation.

9. Are anticoagulants needed for bioprosthetic mitral valves?

Mechanical mitral prostheses require anticoagulation. Bioprosthetic valves are usually considered to require anticoagulants as well, since most such patients are in atrial fibrillation, have large left atria even if sinus rhythm is maintained, or may have had a systemic embolism. These are all common indications for anticoagulation when a prosthetic valve is in place.

10. How does an apparently normally-functioning mitral prosthesis cause recurrent symptoms?
Implantation of a prosthesis in the mitral annulus sometimes causes the prosthesis to project into the outflow tract of the LV, causing obstruction to outflow. This was more common in the past, when prostheses were larger and bulkier. With modern low-profile valves of various types (e.g., Carpentier-Edwards, St. Jude Medical), the problem is less common but occasionally accounts for failure to improve—either acutely at the time of surgery or postoperatively. Careful Doppler echocardiography can document the presence of a gradient across the outflow tract despite a normal aortic valve and septal thickness.

BIBLIOGRAPHY

1. Baumgartner H, Khan S, DeRobertis M, et al: Discrepancies between Doppler and catheter gradients in aortic prosthetic valves in vitro: A manifestation of localized gradients and pressure recovery. Circulation 82:1467–1475, 1990.
2. Bloomfield P, Wheatley DJ, Prescott RJ, Miller HC: Twelve-year comparison of a Bjork-Shiley mechanical heart valve with porcine bioprostheses. N Engl J Med 324:573–579, 1991.
3. Henry WL, Donow RO, Rosing DR, Epstein SE: Observations on the optimum time for operative interventions for aortic regurgitation: II. Serial echocardiographic evaluation of asymptomatic patients. Circulation 61:484–492, 1980.
4. Kotler MN, Mintz GS, Panidis I, et al: Noninvasive evaluation of normal and abnormal prosthetic valve function. J Am Coll Cardiol 2:151–173, 1983.
5. Ross J. Jr: Left ventricular function and the timing of surgical treatment in valvular heart disease. Ann Intern Med 94(pt I): 498–504, 1981.
6. Schwartz SL, Sherif BL, Pandian NG: Guide to cardiology: Doppler echocardiography. Cardiovasc Rev Rep (Dec):44–63, 1989.
7. Schneider RM, Helfant RH: Timing of surgery in chronic mitral and aortic regurgitation. Cardiovasc Clin 16:361–374, 1986.
8. Siemienczuk D, Greenberg B, Morris C, et al: Chronic aortic insufficiency: Factors associated with progression to aortic valve replacement. Ann Intern Med 110:587–592, 1989.
9. Silverman NA, Levitsky S: Current choices for prosthetic valve replacement. Mod Concepts Cardiovas Dis 52:35–39, 1983.
10. Slater J, Gindea AJ, Freedberg RS, et al: Comparison of cardiac catheterization and Doppler echocardiography in the decision to operate in aortic and mitral valve disease. J Am Coll Cardiol 17:1026–1036, 1991.

VI. Cardiovascular Pharmacology

46. ANTIARRHYTHMIC THERAPY

Olivia V. Adair, M.D.

1. What major clinical trials have influenced the management of arrhythmias?

The Cardiac Arrhythmia Suppression Trial (CAST) and studies of beta blockers have had a major impact on attempts to decrease mortality. CAST tested the hypothesis that pharmacologic suppression or abolition of ventricular ectopy reduces the risk of sudden death and improves survival in patients with recent myocardial infarction and left ventricular dysfunction. The trial was stopped before completion of enrollment because of a more than twofold increase in sudden death and increased mortality in the initially treated group (encainide and flecainide, both class IC drugs, and moricizine, class IB, terminated with no benefit). Although the data may not apply directly to management of all arrhythmias, they certainly strengthen the practice of treating the patient rather than the arrhythmia. Pharmacologic suppression of asymptomatic, unsustained ventricular ectopy in patients with infarction is contraindicated. CAST had an important impact not only on physicians but also on patients because of the extensive television and newspaper coverage; most physicians are cautious, if not reluctant, to use antiarrhythmic agents.

Ongoing studies of beta blockers, amiodarone, and sotalol, both oral and intravenous, and their effect on arrhythmia in postinfarction patients (n=> 20), have shown an average reduction of approximately 20% in mortality rates.

2. What information should be gathered to determine if an arrhythmia is the cause of a patient's symptoms?

1. The first essential element in evaluation of a possible arrhythmia is a good **history.** Of special interest are frequency, duration, mode of onset, and mode of cessation, along with associated symptoms and any history of medications.

2. **Physical examination** focuses on blood pressure, peripheral pulses, jugular venous pulsation, heart auscultation for measurement of gallops and variations of first heart sound, and evidence of cardiomegaly, congestive heart failure, or thyroid dysfunction.

3. **Laboratory tests** should include electrolytes, especially calcium and magnesium; antiarrhythmic level; thyroid function; chest radiography; and EKG with a long rhythm strip.

3. In view of the side effects shown in recent studies, what options remain for management of arrhythmias?

1. No therapy
2. Pharmacologic therapy
3. Electrical therapy
    Direct current conversion
    Implantible cardioversion defibrillator
    Radiofrequency ablation
4. Surgical therapy

4. How should treatment of a patient with an arrhythmia be determined?

The decision to treat a patient with an arrhythmia must be individualized with consideration of

1. **Electrocardiographic analysis of the arrhythmia** with evaluation of atrial and ventricu-

lar activation and atrioventricular conduction pattern; whether the arrhythmia is triggering additional arrhythmias; and whether the arrhythmias are sustained.

2. **Assessment of the clinical setting,** including categorization of arrhythmia as acute or chronic, and as transient, persistent, or recurrent. Anatomic and physiological substrate also should be evaluated.

3. **Defining the goal or endpoint of therapy,** which depends on the evaluations in 1 and 2.

Appropriate diagnostic tools in addition to history, physical examination and routine laboratory tests and electrocardiogram include (1) special leads to identify the P waves (esophageal lead, intraatrial electrode, or Lewis leads), (2) Holter monitoring; (3) echocardiography; (4) exercise testing; (5) tilt table test; (6) signal-averaged electrocardiography, and (7) electrophysiologic studies.

5. Discuss the categories of patients who do not require antiarrhythmic therapy.

Because of the risk of proarrhythmia or exacerbation of preexisting arrhythmia by antiarrhythmia drugs, the trend in the 1970s to suppress ventricular ectopy has diminished. Although controversy still surrounds arrhythmic therapy, in specific circumstances, by general agreement, antiarrhythmia therapy is not indicated:

1. Asymptomatic atrial ectopy and unsustained supraventricular tachycardia (SVT)

2. Asymptomatic ventricular ectopy without runs of ventricular tachycardia (VT)

3. Simple ventricular ectopy in acute myocardial infarction, not associated with hemodynamic compromise

4. Asymptomatic, unsustained VT with no structural heart disease or other risk indicators

5. Asymptomatic Wolff-Parkinson-White (WPW) syndrome without known superventricular tachycardia

6. Mildly symptomatic, simple atrial or ventricular ectopy

6. When should programmed electrical stimulation (PES) be used in the management of a suspected arrhythmia?

PES studies use percutaneous catheter electrodes placed in the atria and ventricle (usually right venous) to record intracardiac electrograms and to evaluate SVT and ventricular arrhythmias, including VT and ventricular fibrillation (VF). The primary indications for PES are (1) to identify the tachycardia and its mechanisms; (2) to select appropriate therapy; and (3) to map the substrate of the arrhythmia for ablation or (rarely) surgical intervention. The rate of complications is small: death, 0.06%; perforation, 0.2%; major hemorrhage, 0.05%; atrial injury, 0.1%; and major venous thrombosis, 0.2%. PES is especially accurate in evaluation of SVT with induction in 90–95% of patients with clinical atroventricular nodal reentrant tachycardia or WPW. Ablation is used after the mechanism is defined, with deliverance of radiofrequency current through the catheter positioned at the site of the pathway.

PES is extensively used in VT evaluation; sustained VT/VF is reproducible in 75% of survivors of sudden cardiac death and 95% of patients with sustained monomorphic VT. The efficacy of antiarrhythmic therapy also can be evaluated with PES; a 10% recurrence rate is expected over 2 years compared with 50% recurrence with no therapy identified.

7. How do PES and Holter monitoring compare in evaluation of antiarrhythmic drug efficacy?

The recent Electrophysiologic Study Versus Electrocardiographic Monitoring (ESVEM) trial examined this question in patients with VT. Holter monitoring predicted efficacy in 77% of cases; PES, in only 45%. In addition Holter monitoring required only about one-half the number of hospital days. Thus PES offers no advantage over Holter monitoring in accurate evaluation of drug efficacy. The negative predictive value of PES is good (approximately 90%), but the positive predictive value is weak (25%). Therefore Holter monitoring may offer an alternative to PES in evaluation of antiarrhythmic agents.

8. Are antiarrhythmic drugs still classified according to their electrophysiologic effects?

The Vaughn Williams classification of antiarrhythmic agents is still used despite multiple attempts to develop more clinically oriented system, based, for example, on channels, pumps, and receptors. The Vaughn Williams system serves as a useful means of communication:

Class 1—local membrane-stabilizing activity; blocks the fast sodium channel

Class 2—blocks the beta-adrenergic receptors

Class 3—prolongs duration of cardiac action potential and repolarization; blocks potassium channels

Class 4—blocks the slow calcium channel.

This classification is based on the repolarization/depolarization curve of the action potential.

9. Should lidocaine be initiated in all patients with acute myocardial infarction (AMI)?

Although some data suggest that lidocaine decreases VF in patients admitted within 6 hours of onset of AMI symptoms, the untreated group had no increased risk of death, and all patients were resuscitated. Likewise, two meta-analyses in over 9,000 patients showed a reduction in primary VF but no benefit in survival, perhaps because the toxic effects of lidocaine produce conduction abnormalities and increased asystole, which negate the benefit of decreased VF.

No evidence suggests that routine or prophylactic use of lidocaine in AMI is beneficial. Use of lidocaine in AMI is recommended (1) for frequent, multiform ventricular ectopy, especially R-on-T phenomenon, or short runs of nonsustained VT; (2) after an episode of VT or VF requiring electrical conversion or after cardiopulmonary resuscitation; and (3) for ventricular ectopy so frequent or so timed that it significantly impairs hemodynamics. Treatment of left ventricular failure is essential in the treatment of arrhythmias in patients with AMI. Ischemia, which also may contribute to ectopy, should be aggressively treated. The possibility of drug-induced VT or hypokalemia should always be considered.

10. When is cardioversion indicated? What are the contraindications?

Immediate cardioversion should be attempted if an arrhythmia causes angina, hypotension, or heart failure. Cardioversion should be attempted with the lowest possible energy level to reduce complications. Major complications are infrequent and success is seen in approximately 90% of recent-onset arrhythmias. Atrial fibrillation, the most commonly cardioverted arrhythmia, requires at least 100 Joules (J) and has a higher rate of systemic emboli if the arrhythmia has a > 3-day duration. Atrial flutter is the easiest rhythm to convert to sinus; it requires low energy (approximately 50 J) but may be converted to atrial fibrillation if too little energy is used (5–10 J); reentrant SVT due to atrioventricular nodal pathways can be converted with 25–100 J. VT can be converted with low energy, but in the presence of hemodynamic compromise, 200 J should be delivered immediately, followed by 360 J if the first attempt is not successful.

Relative contraindications to cardioversion include (1) digoxin toxicity (in emergencies cardioversion should be started with low energy levels and prophylactic lidocaine and energy delivery progressively increased); (2) short repetitive runs of VT; (3) multifocal atrial tachycardia; (4) immediately before or after surgery in patients with stable atrial fibrillation; (5) SVT and hyperthyroidism; and (6) SVT with complete heart block.

11. Amiodarone is frequently used in patients with a history of ventricular tachycardia. Why is it so popular? What are its side effects?

Amiodarone has class-3 activity with prolongation of both refractoriness and duration of cardiac action potential as well as antiarrhythmic, beta-blocker, and vasodilator effects. Many authorities believe that amiodarone is the most effective single agent for many arrhythmias, including SVT and VT. Its ability to prolong survival has been studied in various disease states, such as myocardial infarction and congestive heart failure (CHF). Amiodarone is approved by the Food and Drug Administration (FDA) for treatment of life-threatening ventricular arrhythmias when other drugs are ineffective or not tolerated. Amiodarone is quite effective in many cases of SVT, atrial fibrillation conversion and rate control, atrioventricular nodal reentry, and WPW. Long-term therapy is well tolerated hemodynamically in patients with congestive heart failure (CHF) and severe cardiomyopathies. Two recent controlled trials showed an improvement in longevity among survivors of myocadial infarction. Another study suggests that amiodarone therapy prolongs life in patients with CHF and arrhythmias, but a recent short-term study showed no benefit in patients with CHF and ventricular ectopy. An ongoing study is comparing implantable cardioversion-defibrillators with amiodarone in patients with sudden death syndrome or inducible or spontaneous symptomatic VT/VF. The major disadvantage of amiodarone is adverse reactions, which include the potentially lethal interstitial pneumonitis.

12. Sotalol is a relatively new drug. What are its indications and side effects?
Sotalol is a class 3 drug and an unusual beta blocker that prolongs the action potential and increases its refractoriness. It is effective for many superventricular and ventricular arrhythmias, including sustained inducible VT. In the ESVEM study sotalol was more effective than the other antiarrhythmic drugs evaluated (31% vs. 12%). The major side effects are QT prolongation, which may result in torsade de pointes (2%); proarrhythmic events (4.5% at higher doses of 640 mg/day); and worsening heart failure (3%).

13. Procainamide and quinidine are class 1A agents that used to be popular. Are they still used as much as before?
As a result of the CAST study, class 1 agents have fallen into disfavor. Both procainamide and quinidine are effective against supraventricular or ventricular arrhythmias. Procainamide has a high rate of intolerable side effects; 40% of patients stop the drug in the first 6 months. As a class 1A agent, it prolongs QT and may produce torsade de pointes as well as lupuslike syndrome in 20% of patients; agranulocytosis is another possible side effect. Quinidine has been shown in two meta-analyses to increase mortality compared with untreated patients and with other agents, but it is still one of the most widely used antiarrhythmic agents. Most physicians, however, are cautious and stratify risk to justify antiarrhythmic use as well as individualize therapy.

14. How are implantable cardioverter defribrillators (ICD) used in the treatment of arrhythmias?
Monitoring systems have shown that the principal cause of sudden cardiac death in outpatients is VF with > 80% of deaths due to progression of abrupt-onset VT to VF. The mortality rate of out-of-hospital cardiac arrest is high (> 75%), mainly because of delay in effective therapy. The ICD is able to deliver an initial electrical countershock within 10–20 seconds of arrhythmia onset, a delay in which the potential for reversed arrhythmia approaches 100%. Because of this immediate response, ICDs are the most effective method for aborting sudden death due to life-threatening ventricular arrhythmias. The indications for ICS continue to broaden and change with new technology and more experience. There are basically three categories of patient for which ICDs are indicated:
    1. Survivors of cardiac arrest with documented VF or VT
    2. Patients with drug-refractory, clinical, and inducible sustained VT
    3. Patients without documented sustained ventricular arrhythmias at high risk for future life-threatening arrhythmic events because of inducible arrhythmias at electrophysiologic study.

BIBLIOGRAPHY

1. Echr DS, Liebson PR, Mitchell LB, et al: Mortality and morbidity in patients receiving encainide, flecainide, or placebo. The Cardiac Arrhythmia Suppression Trial, N. Engl J Med 324:781–788, 1991.
2. Jackman WM, Wang XZ, Friday KJ, et al: Catheter ablation of accessory atrioventricular pathways (Wolff-Parkinson-White syndrome) by radiofrequency current. N Engl J Med 324:1605–1611, 1991.
3. Lau C, Camm AJ: Rate-responsive pacing: technical and clinical aspects. In El-Sherif N, Samet P, (eds): Cardiac Pacing and Electrophysiology. Philadelphia, W. B. Saunders. 1991, pp. 534–544.
4. Opie LH: In Drugs of the Heart, 3rd ed. Philadelphia, W.B. Saunders, 1991.

5. Myerburg RJ, Kessler KM, Castellanos A: Recognition, clinical assessment, and management of arrhythmias and conduction disturbances. In Schlant RC, Alexander RW (eds): The Heart Arteries and Veins, 8th ed. New York, McGraw-Hill, 1994, pp 705–758.
6. Richards DA, Byth K, Ross DL, Uther JB: What is the best predictor of spontaneous ventricular tachycardia and sudden death after myocardial infarction? Circulation 83:756–763, 1991.
7. Wilber DJ, Olshansky B, Moran JF, Scanlon PJ: Electrophysiological testing and nonsustained ventricular tachycardia. Use and limitations in patients with coronary artery disease and impaired ventricular function. Circulation 82:350–358, 1990.
8. Woosley RL: Antiarrhythmic Drugs. In Schlant RC, Alexander RW (eds): The Heart Arteries and Veins, 8th ed. New York, McGraw-Hill, 1994, pp. 775–805.
9. Zee-Cheng CS, Kouchoukos NT, Connors JP, Ruffy R: Treatment of life-threatening ventricular arrhythmias with nonguided surgery supported by electrophysiologic testing and drug therapy. J Am Coll Cardiol 13:153–162, 1989.

47. BETA-ADRENERGIC RECEPTOR BLOCKERS

John T. Madonna, M.D., Mark E. Dorogy, M.D., and Richard C. Davis, M.D., Ph.D.

1. Name some of the beta-adrenergic receptor blockers (beta blockers) and their important pharmacologic properties.
See table on facing page.

2. What are the mechanisms of action of beta blockers?
Beta blockers are competitive antagonists of beta-adrenergic receptors. There are two receptor classes. **Beta-1 receptors,** located in the heart, lead to increases in heart rate, contractility, and antrioventricular conduction when stimulated. Blockade of beta-1 receptors attenuates these increases, particularly during exercise or stress, but also during rest if resting adrenergic tone is increased. Several beta blockers produce low-level receptor stimulation, offsetting the effects of receptors blockade in the resting state while maintaining antagonism during exercise or stress—this is referred to as **intrinsic sympathomimetic activity** (ISA).

Beta-2 receptors are more widespread than beta-1 receptors. Activation of these receptors results in such diverse actions as bronchodilation, peripheral vasodilation, and lipolysis. Many adverse effects of beta blockers, such as bronchospasm, are due to beta-2 receptor blockade. Agents that are beta-1 specific, or **cardioselective,** have been developed to minimize these adverse effects. This preferential blockade is not complete however, and some beta-2 receptor antagonism can be observed at standard pharmacologic doses.

3. What are the cardiovascular indications for beta-blocker therapy other than hypertension and angina pectoris?

Acute myocardial infarction	Hypertrophic cardiomyopathy
Postinfarction	Mitral valve prolapse
Supraventricular arrhythmias	Prolonged QT syndrome
Ventricular arrhythmias	Heart failure
Aortic dissection	Digitalis-induced ventricular arrhythmius

4. When is the use of beta blockers contraindicated?

Contraindications	**Relative contraindications**
Hypotension	Bradydysrhythmias
Asthma	Atrioventricular conduction disturbances
Chronic obstructive pulmonary disease	Congestive heart failure (LV systolic function)
	Raynaud's phenomenon

5. What are the signs and symptoms of beta-blocker toxicity? How is this best treated?
Beta-blocker toxicity, although rare, should be considered in any patient experiencing the sudden onset of bradycardia and hypotension. Generalized seizures can also occur, especially with use of agents that are both lipophilic and have membrane-stabilizing effects. Other reported symptoms include peripheral cyanosis and coma. A history of hypertension, coronary artery disease, or chronic beta-blocker therapy should heighten the suspicion for this diagnosis.

Glucagon is the most effective agent for treating the hemodynamic disturbances due to beta-blockers; epinephrine should be considered second-line therapy, and atropine and isoproterenol are frequently ineffective. Glucagon exerts both positive inotropic and chronotropic effects on the heart. The inotropic effects are not affected by beta blockade, but the increase in heart rate with glucagon may be blunted by beta blockade, and temporary transvenous pacing may be necessary. The initial dose of glucagon is 3 mg or 0.05 mg/kg given intravenously over 30 seconds followed by a continuous infusion at 5 mg/hr or 0.07 mg/kg/hr. The infusion is tapered slowly as the patient improves.

Pharmacologic Properties of Commonly Used Beta Blockers

	AVERAGE DAILY DOSE (mg)	CARDIOSELECTIVITY	LIPID SOLUBILITY	ISA*	MEMBRANE-STABILIZING ACTIVITY
Acebutolol	400–1200	Yes	Moderate	Yes	Yes
Atenolol	50–200	Yes	Weak	No	No
Esmolol	50–150†	Yes	Weak	No	No
Labetalol	400–800	No	Weak	Possible	No
Metoprolol	100–200	Yes	Moderate	No	No
Nadolol	40–80	No	Weak	No	No
Pindolol	5–30	No	Moderate	Yes	Yes
Propranolol	40–160	No	High	No	Yes
Sotalol	80–320	No	Weak	No	No

*Intrinsic sympathomimetic activity.
†Dose in μg/kg/min, parenteral.

6. How is beta-blocker therapy used following myocardial infarction?
Beta blockers decrease the risk of death in approximately 20% of patients following myocardial infarction. This benefit is due almost entirely to a reduction in cardiovascular deaths, both sudden and nonsudden, and is independent of the timing of drug administration. Administration of beta-blocker therapy within hours after infarction provides the additional benefits of limiting infarct size and reducing the risks of nonfatal reinfarction and recurrent ischemia.

The advantages of long-term therapy may be diminished in low-risk subgroups, but data are lacking on which patients can forgo therapy. For example, a 45-year-old man presenting with his first myocardial infarction who has been treated successfully with thrombolytics, has a normal ejection fraction, inferior location, and single-vessel coronary disease is at low risk and may not benefit from long-term beta-blockade. Characteristics of postinfarction survivors likely to receive maximum benefit from long-term administration include:

Impaired LV function

Persistent ischemia (angina, abnormal postinfarction stress test, significant coronary disease supplying viable myocardium)

Complex ventricular ectopy

Coexisting illness treatable with beta blockade (hypertension, supraventricular tachycardia, anxiety, etc.)

7. A 19-year-old woman is referred for recurrent fainting spells. A head-up tilt test elicits hypotension and bradycardia, and her symptoms are reproducible. Why might beta-blocker therapy be appropriate?
Neurocardiogenic syncope (common faint) is often a cause of temporary loss of consciousness in young people. Syncope follows profound vasodilatation, bradycardia, or a combination of these responses. It seems paradoxical that beta blockers would be effective in treating this disorder. It is postulated that in response to a diminished venous return to the heart, such as from prolonged standing, adrenergic tone is enhanced. This results in vigorous myocardial contraction, which stimulates intramyocardial mechanoreceptors (C fibers). Activation of these fibers may override the normal baroreceptor-mediated reflex and produce bradycardia and vasodilatation, which leads to hypotension and syncope. The negative inotropic effects of beta blockers may diminish C-fiber activation, allowing normal reflex physiology to prevail. A follow-up tilt test on therapy in this patient should be attempted to reproduce her symptoms and ensure the effectiveness of therapy.

8. Beta blockers have demonstrated efficacy in treating *what* ventricular arrhythmias?
Beta blockers are effective in preventing ventricular fibrillation during acute myocardial infarction and sudden cardiac death in the postinfarction period, in treating digitalis-induced ventricular arrhythmias, suppressing torsade de pointes in the long QT syndrome, treating exercise-induced ventricular tachycardia, and suppressing premature ventricular contractions and complex ventricular ectopy. Some recent studies suggest they may be as effective as sole agents in selected patients with sustained ventricular tachycardia or primary ventricular fibrillation.

9. A middle-aged woman with long-standing hypertension is currently on an antihypertensive regimen of clonidine and propranolol. She complains of symptoms referable to the clonidine. What special considerations are needed before you withdraw clonidine?
Rapid withdrawal of clonidine can provoke a **hypertensive rebound** thought secondary to increased catecholamine release. Concurrent beta blocker use may greatly enhance the hypertension as a result of unopposed alpha-adrenergic receptor stimulation. A prolonged clonidine taper or withdrawal of the beta blocker prior to tapering should be considered.

10. A 39-year-old man with hypertension presents to the emergency room with resting chest pressure and a 4-mm ST-segment elevation in the inferior leads on ECG. Both the chest pressure and ECG changes are relieved by nitroglycerin. Cardiac catheterization demonstrates normal coronary arteries, and spasm of the right coronary artery is subsequently

provoked with ergonovine. He currently takes nadolol and a diurectic for hypertension. How should his medical regimen be altered?

This presentation is typical of coronary vasospasm (Prinzmetal's angina). Use of a beta blocker in this disorder has been associated with increased frequency and severity of angina. Discontinuation of the beta blocker and initiation of a calcium channel blocker or nitrate are recommended. When coronary vasospasm occurs in the setting of obstructive coronary disease, beta-blocker administration may be desirable in combination with a calcium channel blocker.

11. A 43-year-old man, referred for management of severe hypertension, was found at the initial visit to have a blood pressure of 190/120 mmHg and tachycardia. He has been followed by a local psychiatrist for several years for episodic anxiety with recurrent spells of apprehension, diaphoresis, nausea, and headache. Antihypertension therapy with a beta blocker was begun. Several days later he returned with pulmonary edema, confusion, and a blood pressure of 260/140 mmHg. What is the most likely diagnosis? Could the accelerated hypertension be related to beta blocker therapy?

This is a classic presentation of pheochromocytoma. Precipitation of the hypertension crisis is directly related to initiating beta blockade. The resultant unopposed α-adrenergic stimulation may cause intense peripheral vasoconstriction. While beta blockers may be beneficial in treating this disorder, they should be withheld until alpha-blocker therapy is started. The diagnosis of pheochromocytoma, although not established definitively in this example, should be suspected and beta-blocker therapy avoided until the appropriate diagnostic tests are performed.

12. A 29-year-old woman with a history of mitral valve prolapse complains of palpitations and light-headedness. A rhythm strip taken during her symptoms is shown below. Would beta blockers be effective in treating this disorder?

Yes. This case is an example of an atrioventricular (AV) nodal reentrant tachycardia. Beta blockers interrupt the reentrant circuit by prolonging AV nodal refractoriness and conduction and provide effective treatment and prevention of this arrhythmia. Beta blockers also are effective in treating other supraventricular arrhythmias, including sinoatrial reentrant tachycardia, AV reciprocating tachycardia, and atrial fibrillation and flutter.

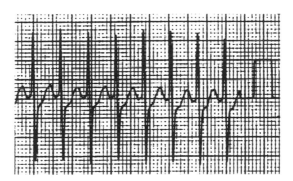

13. What is the proposed mechanism of action for beta blockers in the treatment of heart failure?

Increased adrenergic activity in patients with congestive heart failure can downregulate cardiac beta-adrenergic receptors and cause peripheral vasoconstriction. Beta blockers can attenuate these deleterious effects of chronic catecholamine stimulation. Clinically, this has translated into improvements in hemodynamics, symptoms, exercise tolerance, and left ventricular function. Beta blockers, however, have not been shown to decrease mortality in this setting.

14. In patients with left ventricular (LV) hypertrophy induced by hypertension, do beta blockers reduce LV mass? How do they compare with other agents?
Beta blockers have been shown to cause regression of LV mass in hypertensive patients with LV hypertrophy. In a meta-analysis, LV mass was reduced an average of 8%, as compared to 15% for angiotensin-converting enzyme (ACE) inhibitors, and 8.5% for calcium channel blockers. Diuretics decreased LV mass an average of 11.3%, but this was attributed to a reduction in LV volume and not reversal of wall hypertrophy as seen with the other drug classes.

15. A hypertensive patient presents with an acute aortic dissection. What would proper emergency management include?
While immediate lowering of blood pressure is essential acute therapy for aortic dissection, initial use of nitroprusside may increase the force and velocity (dP/dT) of ventricular contraction, which may increase aortic shear forces and accelerate the propagation of the dissection. By reducing dP/dT, beta blockers decrease aortic shear forces and allow safer introduction of nitroprusside. Labetalol, with its combined beta- and alpha-adrenergic blockade, can be administered intravenously and is a single agent alternative to the more traditional therapy.

The opinions and assertions contained herein are the private views of the authors and are not to be construed as official or reflecting the views of the Department of the Army or Department of Defense.

BIBLIOGRAPHY

 1. Dahlof B, Pennert K, Hansson L: Reversal of left ventricular hypertrophy in hypertensive patients: A metaanalysis of 109 treatment studies. Am J Hypertens 5:95–110, 1992.
 2. Eagle KA, DeSanctis RW: Diseases of the aorta. In Braunwald E (ed): Heart Disease: A Textbook of Cardiovascular Medicine, 4th ed. Philadelphia, W.B. Saunders, 1992, pp 1535–1543.
 3. Engelmeier RS, O'Connel JB, Walsh R, et al: Improvement in symptoms and exercise tolerance by metoprolol in patients with dilated cardiomyopathy: A double-blind, randomized, placebo-controlled trial. Circulation 72:536–546, 1985.
 4. Frishman WH: Beta-adrenergic blockers. Med Clin North Am 72:37–81, 1988.
 6. Frishman WH, Furberg CD, Friedwald WT: Beta adrenergic blockade for survivors of acute myocardial infarction. N Engl J Med 310:830–837, 1984.
 7. Heilbrunn SM, Shah P, Bristow MR, et al: Increased beta-receptor density and improved hemodynamic response to catecholamine stimulation during long-term metoprolol therapy in heart failure from dilated cardiomyopathy. Circulation 79:483–490, 1989.
 8. Kowey PR, Friehling TD, Marinchak RA: Electrophysiology of beta blockers in supraventricular arrhythmias. Am J Cardiol 60:32D–38D, 1987.
 9. Landsberg L, Young JB: Pheochromocytoma. In Wilson JD, Braunwald E, Isselbacher KJ, (eds): Harrison's Principles of Internal Medicine, 12th ed. New York, McGraw-Hill, 1991, pp 1735–1739.
10. Sra JS, Anderson AJ, Sheikh SH, et al: Unexplained syncope evaluated by electrophysiologic studies and head-up tilt testing. Ann Intern Med 114:1013–1019, 1991.
11. Steinbeck G, Andresen D, Bach P, et al: A comparison of electrophysiologically guided antiarrhythmic drug therapy with beta-blocker therapy in patients with symptomatic, sustained ventricular tachyarrhythmias. N Engl J Med 327:987–992, 1992.
12. TIMI Study Group: Comparison of invasive and conservative strategies after treatment with intravenous tissue plasminogen activator in acute myocardial infarction: Results of the thrombolysis in myocardial infarction (TIMI) phase II trial. N Engl J Med 320:618–627, 1989.
13. Weinstein RS: Recognition and management of poisoning with beta-adrenergic blocking agents. Ann Emerg Med 13:1123–1131, 1984.

48. ANTICOAGULANT AND ANTIPLATELET DRUGS

Madeline Jean White, M.D.

1. What anticoagulant and antiplatelet agents are commonly used in cardiology?

The main anticoagulants used are warfarin, given orally, and heparin, given intravenously or subcutaneously. The antiplatelet drug used in the most recent clinical trials is aspirin.

2. How does warfarin work?

The synthesis of several clotting factors (prothrombin, factors VII, IX, and X) depends on the availability of the hydroquinone form of vitamin K for the final carboxylation. Without carboxylation, the factors are biologically inactive. Warfarin is able to inhibit enzymes in the recycling process of vitamin K, thereby decreasing levels of the required hydroquinone form. The anticoagulant effect of warfarin results from the decline and depletion of carboxylated clotting factors. Because synthesis and clearance play a role, it takes 4–5 days to achieve a therapeutic level, in contrast to heparin's instantaneous effect.

3. What is the INR value?

In the past, warfarin therapy was monitored with the prothrombin time (PT). Problems with standardization of anticoagulant intensity arose because the thromboplastin used in the PT test varied among batches in its ability to facilitate coagulation. Now, commercial producers assign each lot an ISI (International Sensitivity Index) which relates the preparation's activity to that of an international reference thromboplastin. Individual laboratories then calculate an INR value (International Normalized Ratio) to relate the patient's PT to the intensity of actual anticoagulation:

$$INR = \left(\frac{Patient\ PT}{Mean\ Normal\ PT} \right)^{ISI}$$

Results are reported with both the PT (in seconds) and INR value. The INR is variable in the initial stages of treatment and is most useful once stable dosing is achieved.

4. Which factor level drops the fastest with warfarin therapy?

Factor VII has the shortest half-life (6 hrs) and falls the fastest. Factors X and IX have half-lives of about 24 hours. Thus, the PT/INR may prolong before all the critical clotting factors have fallen and before full anticoagulation is achieved.

5. List the guidelines for starting and following warfarin therapy.

Many indications for chronic anticoagulation are being developed. Maintain sanity by sticking with a few rules:

    1. Start with 5 mg orally each day.

    2. Large loading doses are not recommended. Use 10 mg for 1–2 days if there is some urgency.

    3. Check the PT/INR daily until a therapeutic level is reached for that clinical setting.

    4. After 4–6 days, the dosage may need adjusting as the individual's sensitivity to warfarin is established.

    5. Monitor the PT/INR twice weekly for 2 weeks, then weekly for 2 months.

    6. Once the dose is stable, check the PT/INR every 4–6 weeks.

    7. Never go > 8 weeks for a PT/INR check with therapeutic doses. Many factors can influence the anticoagulant intensity and increase the risk of bleeding unpredictably.

8. For patient convenience, if the patient needs < 1 tablet on a given day of the week, make it 1/2 or 0 tablets, not 1/4.

9. If the patient is on dose "*x*" on certain days of the week and dose "*y*" on the rest, always use dose "*x*" on the same days. For example:

Dose "*x* mg" once a week—Monday

Dose "*x* mg" twice a week—Monday and Friday

Dose "*x* mg" three times a week—Monday, Wednesday, and Friday

10. To make adjustments, look at the total weekly warfarin dose. Go up or down by 1/7 of the total weekly dose distributed over the week. For example, if the week's dose will be decreased by 1 tablet, reduce the dose on Mondays and Fridays by 1/2 tablet rather than eliminate 1 tablet on Mondays.

11. If the dose is adjusted, check the PT/INR at 2–3 weeks depending on the magnitude of the change.

6. How do you avoid the possible development of relative protein C deficiency?

Because protein C, a clot inhibitor protein, has a short half-life, a relative deficiency can result on the first few days of warfarin use. Most warfarin is started concurrently with intravenous heparin, so the concern for relative protein C deficiency is addressed. If the use of warfarin is planned without full heparin anticoagulation (i.e., in atrial fibrillation), the first 5–7 days should be covered with subcutaneous heparin.

7. List some drugs that alter the PT.

Drugs that Alter Prothrombin Time by Interacting with Warfarin

PHARMACOKINETIC (Drugs that change warfarin levels)	PHARMACODYNAMIC (Drugs that do not change warfarin levels)	MECHANISM UNKNOWN (Drugs whose effect on warfarin levels is unknown)
Prolongs prothrombin time	**Prolongs prothrombin time**	**Prolongs prothrombin time**
Stereoselective inhibition of *S* isomer clearance*	Inhibits cyclic interconversion of vitamin K (2nd- and 3rd-generation cephalosporins)	Evidence for interaction convincing
Phenylbutazone		Erythromycin
Metronidazole	Other mechanisms	Anabolic steroids
Sulfinpyrazone	Clofibrate	Evidence for interaction less
Trimethoprim-sulfamethoxazole	Inhibits blood coagulation	convincing
Disulfiram	Heparin	Ketoconazole
Stereoselective inhibition of *R* isomer clearance	Increases metabolism of coagulation factors	Fluconazole
Cimetidine†	Thyroxine	Isoniazid
Omeprazole†		Piroxicam
Nonstereoselective inhibitions of *R* and *S* isomers clearance		Tamoxifen
Amiodarone		Quinidine
		Vitamin E (megadose)
		Phenytoin
Reduces prothrombin time	**Inhibits platelet function**	**Reduces prothrombin time**
Reduces absorption	Aspirin	Penicillins
Cholestyramine	Other nonsteroidal anti-inflammatory drugs	Griseofulvin‡
Increases metabolic clearance	Ticlopidine	
Barbiturates	Moxalactam	
Rifampin	Carbenicillin and high doses of other penicillins	
Griseofulvin		
Carbamazepine		

*Warfarin is a racemic mixture of *S* and *R* isomers, which have different metabolisms.

†Causes minimal prolongation of the prothrombin time.

‡May cause increased metabolic clearance.

Adapted from Hirsh J: Oral anticoagulant drugs. N Engl J Med 324:1865, 1991.

8. What clinical conditions can alter warfarin effects?

High vitamin K intake with diets rich in green vegetables or food supplements can antagonize warfarin's action. Situations that decrease vitamin K availability, such as fat malabsorption and starvation, can enhance the drug's effect. Increased catabolism with fever or hyperthyroidism causes increased clearance of clotting factors, and hepatic dysfunction can reduce synthesis—both of these situations increase sensitivity to warfarin.

9. What are the recommended INR ranges?

Once the PT/INR has reached therapeutic levels for a specific clinical situation, the dose of warfarin should be adjusted to keep within the INR ranges recommended. For most conditions of anticoagulation, INR values of 2.0–3.0 are adequate. High-risk situations may call for greater intensity:

INR 3.0–4.5:

Mechanical mitral valve prosthesis,

Systemic embolization at less intensive levels of anticoagulation

Following acute myocardial infarction when aspirin is contraindicated.

INR 2.5–3.5:

Mechanical valves other than mitral.

If aspirin can be used at 100 mg/day, an INR of 2.0–3.0 may be as effective as the higher intensities.

10. How long should anticoagulation be maintained?

In situations in which the risk of embolization is **chronic,** such as mechanical valves, atrial fibrillation, dilated cardiomyopathy with heart failure, and recurrent deep venous thrombosis, anticoagulation should be lifelong unless contraindications exist.

Duration after **acute events** (pulmonary embolism, deep venous thrombosis, acute anterior myocardial infarction) is controversial, but most clinicians maintain therapy for 4–6 months. **Prophylactic** use usually covers just the period of risk.

11. What factors increase the risk of bleeding during warfarin therapy?

a. **Intensity of dose:** INR values > 3.0 have increased risk.

b. **Age:** Risk rises with increased age, but some find age *not* to be an independent risk factor.

c. **Duration of therapy:** The risk of bleeding is highest in the first several weeks of therapy: 3% risk in the first month, 0.8% risk per month in the first year, and 0.3% risk monthly for subsequent years. Cumulative risk increases with the duration of therapy.

d. **Comorbid conditions:** Cerebrovascular, renal, heart, and liver disease are associated with more bleeding complications.

e. **Concurrent medications:** Some drugs can predictably alter the PT/INR, but variability is the norm. When adding any new chronic medication, increase monitoring of PT/INR until a stable state is achieved.

f. **Compliance:** Safe, effective, outpatient warfarin use demands regular monitoring and systematic dose adjustments. Patient compliance is critical.

12. How does heparin work?

Heparin is a highly sulfated, natural glycosaminoglycan. Commercial preparations are derived from porcine intestine or bovine lung. Its anticoagulant affect is mediated through antithrombin III, which has a native ability to inhibit thrombin, activated Factor X (Xa), and activated Factor IX (IXa). Once heparin binds to antithrombin III, this inhibition is increased up to 1000 times. Anticoagulation is almost instantaneous.

13. Before starting therapy with heparin, what baseline tests should you obtain?

Hematocrit, platelet count, activated partial thromboplastin time (aPTT), and prothrombin time (PT—with INR). The aPTT serves as a baseline value to gauge the therapeutic dose of heparin;

the PT/INR is the baseline for anticipated warfarin therapy. The hematocrit and platelet count provide pretreatment values if complications arise.

14. How do you achieve and monitor the therapeutic level of heparin?
Heparin therapy is very empirical, and there are many patterns for initiating and monitoring it. Most clinicians give an **intravenous** bolus of 5000 U (or 80 U/kg), then start a continuous infusion of 1000 U/hr (or 18 U/kg/hr). The aPTT is checked at 4–6 hours. If it is not within the goal of 1.5–2.5 times baseline, the rate is adjusted up or down (100–200 U/hr). Minimally prolonged aPTT may require a re-bolus of 5000 U. If the aPTT is markedly prolonged, the infusion is held for 1 hour and then a reduced rate resumed. The aPTT is rechecked at 4–6 hours.

The body-weight dosing schedule reaches the therapeutic threshold (aPTT 1.5 times control) in more cases (90 % vs. 77%) than the standard dosing schedule. In life-threatening situations, achieving a therapeutic level promptly is very important. With interpatient variability, the clinician must be alert and *not* assume that the dose selected is correct without laboratory confirmation. Once an adequate rate is achieved, the aPTT should be checked each day.

Brill-Edwards et al. have pointed out a considerable variation among aPTT reagents. A therapeutic range using protamine titrated heparin levels of 0.2–0.4 U/ml would be more accurate than relying on prolongation of aPTT vs control.

Subcutaneous heparin, used prophylactically is started at 5000 U every 8–12 hours. It is not monitored because therapeutic goals are achieved at levels that may not prolong the aPTT.

15. What are the complications of heparin therapy?
In any anticoagulant therapy, the major risk is bleeding. Estimates range from 0.8% per day to about 5% overall in recent surveys. Dose seems to be the most important factor, hence the vigilance regarding the aPTT. Bleeding risk also increases with intermittent subcutaneous use, duration of therapy, and concurrent use of aspirin and thrombolytic agents.

Heparin can cause mild or severe **thrombocytopenia.** The mild form is due to heparin-induced platelet aggregation and occurs after 2 days to 2 weeks of full-dose heparin in about 15–25% of cases. The platelet counts usually stabilize above 100,000/μl, even with continued heparin therapy. In the severe form, immune mechanisms cause a marked fall in platelet count (< 50,000/μl) and arterial thrombi can occur. Bovine-derived heparin is more commonly involved than the porcine product. Platelet counts should be checked daily; if they drop below 100,000, heparin should be discontinued. Switching from bovine to porcine heparin, adding antiplatelet drugs, or using the new low molecular weight heparin may be options.

At 5–10 days of therapy, transient abnormalities of **liver function** tests can occur. Rarely, anaphylaxis, skin necrosis, local urticaria, or hyperkalemia is seen. Long-term heparin use can cause osteoporosis.

16. What are some contraindications to heparin therapy?
Contraindications
    Severe active bleeding
    Allergic reactions
    Heparin-induced thrombocytopenia and thrombosis
Relative contraindications
    Central nervous system hemorrhage
    Intracranial metastases
    Severe hypertension
    Retinopathy
    Pericarditis
    Endocarditis
    Recent surgery
    Trauma

17. Is heparin "resistance" real?
Massive pulmonary embolism can be associated with increased clearance of heparin, giving a picture of relative resistance. Antithrombin III, which is required for heparin's action, can be the key to heparin "resistance." Congenital antithrombin III deficiencies usually reduce antithrombin III levels to 40–60%, sufficient for anticoagulation with heparin. In acquired deficiencies from hepatic cirrhosis, nephrotic syndrome, or disseminated intravascular coagulation, antithrombin III levels can fall to lower levels (< 25%), where heparin activity is impaired.

18. If long-term anticoagulation is anticipated, how do you combine heparin and warfarin?
Start warfarin on day 1 of heparin therapy. This allows depletion of vitamin K–dependent factors while the patient is fully anticoagulated with heparin. After 5–6 days of heparin and with at least 2 days of a therapeutic PT/INR, heparin can be discontinued. A minor decrease in PT/INR may be seen as the heparin effect wanes.

19. How does aspirin work?
Aspirin acetylates platelet cyclo-oxygenase irreversibly, thereby inhibiting the formation of thromboxane A_2. Platelet reactivity is diminished. Aspirin also inhibits the endothelium's production of prostaglandin I_2, which decreases platelet aggregation and induces vasodilatation.

20. Are any baseline studies needed before starting aspirin therapy?
A good history is needed to evaluate possible allergies, ulcer tendencies, coagulation disorders, and medication interactions. Risk/benefit issues guide the clinician's decision regarding use, dose, and enteric coating. Specific laboratory tests are not routinely needed.

21. Should the effect of aspirin therapy be monitored?
No. Clinical trials have used outcomes (morbidity and mortality) to evaluate aspirin's benefit in populations. Platelet function texts are not followed in the individual patient.

BIBLIOGRAPHY

1. Brill-Edwards P, Ginsberg JS, Johnston M, Hirsh J: Establishing a therapeutic range for heparin therapy. Ann Intern Med 119:104, 1993.
2. Dalen JE, Hirsh J (eds): Third ACCP consensus conference on anti-thrombotic therapy. Chest 102 (Suppl):303S, 1992.
3. Goodnight SH, Coull BM, McAnulty JH, Taylor LM: Anti-platelet therapy: Parts I and II. West J Med 158:385, 506, 1993.
4. Hirsh J: Oral anticoagulant drugs. N Engl J Med 324:1865, 1991.
5. Hirsh J, Dalen JE, Deykin D, Poller L: Oral anticoagulants: Mechanism of action, clinical effectiveness, and optimal therapeutic range. Chest 102:312S, 1992.
6. Hirsh J, Dalen JE, Deykin D, Poller L: Heparin: Mechanisms of action, pharmacokinetics, dosing considerations, monitoring, efficacy, and safety. Chest 102:337S, 1992.
7. Hirsh J, Dalen JE, Fuster V, et al: Aspirin and other platelet-active drugs: The relationship between dose, effectiveness, and side effects. Chest 102:327S, 1992.
8. Hoffman R, Benz EJ, Shattil SJ, et al (eds): Hematology: Basic Principles and Practice. New York, Churchill Livingstone, 1991.
9. Kearon C, Hirsh J: Optimal dose for starting and maintaining low dose aspirin. Arch Intern Med 153:700, 1993.
10. Landenfeld CS, Beyth RJ: Anticoagulant related bleeding: Clinical epidemiology, prediction, and prevention. Am J Med 95:315, 1993.
11. Landefeld CS, Rosenblatt MW: Major bleeding in out-patients treated with warfarin: Incidence and prediction by factors known at the start of out-patient therapy. Am J Med 87:144, 1989.
12. Levine MN, Hirsh J, Landefeld S, Raskob G: Hemorrhagic complications of anticoagulant treatment. Chest 102:352S, 1992.
13. Raschke RA, Reilly BM, Guidry JR, et al: The weight-based heparin dosing nomogram compared with a "standard care" nomogram. Ann Intern Med 119:874, 1993.
14. Reilly BM, Raschke R, Srinivas S, Neiman T: Intravenous heparin dosing: Patterns and variations in internists' practices. J Gen Intern Med 8:536, 1993.

49. DIURETICS AND NITRATES

Jennifer L. Calagan, M.D., David T. Schachter, M.D., Mitchel Kruger, M.D.,
and Robert W. Cameron, M.D.

1. Discuss the mechanism of action of the five groups of diuretics?
All diuretics interfere with sodium chloride resorption, but each class of diuretics has a distinct
site of action in the nephron. The site of inhibition of sodium chloride resorption partially dictates
the efficacy and side effects of each drug class.

Mechanism of Action of the Diuretics

CLASS	DRUGS	SITE OF ACTION
Thiazide diuretics	Hydorchlorothiazide Indapamide Chlorthalidone	Cortical thick ascending loop of Henle Cortical diluting segment
Loop diuretics	Furoscmide Bumetanide Ethacrynic acid	Medullary and cortical portions of the thick ascending limb of loop of Henle
Osmotic diuretics	Mannitol	Proximal tubule Loop of Henle Distal tubule Collecting tubule
Potassium sparing diuretics	Spironolactone Triamterene Amiloride	Distal tubule
Carbonic anhydrase inhibitors	Acetazolamide	Proximal tubule

**2. A patient presented to the emergency department with pulmonary edema and was
treated with intravenous furosemide and oxygen, with clinical improvement. The pulmonary congestive symptoms were alleviated without a significant increase in urine output.
Can you explain why this patient improved?**
This early effect of furosemide is believed to be due to direct pulmonary venous dilation. It may
also redistribute pulmonary blood flow away from fluid-filled alveoli to well-aerated alveoli. This
improves blood oxygen saturation and alleviates symptoms of congestive heart failure. Taken
orally, furosemide has an onset of action within 1 hour, and its diuretic effect lasts for 6–8 hours.
Administered intravenously, it has a diuretic effect beginning within minutes and lasting
approximately 2 hours.

3. What are some adverse metabolic effects of diuretics?
Thiazide and loop diuretics cause **hyperglycemia.** The exact mechanism is unknown, but two
theories are proposed. One states that diuretic-induced hypokalemia impairs insulin release from
the pancreas. Correction of hypokalemia in some patients improves carbohydrate tolerance. The
other theory is that diuretics cause peripheral insulin resistance. This may explain why serum
insulin levels are increased in patients taking diuretics.

Diuretics elevate serum **cholesterol** and **triglycerides.** The mechanism for this is also
unknown. The elevation is mild and can be overcome by maintaining a diet low in saturated fat
and cholesterol. α-Antagonists such as prazosin appear to block or reverse the hyperlipidemic
effects of thiazides.

All diuretics cause **hyperuricemia** by inhibition of the organic acid secretory pathway in the
proximal tubule and by enhanced resorption of uric acid in the proximal and distal tubules.

4. Do diuretics have an effect on calcium excretion?

Yes. Thiazide diuretics increase serum calcium concentrations by promoting tubular resorption of calcium. They are contraindicated in acute hypercalcemic states. Thiazides are useful in preventing calcium-containing renal calculi or urolithiasis since they diminish the calcium concentration of urine. Thiazides may cause hypercalcemia in patients with renal insufficiency who take calcium-containing medications or vitamin D.

5. What complications of diuretic use are potentially life-threatening?

The thiazide diuretics and loop diuretics can cause **pancreatitis.** With loop diuretics, the mechanism is unknown but may involve excessive pancreatic secretion because of amplified secretin release. With thiazides, the inciting factor is thought to be hypercalcemia caused by the medication. Diuretic-induced pancreatitis is uncommon.

In patients prone to **ventricular arrhythmias,** such as those with congestive heart failure, hypokalemia may help precipitate ventricular tachycardia or ventricular fibrillation. This is especially important when digoxin is being used concurrently.

6. Diabetes insipidus is characterized by an inappropriate increase in urine production. Why are diuretics used to treat this disorder?

Thiazide drugs, by inducing mild sodium and extracellular volume depletion, invoke a compensatory increase in proximal tubule sodium and water resorption. The amount of filtrate delivered to the distal diluting segment is thereby reduced and urine output is diminished.

7. A patient is vacationing in Colorado to ski. On prior trips, he experienced headaches, nausea, and insommia. His doctors advised him to take a "water pill" prior to skiing, but he forgot the medication and cannot remember its name. What medication would you prescribe?

This patient's history and symptoms are consistent with high-altitude sickness. Acetazolamide, a carbonic anhydrase inhibitor, has been used to treat this condition. Its mechanism of action is the induction of a metabolic acidosis which stimulates the respiratory drive and diminishes altitude-induced hypoxemia. It cannot, however, be relied upon to prevent the life-threatening complications of pulmonary or cerebral edema or reduce the incidence of retinal hemorrhage. Descent is the only effective treatment for these problems.

8. What is the role of diuretics in treating hypertension?

Thiazides frequently are still a first-choice therapy for hypertension, especially when cost and compliance are important. They are also effective in the elderly with isolated systolic hypertension. Diuretics are often still required in controlling severe hypertension when multiple classes of drugs at maximal doses are being used without complete success. Loop diuretics are effective in patients with renal failure, and in those with congestive heart failure or others in whom edema is a major complaint.

9. What are the indications for chronic nitrate therapy?

Nitrates are used to treat angina related to atherosclerotic coronary artery disease and coronary artery spasm. They also lessen symptoms of chronic congestive heart failure and, in combination with hydralazine, improve survival and delay progression of left ventricular dysfunction (though not as well as angiotensin-converting enzyme inhibitors).

10. How do nitrates achieve their antianginal affects?

Nitrates dilate epicardial coronary arteries and coronary resistance vessels. Atherosclerotic coronary arteries respond to nitroglycerin even in areas of significant stenosis. Collateral vessels also dilate. Both result in an increase in O_2 delivery to ischemic myocardium. Nitrates also affect systemic arteries and veins. Venodilation, by reducing preload, decreases diastolic volume, wall stress, and O_2 consumption. Dilatation of systemic arteries decreases myocardial O_2 consumption by decreasing afterload. Angina is relieved as O_2 delivery to ischemic regions is increased and O_2 consumption is decreased. In coronary spasm, nitrates relieve angina by their direct ability to dilate epicardial vessels at the sites of spasm.

11. By what additional mechanism may nitrates be beneficial in unstable angina or acute myocardial infarction?
Nitroglycerin has antiplatelet effects which inhibit thrombus formation. This antiplatelet effect may contribute to the improved survival seen when intravenous nitroglycerin is used during myocardial infarction, and it may decrease recurrent ischemic episodes in patients with unstable angina.

12. What kinds of nitrate therapy are available?
Nitroglycerin is available as a sublingual tablet or spray, a buccal preparation, long-acting oral tablets, topical preparations (ointment or patch) and intravenous preparations. **Isosorbide dinitrate** can be used sublingually or orally. **5-Isosorbide mononitrate** is available for oral administration only.

13. What are the mechanisms of action of organic nitrates on the cellular level?
Organic nitrates act as prodrugs which must be converted inside vascular smooth muscle cells to nitric oxide. This conversion is accomplished by a reduction reaction using sulfhydryl groups from cysteine within the cytosol as follows:

$$NO_2 + 2\ SH \rightarrow NO + S{=}S + H_2O$$
$$(\text{nitrate} + \text{cysteine} \rightarrow \text{nitric oxide})$$

Nitric oxide (NO) directly stimulates guanylate cyclase (GC), resulting in increased levels of intracellular cyclic GMP. GMP acts through phosphorylation of cellular proteins via protein kinases to decrease the availability of calcium to contractile proteins. This results in relaxation.

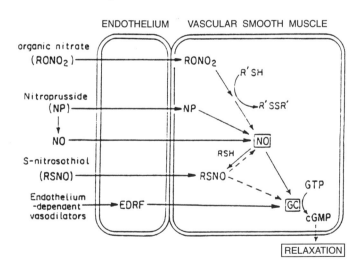

14. How is nitrate tolerance manifested?
Tolerance was first noted nearly 100 years ago in munitions workers, who suffered headache, fatigue, and orthostatic symptoms on returning to work after short holidays. Their symptoms resolved after hours to days of continued exposure.

Tolerance today is manifested by loss of efficacy in treating symptoms of angina or congestive heart failure with long-acting preparations used without a nitrate-free interval. Tolerance is also seen when increasing doses of intravenous nitroglycerin are needed over time to achieve a specific hemodynamic response or antianginal effect.

15. A 64-year-old man with stable exertional angina has been doing well on isosorbide dinitrate, 20 mg twice daily. Recently, he increased his dose to four times daily, thinking "more is better." Soon after, he noted worsening angina. Why might this occur?

This patient could have worsening angina secondary to progression of his coronary artery disease or it may be the development of nitrate tolerance. Studies in patients with stable angina have shown persistent antianginal effects when a nitrate-free interval of 10–12 hours is provided. Many patients experience an attenuation or complete loss of anti-anginal effects when long-acting agents are used three or four times daily. Similarly, long-acting nitroglycerin patches should be removed for 10–12 hours daily.

16. Name some possible mechanisms of nitrate tolerance.

1. Sulfhydryl depletion—Inadequate generation of sulfhydryl groups necessary for transformation of organic nitrates to nitric oxide.

2. Chronic stimulation by nitric oxide causes desensitization of guanylate cyclase.

3. Activation of counter-regulatory neurohumoral mechanisms—Increased catecholamines, arginine vasopressin, plasma renin, aldosterone, and angiotensin II.

4. Increased intravascular volume—Starting forces favor net movement of fluid from tissues into the vascular space when capillary pressure is reduced by vasodilation.

17. How do nitroglycerin and heparin interact?

Nitroglycerin may interfere with the anticoagulant activity of heparin, necessitating increased heparin doses to achieve therapeutic results. When nitroglycerin is discontinued, excessive anticoagulation may occur.

18. A patient is admitted with unstable angina. Cardiac catheterization demonstrates triple-vessel coronary artery disease. He subsequently develops several episodes of chest pain at rest treated with increasing high doses of intravenous nitroglycerin, calcium blockers, heparin, and aspirin. On rounds the following morning, he appears cyanotic and also complains of weakness, headache, and shortness of breath. His lungs are clear, he has no murmurs, and his chest x-ray is normal. How would you treat this syndrome? Are these findings related to his therapy?

High doses of nitroglycerin can result in clinically significant methemoglobinemia. Cyanosis occurs when the level of methemoglobin ($HbFe^{+3}$) exceeds 10%. When the level exceeds 35%, symptoms of dyspnea, headache, and weakness appear. The treatment for toxic methemoglobinemia is intravenous methylene blue at 2 mg/kg. Methemoglobin levels become significantly reduced, and symptoms substantially improve within 1 hour.

BIBLIOGRAPHY

1. Abrams J: Use of nitrates in ischemic heart disease. Cur Probl Cardiol 17:483–542, 1992.
2. Amsterdam, EA: Rationale for intermittent nitrate therapy. Am J Cardiol 70:556–606, 1992.
3. Bell D: Insulin resistance. Postgrad Med 93(7):99–107, 1993.
4. Elkayam U, Mehra A, Avraham S, Osprzega E: Possible mechanisms of nitrate tolerance. Am J Cardiol 70:496–546, 1992.
5. Folts JD: Inhibition of platelet function in vivo or in vitro by organic nitrates. J Am Coll Cardiol 18:1537–1538, 1991.

6. Fung H, Chung S, Bauer J, et al: Biochemical mechanism of organic nitrate action. Am J Cardiol 70:4B–10B, 1992.

7. Greene MK, et al: Acetazolamide in prevention of acute mountain sickness: Double-blind controlled crossover study. BMJ 283:811–813, 1991.

8. Habbab J, Haft J: Heparin resistance induced by intravenous nitroglycerin. Arch Intern Med 147:857–860, 1987.

9. Kaplan N: Treatment of hypertension: Drug therapy. In Kaplan N (ed): Clinical Hypertension, 4th ed. Baltimore, Williams & Wilkins, 1986, pp 180–204.

10. Pollare T, Lithell H, Berne C: A comparison of the effects of hydrochlorothiazide and captopril on glucose and lipid metabolism in patients with hypertension. N Engl J Med 321:868, 1989.

11. Sinoway L, Minotti J, Musch T: Enhanced metabolic vasodilation secondary to diuretic therapy in decompensated congestive heart failure secondary to coronary artery disease. Am J Cardiol 60:107, 1987.

12. Smith TW, Braunwald E, Kelly R: The management of heart failure. In Braunwald E (ed): Heart Disease: A Textbook of Cardiovascular Medicine, 4th ed. Philadelphia, W.B. Saunders, 1992, pp 464–479.

50. ANGIOTENSIN-CONVERTING ENZYME INHIBITORS AND OTHER VASODILATORS

Talley F. Culclasure, M.D., Christopher M. Kozlowski, M.D., and William T. Highfill, M.D.

1. What vasodilators are in common clinical use?

Vasodilators in Clinical Use

MECHANISM	DRUGS
Angiotensin-converting enzyme (ACE) inhibitors	Captopril, enalapril, lisinopril, quinapril, ramipril, benazepril, fosinopril
Direct smooth muscle relaxants	Nitroprusside, nitrates, hydralazine, minoxidil
Alpha-adrenergic blockers	Prazosin, terazosin, doxazosin
Calcium channel blockers	Nifedipine, isradipine, amlodipine, felodipine, nimodipine, verapamil

2. Why are vasodilators useful in congestive heart failure due to left ventricular systolic dysfunction?

In patients with low cardiac output, the arterial and venous beds are inappropriately constricted. This is the body's response to a low flow state in order to maintain adequate blood flow to vital organs. Some compensatory mechanisms responsible for this constriction are increased catecholamine levels, increased sympathetic tone, and increased activity of the renin-angiotensin aldosterone system. These compensatory mechanisms work against the failing heart, causing a vicious cycle of decreasing cardiac output and increasing vasoconstriction. Vasodilators break this cycle by decreasing vascular resistance, thus improving cardiac output.

3. What effects do vasodilators have on fluid and electrolyte metabolism?

Non-ACE inhibitor vasodilators are potent stimulators of the renin-angiotensin-aldosterone system. This response is the result of lowering the mean systemic blood pressure and decreasing renal perfusion. Activation of the renin-angiotensin-aldosterone system increases aldosterone levels which, in turn, act at the distal renal tubule to cause sodium resorption and water retention. The result of this process is increased intravascular volume and progressive edema.

ACE inhibitors, on the other hand, exert a direct effect on the renin-angiotensin-aldosterone system by blocking the conversion of angiotensin I to angiotensin II. Because angiotensin II stimulates aldosterone production, circulating levels of aldosterone are reduced. Diminished aldosterone levels decrease sodium resorption and potassium secretion in the distal renal tubule. Thus, increased intravascular volume and edema are not side effects of ACE inhibition. Hyperkalemia can occur, and care should be taken when ACE inhibitors are used in conjunction with potassium-sparing diuretics or potassium supplements.

4. Do these fluid and electrolyte differences translate into clinical differences?

Yes. In patients with congestive heart failure, inhibitors of the renin-angiotensin system are more effective than other vasodilators for lowering long-term mortality. They lower mortality more than the combination of hydralazine and isosorbide dinitrate does. This combination, in turn, lowers mortality more than does prazosin, which is no better than placebo.

5. What are some other beneficial clinical effects of ACE inhibitors?

1. In patients with reduced ejection fraction (<40%) following myocardial infarction, captopril reduces mortality by favorably altering left ventricular remodelling, thus reducing left ventricular dilation and hypertrophy.

2. Many clinicians believe ACE inhibitors are more effective than other agents for reducing ventricular mass and improving diastolic dysfunction in patients with left ventricular hypertrophy due to hypertension.

3. Captopril provides more protection against decline in renal function in insulin-dependent diabetics than other antihypertensives provide.

4. ACE inhibitors that contain a sulfhydryl group, such as captopril, may have a mild antiplatelet effect and may increase insulin receptor sensitivity.

6. Ten days after initiation of an ACE inhibitor for hypertension, a 71-year-old patient with a history of coronary disease returns complaining of malaise, progressive edema, diminished urine output, and a 15-lb weight gain. His serum creatinine has risen to 4.8 mg/dl. What happened?

ACE inhibitors can cause acute renal failure in patients with bilateral renal artery stenosis. ACE inhibition causes dilation of the efferent glomerular arterioles, resulting in decreased glomerular filtration and acute renal failure. Because of this potential complication, renal function should be evaluated prior to and monitored 1–2 weeks after the initiation of ACE inhibitors in high-risk patients. In this patient, the ACE inhibitor should be discontinued.

7. In the same patient, the ACE inhibitor was discontinued and renal function returned to baseline. What vasodilator regimen might now be substituted?

Hydralazine in combination with isosorbide dinitrate.

8. A patient with congestive heart failure due to a dilated cardiomyopathy returns 1 month after the initiation of an ACE inhibitor complaining of a persistent dry cough. Should the ACE inhibitor be discontinued?

Cough is a bothersome side effect in 10–20% of patients started on ACE inhibitors. The cough is almost invariably nonproductive and usually begins within 1–6 weeks after initiation of therapy. It is seen most frequently with longer-acting preparations. Changing to another ACE inhibitor is rarely helpful, though a trial of antitussive therapy may allow continuation in patients where ACE inhibition is essential. Occasionally, the cough is a manifestation of worsening heart failure.

9. What other side effects are seen with ACE inhibitors?

Other less common side effects of ACE inhibitors, most often seen with captopril, include rash, dysgeusia, angioedema, and reversible neutropenia.

10. In asymptomatic patients with severe chronic left ventricular volume overload lesions, aortic insufficiency, and mitral regurgitation, ACE inhibitors and other vasodilators have been utilized to attempt to slow or reverse left ventricular dilation and systolic dysfunction. However, some cardiologists have voiced concerns over the routine use of these agents for these conditions. Why?

Chronic left ventricular volume overload lesions are typically well tolerated for many years, though about one-fourth of patients will develop left ventricular dysfunction prior to onset of symptoms. Once the ventricle begins to fail, 20–30% of patients continue to deteriorate despite valve repair. Left ventricular function is an important marker used to time valve repair. Vasodilators improve left ventricular function, but there are few clinical data on how vasodilators might affect the timing of valve surgery. For example, if an asymptomatic patient with severe chronic aortic insufficiency would normally undergo valve replacement when the left ventricular ejection fraction fell to 50%, at what ejection fraction should the valve be replaced in the same patient being managed with hydralazine? Conversely, aggressive vasodilation may improve the failing heart enough to allow valve repair in patients once thought to be inoperable. Vasodilators may be used in other nonsurgical candidates to relieve symptoms and postpone surgery indefinitely.

11. What are some cardiovascular diseases in which arterial vasodilators may be contraindicated?

Most contraindications to the use of arterial vasodilators are relative. For example, in **severe aortic stenosis,** blood pressure may be dependent on arterial vasoconstriction due to a relatively fixed stroke volume; thus, arterial vasodilators should be used cautiously. However, in patients with severe aortic stenosis and congestive heart failure who were not considered candidates for aortic valve replacement, careful use of arterial vasodilators has provided symptomatic improvement. Similar concerns apply in **hypertrophic cardiomyopathy** and **severe pulmonary hypertension.** Many patients with left ventricular dysfunction are relatively hypotensive (systolic blood pressure < 100 mmHg); however, because this group of patients derives symptomatic and survival benefits from ACE inhibition, cautious use of ACE inhibitors is still indicated in such circumstances.

12. In what acute conditions can the prompt initiation of vasodilator therapy be life-saving?

Vasodilators can be life-saving in several situations that require acute afterload reduction and/or systemic blood pressure reduction.

Severe acute **mitral regurgitation** from any cause results in a sudden rise in left atrial and pulmonary venous pressure, leading to pulmonary edema. Emergent use of sodium nitroprusside lowers systemic blood pressure and afterload, which favors forward ejection of the left ventricular volume, lowers the regurgitant volume, and reduces pulmonary venous pressure. Severe acute **aortic insufficiency** causes a sudden elevation in left ventricular diastolic pressure, leading to pulmonary congestion and systemic hypoperfusion. As in acute mitral regurgitation, the regurgitant volume can be reduced by lowering the systemic blood pressure by acute vasodilation with nitroprusside. Aggressive vasodilation in these instances can stabilize a significant number of patients and allow valve replacement under less emergent circumstances. **Hypertensive emergency** and **aortic dissection** are two other examples.

13. How are vasodilators used in the treatment of hypertensive crisis?

Hypertensive crisis requires rapid lowering of the systolic and diastolic blood pressure to prevent ongoing end-organ damage. Nitroprusside, a fast-acting intravenous drug with a short half-life, is the most-effective and easily-titrated drug for the treatment of this process. The initial dose is 0.5 μg/kg/min and is increased until blood pressure control is attained, usually at a systolic blood pressure of 140–160 mmHg. If hypotension occurs, the dose should be decreased or discontinued, and the patient should be placed in the Trendelenburg position. Prolonged use of high doses of nitroprusside can produce high thiocyanate levels which interfere with oxygen transport. Once blood pressure is controlled, oral antihypertensives should be initiated.

14. Which vasodilator was largely abandoned because of a specific side effect which later proved to be its major clinical indication?

Minoxidil (Rogaine) is a potent arterial vasodilator that is effective in patients with refractory hypertension. Minoxidil proved to have a unique side effect, hirsutism, which caused it to fall into disfavor, especially among female patients. Subsequently, minoxidil was introduced in a topical form to promote hair growth.

15. What is your initial management strategy for a patient with dissection of the descending thoracic aorta?

Although the definitive therapy for many types of aortic dissection remains controversial, most agree that the initial therapy for an uncomplicated dissection of the descending aorta should be medical. Aortic dissections are propagated by the absolute blood pressure and rate of pressure rise (dP/dt) in the aorta. Intravenous sodium nitroprusside allows rapid lowering of the systolic blood pressure to the desired level of 100–120 mmHg. Vasodilators lower the blood pressure but cause a significant rise in dP/dt; thus, concomitant use of beta blockers, initially intravenously, is recommended since beta blockers reduce dP/dt in the aorta.

16. What patient warning is necessary when initiating terazosin?

Terazosin and prazosin are arterial vasodilators that produce their antihypertensive effect through peripheral alpha-receptor blockade. Their use is complicated by significant first-dose hypotension and syncope, most commonly in the elderly. Patients taking this medication should be warned about this possibility, instructed to take the initial dose at bedtime, and to exercise extreme care should they need to get out of bed at night.

The opinions and assertions contained herein are the private views of the authors and are not to be construed as official or reflecting the views of the Department of the Army or Department of Defense.

BIBLIOGRAPHY

1. Braunwald E: Aortic dissection. In Braunwald E (ed): Heart Disease: A Textbook of Cardiovascular Medicine. Philadelphia, W.B. Saunders, 1992.
2. Braunwald E: Vasodilators. In Braunwald E (ed): Heart Disease: A Textbook of Cardiovascular Medicine. Philadelphia, W.B. Saunders, 1992.
3. Cohn JN, Archibald DG, Ziesche S, et al: Effect of vasodilator therapy on mortality in chronic congestive heart failure: Results of a Veterans Administration cooperative study. N Engl J Med 314:1547–1552, 1986.
4. Cohn JN, Johnson G, Ziesche S, et al: A comparison of enalapril with hydralazine-isosorbide dinitrate in the treatment of chronic congestive heart failure. N Engl J Med 325:303–310, 1991.
5. CONSENSUS Trial Study Group: Effects of enalapril on mortality in severe congestive heart failure; Results of the Cooperative North Scandinavian Enalapril Survival Study (CONSENSUS). N Engl J Med 316:1429–1435, 1987.
6. Lewis EJ, Hunsicker LG, Bain RP, et al: The effect of angiotensin-converting-enzyme inhibition on diabetic nephropathy. N Engl J Med 329:1456–1462, 1993.
7. Pfeffer MA, Braunwald E, Moyé LA, et al: Effect of captopril on mortality and morbidity in patients with left ventricular dysfunction after myocardial infarction: Results of the survival and ventricular enlargement trail. N Engl J Med 327:669–677, 1992.
8. Simon SR, Black HR, Moser M, Berland WE: Cough and ACE inhibitors. Arch Intern Med 152:1698–1700, 1992.
9. The SOLVD Investigators: Effect of enalapril on mortality and the development of heart failure in asymptomatic patients with reduced left ventricular ejection fractions. N Engl J Med 327:685–691, 1992.

51. DIGOXIN AND OTHER POSITIVE INOTROPIC DRUGS

Mohamed Chebaclo, M.D., FACC

1. How many classes of inotropic agents are available clinically?

There are two classes of inotropic agents:

1. **Glycosides** include digoxin and digoxin-like agents.
2. **Nonglycosides** are divided into two large groups:
   a. *Sympathomimetic amines* include dopamine, dobutamine, epinephrine, norepinephrine, isoproterenol, and methoxamine.
   b. *Phosphodiesterase inhibitors* comprise amrinone and milrinone.

2. Do the classes of inotropic agents differ in their endpoint effect?

No. They both increase the availability of Ca^{2+} to the contractile element at the time of excitation-contraction coupling, although the endpoint effect is reached through different mechanisms.

3. What is the mechanism of action of the glycosides at the cellular level?

Digoxin and other glycosides increase inotropy at the cellular level by inhibiting the Na^+–K^+ ATPase pump. The glycosides bind to the Na^+–K^+ ATPase pump, which is responsible for active transport of Na^+ across the myocardial cell membrane. This blockage leads to an increase in intracellular Na^+ which, in turn, enhances Na^+–Ca^{2+} exchange. This leads to an increase in intracellular Ca^{2+} which, in turn, contributes to an increase in inotropy.

4. By what mechanism do the beta-adrenergic sympathomimetic drugs increase calcium that leads to increased inotropy?

The beta-adrenergic agents stimulate adenylate cyclase which results in an increase in cyclic AMP. cAMP phosphorylates a protein kinase which, in turn, increases the Ca^{2+} influx through the calcium channel.

5. Does the positive inotropic action of digoxin persist in the presence of full beta-adrenergic blockade?

Yes. The inotropic functions of digoxin are not mediated by catecholamine release or through increased sensitivity to catecholamines. Adenylate cyclase activity which is responsible for the positive inotropic effects of beta-adrenoreceptor agents is not influenced by digoxin.

6. Does the same increase in oxygen consumption during the use of an inotropic agent like digoxin occur in the failing heart as well?

No. Digoxin decreases heart size when administed to a patient in congestive heart failure. There is a reduction in oxygen consumption, heart size, and wall tension, as explained by Laplace's law.

7. How is digoxin excreted?

Digoxin is excreted through the kidney. Its half-life is 35–48 hours in the normally functioning kidney, so that one-third of the stores are excreted daily. Renal excretion is proportional to the glomerular fitration rate.

8. Do patients with digoxin toxicity benefit from dialysis?

Dialysis is not effective because of the high tissue binding of digoxin.

9. Should the digoxin maintenance dose be changed if you add quinidine?
Yes. An approximately twofold increase in serum digoxin concentration occurs when conventional quinidine doses are added to standard maintenance doses of digoxin.

10. What happens to the inotropic effect of digoxin in doses above its therapeutic range?
The therapeutic range for digoxin 1.5–2 ng/ml, but we usually titrate it in our patients. The inotropic effect of digoxin increases in a graded manner with increasing doses, nevertheless, above 2 ng/ml, the risk of toxicity becomes far greater than the additional therapeutic benefit for patients in congestive heart failure and sinus rhythm.

11. Is digoxin indicated in every patient with heart failure?
No. Congestive heart failure with dilated left ventricle, impaired systolic function, and an S_3 gallop are the prime candidates. Congestive heart failure due to diastolic dysfunction and preserved systolic function are not candidates unless supraventricular tachycardia is a concomitant problem. The effect of digoxin is cumulative on the effect of angiotensin-converting enzyme (ACE) inhibitors and diuretics, and therefore an added benefit can be seen with their combination.

12. Is digoxin indicated and safe in acute myocardial infarction?
This issue has been long debated. There appears to be no convincing evidence for an increased incidence of arrhythmias complicating digitalis use in patients with acute myocardial infarction when serum levels do not exceed the conventional therapeutic range. Still, the clearest indication for digoxin is atrial fibrillation with fast response. Electrical cardioversion is preferred for other supraventricular arrhythmias or atrial fibrillation in hemodynamically unstable patients. The available data do not support the assertion that digoxin therapy is excessively hazardous after infarction. However, a randomized study is not available to confirm this belief. In summary, digoxin use has no place in myocardial infarction without congestive heart failure or supraventricular arrhythmias.

13. What are the electrocardiographic (ECG) findings in digoxin toxicity?
An array of ventricular and supraventricular arrhythmias and blocks can result from digoxin toxicity—e.g., atrail, ventricular, atrioventricular (AV) node arrhythmias, AV junctional escape, nonparoxysmal AV junctional tachycardia, paroxysmal atrial tachycardia, ventricular tachycardia, sinus arrest, Mobitz type I and II block. Most commonly seen are premature ventricular contractions.

An ECG rhythm combining increased automaticity and escape ectopic pacemakers with impaired conduction suggests digoxin toxicity. A typical example is paroxysmal atrial tachycardia with block.

14. What are some of the clinical symptoms of digoxin toxicity?
- Gastrointestinal symptoms: nausea and vomiting.
- Neurologic symptoms: headache, fatigue, confusion.
- Visual symptoms: scotomas, halos, change in color perception.

15. How do you treat digoxin toxicity?
- There is no role for dialysis in treating digoxin toxicity.
- For ventricular arrhythmias, phenytoin and lidocaine are helpful.
- Correction of hypokalemia is vital.
- Beta-blockers are useful for ventricular or supraventricular arrhythmias, especially short-acting beta-blockers like esmolol, which are easy to titrate.
- On occasion, direct countershock is necessary in hemodynamically unstable arrhythmias.
- For potentially life-threatening arrhythmias, Digibind, an Fab-specific digoxin antibody, is helpful.

16. What would you do for a digoxin level of 56 ng/ml after Digibind?

Nothing. The typical scenario is a patient who has runs of ventricular tachycardia and episodes of high-grade AV block with a digoxin level of 56. The use of Digibind would successfully control the arrhythmias and AV block, but a repeat digoxin measurement would remain above 50. No therapy is needed, because digoxin levels are usually elevated after Digibind due to the binding of Fab to digoxin from body stores which has not yet been excreted by the kidney. The digoxin is not active in this bound state. Digoxin levels measured post-Digibind are not clinically helpful and should not be obtained.

17. On what receptors are the sympathetic amines active, and what is their effect?

Sympathetic amines exert effects on four different receptors:

1. **Alpha-receptors** provoke vasoconstriction of peripheral arteries when stimulated.

2. **Beta-receptors** increase atrial and ventricular contraction, increase heart rate by stimulating the sinus node, and enhance AV conduction.

3. **Beta$_2$-receptors** promote bronchodilation and vasodilation.

4. **Dopaminergic receptors,** found in various tissues including blood vessels and nervous system tissues, are of two types: The activation of dopamine-1 receptors causes vasodilation in coronary, renal, mesenteric, and cerebral vascular beds, by stimulating adenylate cyclase and increasing cAMP. The activation of dopamine-2 receptors causes vasodilation, but by inhibiting transmission of sympathetic nerve endings.

18. What amines are alpha or beta selective?

Isoproterenol has practically no alpha-stimulating effect, with relatively pure beta-stimulation. It is clinically valuable in stimulating the sinus node and enhancing AV conduction in bradyarrhythmias. Its limitation in this setting is its hypotensive effect through its beta$_2$ properties.

Methoxamine is a practically a pure alpha-stimulant, helpful in hypotension in the cardiac catheterization laboratory.

Norepinephrine is predominantly alpha- and beta-stimulant and is valuable in cardiogenic shock following bypass surgery for stunned myocardium, and in hypotension.

19. What are the effects of dopamine at different dosages?

Dopamine has different effects at different dosages which can create a conflicting clinical response if not known.

≤ 2 µg/kg/min: Stimulate the dopamine receptors; promote renal perfusion; and promote cerebral, coronary, and mesenteric circulation.

2–5 µg/kg/min: Have a predominantly positive inotropic effect manifested by an increase in cardiac output and cardiac contractility with little change in heart rate.

5–10 µg/kg/min: Increase in blood pressure, peripheral vascular resistance, and heart rate; and a decrease in renal blood flow.

20. How do you reduce the vasoconstrictive effect of high-dose dopamine in patients with shock?

When high doses of dopamine are required for inotropic effects it may be infused together with nitroprusside and/or nitroglycerin to counteract the vasoconstrictive action.

21. How does prolonged administration of sympathomimetic drugs affect the failing myocardium?

Ventricle obtained from patients with congestive heart failure demonstrate marked reduction in beta-adrenoreceptor density and in myocardial contractility. This is consistent with an increase in norepinephrine that downregulates beta-receptors. The decrease in receptor density is proportional to the severity of heart failure and involves beta$_1$, but not beta$_2$-receptors. This might be the basis for use of low doses of beta-blockers to reverse the downregulation of beta-receptors and restore responsiveness to adrenergic inotropic stimulation. In sum, the failing myocardium becomes tolerant to prolonged exposure to catecholamines.

22. What is the mechanism of action of the phosphodiesterase inhibitors?

This positive inotropic agent increases availability of Ca^{2+} to the intracellular compartment. The beta-adrenergic mimetic drugs stimulate adenylate cyclase that then increases cAMP. cAMP phosphorylates the protein kinase which, in turn, increases the Ca^{2+} influx through the calcium channel. The phosphodiesterase inhibitors inhibit the degradation of cAMP, thereby limiting Ca^{2+} influx through the calcium channel.

23. What are the indications for use of amrinone?

Amrinone causes a dose-dependent increase in cardiac output and a decrease in right and left filling pressure and systemic vascular resistance.

Its effects are similar, in ways, to a combination of sympathomimetics and vasodilators. The effect of amrinone is additive to the effect of digoxin and other mimetic agents, and there is no tolerance problem as seen in other amines. Intravenous infusions are indicated for treatment for congestive heart failure refractory to digoxin and furosemide and for post-myocardial depression, for left ventricular failure in myocardial infarction, and in patients awaiting cardiac transplantation.

BIBLIOGRAPHY

1. Akerman GL, et al: Peritoneal dialysis and hemodialysis of tritiated digoxin. Ann Intern Med 67:718; 1967.
2. Braunwald E, et al: Effects of digitalis on the normal and the failing heart. J Am Coll Cardiol 5:51A, 1985.
3. Braunwald E, et al: A symposium on amrinone. Am J Cardiol 56:113, 1985.
4. Heitbrunn S, et al: Increased beta-receptor density and improved hemodynamic response to catecholamine stimulation during long-term metoprolol: Therapy in heart failure from dilated cardiomyopathy: Circulation 79:483, 1989.
5. Leahy EB, Retffel JA, et al: Interaction between quinidine and digoxin. JAMA 240:533, 1978.
6. Maskin CS, et al: Comparative systemic and renal effects of dopamine and angiotensin converting enzyme inhibition with enalapril in patients with heart failure. Circulation 72:846, 1985.
7. Miller R, Awan M: Combined dopamine and nitroprusside in therapy in CHF. Circulation 55:881, 1977.
8. Muller JE, Turt Z, et al: Digoxin therapy and mortality after myocardial infarction: Experience in the Millis study. N Engl J Med 314:265, 1986.
9. Sonnenblick E, et al: Dobutamine: A new sympathetic cardioactive sympathomimetic amine. N Engl J Med 300:18, 1979.

52. CALCIUM CHANNEL ANTAGONISTS

Querubin P. Mendoza, M.D., and Arvo J. Oopik, M.D.*

1. What are some of the important pharmacologic properties of calcium channel antagonists?
There are important pharmacologic differences among calcium channel antagonists. Knowledge of these properties is helpful when selecting a drug for a given patient, and for avoiding potential toxicities.

Pharmacologic Properties of Calcium Channel Antagonists

	VERAPAMIL	NIFEDIPINE (AND OTHER DIHYDROPYRIDINES)	DILTIAZEM
Heart rate	↓↓	↑	↓
AV nodal conduction	↓↓	—	↓
Myocardial contractility	↓↓	↓	↓
Arterial vasodilatation	↑↑	↑↑↑	↑

2. Are the calcium channel antagonists interchangeable?
No. Although they belong to the same broad category, there are distinct subclassifications. The major approved indications for these agents are summarized in the table below. The sustained-release preparations often do not have the same indications as the shorter-acting preparations.

Therapeutic Uses of Calcium Channel Blockers

CHEMICAL CLASS AND DRUG	VASOSPASTIC	ANGINA STABLE	UNSTABLE	HYPERTENSION	ATRIAL FIBRILLATION OR FLUTTER	PSVT
Diphenylalkylamine Verapamil	+	+	+	+	+	+
Benzothiazepine Diltiazem	+	+	+	+	+	+
Dihydropyridine Nifedipine	+	+	+	+		
Amlodipine	+	+	+	+		
Nicardipine	+	+	+	+		
Other Bepridil			+			

PSVT = paroxysmal supraventricular tachycardia.

3. Name some contraindications to the use of calcium channel antagonists.
In addition to known hypersensitivity reactions, contraindications are related to the pharmacologic properties of the various subclasses, including hypotension, congestive heart failure, sick-sinus syndrome, and second- or third-degree atrioventricular (AV) block. Because of significant vasodilatation and lowering of vascular resistance, the dihydropyridine subclass is avoided in patients with severe aortic stenosis and hypertrophic cardiomyopathy. Bepridil prolongs QT intervals, is contraindicated in patients with a history of serious ventricular arrhythmias, and is reserved for patients with angina that does not respond to other medications.

---

*Deceased.

4. Why is nifedipine potentially deleterious when used in unstable angina?

By lowering arterial pressure with subsequent reflex tachycardia, nifedipine may aggravate angina. This problem can be avoided with simultaneous use of beta blockers. Withdrawal of beta blockade in some patients taking nifedipine may worsen angina.

5. What are some of the important drug interactions of calcium channel antagonists?

Drug Interactions of Calcium Channel Antagonists

Beta-adrenergic blockers	Negative inotropic and chronotropic effects; heart block
Digoxin	Increased plasma digoxin levels
Alpha blockers (prazosin)	Excessive hypotension
Quinidine	Hypotension, bradycardia, decreased quinidine level
Carbamazepine	Increased carbamazepine levels
Cimetidine	Increased plasma level of calcium channel antagonist
Cyclosporine	Increased cyclosporine levels
Enzyme inducers (rifampin, sulfinpyrazone, phenobarbital)	Decreased effects of calcium channel antagonists

6. What are the signs and symptoms of calcium channel antagonist toxicity?

The most common toxic effects are hypotension and bradydysrhythmias. Of the latter, most common are AV block and sinus bradycardia with junctional escape rhythms. Rarely, one sees a slow idioventricular rhythm and prolonged QRS duration.

7. How are these toxicities treated aside from discontinuing the drug?

Treatment is primarily supportive. For severe cardiotoxicity, such as seen with large ingestions in suicide attempts, cathecholamines with chronotropic activity (dopamine, epinephrine, norepinephrine) should be used. Isoproterenol is effective in this regard but may potentiate vasodilation. Atropine is inconsistently effective. Temporary pacing should be considered. Whereas intravenous administration of calcium may improve contractility, this maneuver is less effective in managing heart block or excessive vasodilation. Oral charcoal should be given for acute ingestion. Hemoperfusion, however, is ineffective in clearing these drugs because of their large volume of distribution and high endogenous clearance. Glucagon has been felt to be useful in a few cases. The mechanism is thought to be improvement in myocardial contractility through increased cyclic AMP in myocardial cells.

8. Are calcium channel antagonists indicated in patients with acute Q-wave myocardial infarctions?

No. Most studies of the calcium channel antagonists have not demonstrated any definitive benefits in patients with acute myocardial infarction. In a meta-analysis of 22 trials, no improvement in mortality, reduction of infarct size, or reduction in incidence of reinfarction was documented. One trial explored administration of verapamil starting 1 week after the acute event and showed a significant reduction in mortality. In another trial, nifedipine was associated with increased mortality and reinfarction rate.

9. Are calcium antagonists indicated in non-Q-wave myocardial infarctions?

Calcium channel antagonists may have a role in patients without evidence of left ventricular failure. Diltiazem decreases the short term reinfarction rate and the incidence of postinfarction angina but does not improve overall survival. In patients with pulmonary congestion, however, use of diltiazem was associated with increased mortality.

10. Is there a role for calcium-channel antagonists in the treatment of heart failure due to left ventricular systolic dysfunction?

In general, no. Most studies have not shown sustained clinical benefit. Because of significant negative inotropic effect, calcium channel blockers may, in fact, worsen heart failure due to systolic dysfunction. Even those agents selective for vascular smooth muscle–relaxant effects have competing negative inotropic effects.

11. Do patients with hypertrophic cardiomyopathy benefit from calcium channel antagonists?
Yes. Most experience has been with verapamil. By depressing myocardial contractility, verapamil can decrease the left ventricular outflow gradient. It also improves diastolic filling by improving myocardial relaxation. Exercise capacity and overall symptoms are often improved.

12. Are calcium channel blockers useful in the reduction of left ventricular hypertrophy caused by hypertension?
Yes. Numerous studies have shown that calcium channel antagonists reduce left ventricular mass and improve pathophysiologic sequelae, such as ventricular dysrhythmias, impaired ventricular filling, and coronary reserve, while maintaining left ventricular pump function. It remains to be seen, however, whether a reduction in the degree of left ventricular hypertrophy will ultimately reduce the risks of sudden death, acute myocardial infarction, and congestive heart failure associated with hypertensive heart disease.

13. Why are calcium channel antagonists frequently used in patients undergoing percutaneous transluminal coronary angioplasty (PTCA)?
Calcium channel antagonists may prevent coronary spasm which is frequently seen during and shortly after PTCA and other percutaneous coronary interventions. They have not been shown, however, to reduce the incidence of restenosis, which usually occurs within the first 6 months after PTCA.

14. Are there any studies suggesting benefit of calcium channel antagonists in the prevention of coronary atherosclerosis?
Yes. Some preliminary information suggests that calcium blockers may affect the atherosclerotic process. The Montreal Heart Institute Trial with nicardipine showed less progression of stenotic lesions that are ≤20% in severity. In the International Nifedipine Trial on Antiatherosclerotic Therapy (INTACT), nifedipine reduced the rate of appearance of new coronary lesions. In both trials, however, no effect was seen on the overall progression or regression of atherosclerosis. Other preliminary data also suggest that diltiazem may slow the development of accelerated coronary atherosclerosis often seen in heart transplant recipients. At this time, there is not general agreement on the use of calcium channel blockers for this indication.

15. Do the calcium channel antagonists have long-term benefits in patients with primary (unexplained) pulmonary hypertension?
Maybe. High doses of nifedipine or diltiazem produce reductions in pulmonary artery pressure and pulmonary vascular resistance in some patients. However, no clinical trial of calcium channel antagonists in primary pulmonary hypertension has demonstrated a survival benefit.

16. A patient with known Wolff-Parkinson-White syndrome presents with atrial fibrillation with a rapid ventricular response. He is given intravenous verapamil, but then becomes hypotensive and develops ventricular fibrillation. What is the likely mechanism for this deterioration?
This case illustrates the potential danger of using calcium channel antagonists in patients with accessory bypass tracts who present with atrial fibrillation. Calcium channel antagonists may depress conduction through the AV node and enhance conduction through accessory bypass tracts, resulting in acceleration of the ventricular response. Very rapid ventricular rates may lead to hypotension and syncope and may cause rhythm degeneration to ventricular fibrillation.

The opinions and assertions contained herein are the private views of the authors and are not to be construed as official or reflecting the views of the Department of the Army or Department of Defense.

BIBLIOGRAPHY

 1. Garrat C, Antoniou A, Ward D, Camm AJ: Misuse of verapamil in pre-excited atrial fibrillation. Lancet 1:367–369, 1989.
 2. Held PH, Yusuf S, Furberg CD: Calcium channel blockers in acute myocardial infarction and unstable angina: An overview. BMJ 299:1187–1192, 1989.
 3. Hermans WRM, Rensing BJ, Strauss BH, Serruys PW: Prevention of restenosis after percutaneous transluminal coronary angioplasty: The search for a "magic bullet." Am Heart J 122:171–187, 1991.
 4. Messerli FH, Aristizabal D, Soria F: Reduction of left ventricular hypertrophy: How beneficial? Am Heart J 125:1520–1524, 1993.
 5. Morris AD, Meredith PA, Reid JL: Pharmacokinetics of calcium antagonists: Implications for therapy. In Epstein M (ed): Calcium Antagonists in Clinical Medicine. Philadelphia, Hanley & Belfus, 1992, pp 49–67.
 6. Multicenter Diltiazem Postinfarction Trial Research Group: The effect of diltiazem on mortality and reinfarction after myocardial infarction. N Engl J Med 319:385–392, 1988.
 7. Pentel PR, Salerno DM: Cardiac drug toxicity: Digitalis glycosides and calcium-channel and beta-blocking agents. Med J Aust 152:88–94, 1990.
 8. Rich S, Brundage BH: High-dose calcium channel-blocking therapy for primary pulmonary hypertension: Evidence for long-term reduction in pulmonary arterial pressure and regression of right ventricular hypertrophy. Circulation 76:135–141, 1987.
 9. Rutherford JD, Braunwald E. Chronic Ischemic heart disease. In Braunwald E (ed): Heart Disease: A Textbook of Cardiovascular Medicine, 4th ed. Philadelphia, W.B. Saunders, 1992, pp 1310–1316.
10. Waters D, Lesperance J: Interventions that beneficially influence the evolution of coronary atherosclerosis: The case for calcium channel clockers. Circulation 86(Suppl III):III-111–III-116, 1992.

53. THROMBOLYTIC AGENTS

James C. Lafferty, M.D., Donald A. McCord, M.D., and Ali R. Homayuni, M.D.

1. Describe the usual pathogenesis of acute myocardial infarction.

Most acute myocardial infarctions are caused by the occlusion of a coronary artery by a thrombus at the site of a ruptured atheromatous plaque. Total occlusion of an infarct-related artery has been seen in up to 87% of patients undergoing cardiac catheterization within 4–6 hours of acute myocardial infarction.

2. What is the final common pathway in the development of thrombosis?

Whatever the initiating cause, the final pathway involves the conversion of prothrombin to thrombin. Thrombin subsequently converts fibrinogen into fibrin which, together with red blood cells, platelets, and plasminogen, can produce a thrombus.

3. Describe the final common pathway in thrombolysis.

The endogenous thrombolytic system can be activated by thrombus and endogenous or exogenous plasminogen activators. The activation proceeds by converting plasminogen into plasmin. Plasmin, in turn, lyses stable fibrin clots and degrades circulating fibrinogen, both which result in the formation of fibrinogen split products which further inhibit fibrin formation. This process may also be termed **fibrinolysis.**

4. Why would lysing a thrombus potentially alleviate the effect of a myocardial infarction?

A myocardial infarction is not an all-or-nothing phenomenon. Instead, it is a dynamic process known as a wave-front phenomenon that generally progresses over several hours. Thus, there is a window of opportunity to lyse a thrombus and restore flow to the jeopardized myocardium and potentially limit infarct size.

5. Does the endogenous fibrinolytic system lay a role in spontaneous fibrinolysis to produce reperfusion?

Yes. This was demonstrated by DeWood and others who noted that the incidence of total occlusion of an infarct-related artery tends to decrease the longer the time from the development of a myocardial infarction to the time of catheterization. This spontaneous process generally appears to fall outside the window of opportunity for myocardial salvage. For this reason, activating agents have been developed to accelerate the course of thrombolysis.

6. What are the thrombolytic agents available, and how do they differ?

Thrombolytic Agents

	SOURCE	ROUTE
Tissue plasminogen activator (tPA)	Endogenous (human)	Intravenous
Urokinase	Endogenous (human)	Intracoronary
Streptokinase	Exogenous	Intravenous, intracoronary
APSAC*	Exogenous	Intravenous

*APSAC = anisoylated plasminogen–streptokinase activator complex.

Streptokinase acts indirectly by combining with plasminogen to form an activation complex which, in turn, converts plasminogen to plasmin both at the site of a thrombosis and systemically. Streptokinase is antigenic and can cause an early anaphylactic or late serum sickness-like reaction. It has a 50–60% infarct artery patency rate when used intravenously. It is the cheapest agent available and has the lowest incidence of intracerebral bleeds.

tPA directly converts plasminogen to plasmin but only in the presence of fibrin. This allows for increased, but not absolute, clot specificity. It is the most expensive agent but has the highest patency rates (75–85%). It also carries an increased risk for intracerebral bleeding.

APSAC is inactive (due to the acyl group) until exposed to fibrin, when decylation occurs and culminates in an activity similar to that of streptokinase. The patency rates and antigenic activity are similar to that of streptokinase. The acyl group only mildly improves the drug's clot-specific activity. APSAC is very similar to streptokinase but also more expensive.

7. Does the use of thrombolytic agents translate into improved clinical results?
Yes. Early mortality (within the first few weeks) after Q-wave myocardial infarction has been reduced by 33%, from 10–15% to approximately 5–10%. Thrombolytic agents often lead to better recovery of left ventricular function, less ventricular dilatation or remodeling, fewer arrhythmias, and presumably improved long-term survival.

8. What are the indications for intravenous thrombolytic agents?
The are used to treat, within 6 hours of onset, newly developed chest pain consistent with **acute myocardial infarction,** along with ST elevations > 0.1 mV in at least two contiguous leads or the development of a new left bundle branch block. Administration between 6 and 12 hours after onset may show less benefit but is still deemed important. Time frames > 12 hours but < 24 hours yield diminishing benefits but may be useful in certain situations.

Thrombolytic agents may also be considered with ST-segment depression in leads V_2 and V_3; along with the development of an R wave in similar leads, that are thought to represent a **posterior wall myocardial infarction** and not unstable angina.

9. What are the contraindications to thrombolysis?

1. Absolute contraindications

Prolonged trauma or cardioplumonary resuscitation (CPR)
Major trauma or surgery in last 6 wks
GI or GU bleeding in last 6 months
Bleeding diathesis
Known or suspected aortic dissection
Possible pericarditis
Intracranial tumor
Prior neurosurgery
Stroke in last 6 months
Head trauma (< 1 month)
Prior use of streptokinase (if streptokinase or APSAC is being considered)
Previous drug allergy (to streptokinase or APSAC)

2. Relative contraindications

MAJOR	MINOR
Prolonged CPR (> 10 min)	Diabetic retinopathy
Puncture of a noncompressible vessel	CPR < 10 min
Acute severe hypertension	Older age
Recent transient ischemic attack	Female sex
Stroke > 6 months ago	Obesity
Current use of anticoagulation	Small body size
History of peptic ulcer disease	
Pregnancy	
History of bleeding diathesis	
Cancer	
Severe hepatic dysfunction	

10. How are bleeding complications managed?

Bleeding is a major drawback to thrombolytic therapy. It is usually mild and easily treatable, but occasionally it can be devastating, especially intracerebral bleeding, which occurs in 0.2–0.6% of cases. Age, hypertension, prior stroke and prior use of tPA may predispose to bleeding.

Most bleeding occurs at vascular puncture sites, so the initial management is wound compression. If bleeding cannot be controlled or if it involves an intracranial site, all thrombolytic agents, heparin, and aspirin should be discontinued. Protamine can be given to reverse heparin's effects. Because thrombolytic agents cause a depletion of clotting factors, cryoprecipitate infusion can replace fibrinogen and fresh frozen plasma can replace Factors V and VIII. Aspirin causes platelet dysfunction, and a platelet infusion may be considered. Additional antifibrinolytic agents, such as ε-amino caproic acid, that prevent the binding of tPA and plasmin to fibrin may be useful. Even with this management, intracerebral bleeding still yields a poor prognosis.

11. What are the markers of reperfusion?

The gold standard for measuring reperfusion or coronary artery patency is coronary angiography. Bedside markers of reperfusion include the resolution of chest pain, reduction in ST-segment elevations, reperfusion arrhythmia, and early peaking creatine phosphokinase level. These markers, however, are extremely insensitive and lack specificity unless all occur together. Other available tests include early myoglobin peaking, thallium or sestamibi redistribution, improvement of wall motion abnormality on echocardiography, gated blood pool or magnetic resonance imaging, as well as signal average parameters and ultrasound tissue characterization. These tests have different availabilities, various advantages, and disadvantages. Their usefulness may depend on the institution as well as the clinical setting.

12. Does any thrombolytic agent confer improved survival benefit over the others?

Although tPA has higher patency rates than streptokinase or APSAC, there were no difference noted in survival until the recent GUSTO trial. This trial, using an accelerated tPA dosing schedule along with intravenous heparin, provided an approximately 14% survival benefit when compared to streptokinase combined with subcutaneous heparin, intravenous heparin, or tPA. An increased risk of intracerebral bleeding also was noted in the tPA group.

13. What adjunctive therapies are used to prevent reocclusion and potentiate thrombolysis?

Antiplatelet therapy with aspirin is an essential adjunct and has been recommended ever since ISIS II demonstrated its efficacy with or without a thrombolytic agent. Agents that bind or competitively inhibit glycoprotein receptors (glycoprotein IIB–IIIA) and prevent platelet cross-linking are under investigation. Inhibitors of the binding site for von Willebrand factor are also under investigation. Heparin accelerates the formation of antithrombin III complexes which, in turn, impede thrombin activity. Hirudin is a more specific direct inhibitor of thrombin and is currently being evaluated in the GUSTO II trial.

14. Do thrombolytic agents work in unstable angina?

Because coronary thrombosis plays a role in unstable angina, one would expect lytic agents to be useful in unstable angina. Although this makes sense intuitively, it has yet to be shown. On angiography, the coronary artery appears to improve with the thrombolytic agent, but such therapy does not seem to alter the clinical outcome and may just expose the patient to the risk of bleeding.

15. Compare the benefit of immediate angioplasty versus intravenous thrombolytic therapy.

Contraindications may prevent the use of intravenous thrombolytic therapy in 60–70% of patients presenting with acute myocardial infarction. Clearly, in this group, direct angioplasty presents a therapeutic option.

Recently, a study compared direct angioplasty to tPA (although not in accelerated dosing forms), and noted that percutaneous coronary angioplasty (without prior use of thrombolytic therapy) reduced the combined occurrence of reinfarction, death, and intracranial bleeding.

BIBLIOGRAPHY

 1. Anderson HV, Willerson JT: Thrombolysis in acute myocardial infarction. N Engl J Med 329:703–709, 1993.
 2. Arnold AZ, Topol EJ: Assessment of reperfusion after thrombolytic therapy for myocardial infarction. Am Heart J 124:441–447, 1992.
 3. Bar FW, Verheugt FW, Col J, et al: Thrombolysis in patients with unstable angina improves the angiographic but not clinical outcome. Circulation 86:131–137, 1992.
 4. Dewood MA, Spores J, Notske R, et al: Prevalence of total coronary occlusion during the early hours of transmural myocardial infarct. N Engl J Med 303:897–902, 1980.
 5. Fry TA, Sobel BE: Coronary thrombolysis. In Zipes DP (ed): Progress in Cardiology. Philadelphia, Lea & Febiger, 1990.
 6. Fuster V: Coronary thrombolysis—A perspective for the practicing physician. N Engl J Med 329:723–725, 1993.
 7. Grimes CL, et al: A comparison of immediate angioplasty with thrombolytic therapy for acute myocardial infarction. N Engl J Med 328:673–691, 1993.
 8. GUSTO Investigators: An international randomized trial comparing four thrombolytic strategies for acute myocardial infarction. N Engl J Med 329:673–682, 1993.
 9. Handin RI, Loscalzo J: Thrombolytic therapy. In Braunwald E (ed): Heart Disease: A Textbook of Cardiovascular Disease. Philadelphia, W.B. Saunders, 1992.
10. ISIS-2 Collaborative Group: Randomized trial of intravenous streptokinase, oral aspirin, both, or neither among 17,187 cases of suspected acute myocardial infarction: ISIS-2. Lancet 2:349–360, 1988.
11. Pasternak RC, Braunwald E: Coronary thrombolysis. In Braunwald E (ed): Heart Disease. Philadelphia, W.B. Saunders, 1992.
12. Reimer KA, et al: The wavefront phenomenon of ischemic cell death: 1. Myocardial infarct size versus duration of coronary occlusion in dogs. Circulation 56:786–794, 1977.
13. Sane DC, Califf RM, Topol EJ, et al: Bleeding during thrombolytic therapy for acute myocardial infarction: Mechanism and management. Ann Intern Med 111:1010–1022, 1989.
14. Wasserman AG, Ross AM: Coronary thrombolysis. Curr Probl Cardiol 14:5–54, 1989.

VII.   Other Medical Conditions with Associated Cardiac Involvement

54. HEART DISEASE IN PREGNANCY

Jeffrey Pickard, M.D.

1. What is peripartum cardiomyopathy?

A dilated cardiomyopathy that first presents during the last month of pregnancy or the first 6 months postpartum. The etiology is unclear, although by definition it is idiopathic, thereby eliminating hypertension, ischemic heart disease, viral myocarditis, and valvular heart disease.

It is characterized clinically by fatigue, dyspena, edema, cough, jugular venous distention, and S_3. Treatment includes bedrest, oxygen, and diuretics. Digitalis and afterload reduction may also be needed. Prognosis is excellent if complete recovery occurs within the first 6 months. Future pregnancies are generally discouraged, although the actual risk of recurrence is unclear.

2. What changes in cardiovascular physiology occur during normal pregnancy?

Cardiac output starts to rise by about 10 weeks' gestation and plateaus at about 40% above baseline during the second trimester. Blood volume increase to nearly 50% above baseline by around 32 weeks, while erythrocyte mass increases to about 30% above baseline. This accounts for the "physiologic anemia" of pregnancy. Despite the significant increase in cardiac output, blood pressure falls because of a marked diminution in systemic vascular resistance. Pulmonary vascular resistance also decreases.

3. How is this increase in cardiac output distributed to various organs?

The most dramatic increase in blood flow is to the uterus, which receives about 10 times the normal flow. However, this still accounts for a small proportion of the overall increase. Flow to the kidney increases 20–30% above baseline, the skin receives 2–3 times its normal flow, and the breasts receive 3–5 times their normal blood flow.

4. What cardiac signs and symptoms occur during normal pregnancy that may simulate disease?

Dyspnea, chest pains, easy fatigability, palpitations, light-headedness, and dizziness are symptoms that may be felt by the normal pregnant woman. On examination, edema, basilar rales, a loud pulmonic closure sound, S_3, and systolic murmur may be found during normal pregnancy.

5. How should mitral valve prolapse be managed during pregnancy?

Pregnancy has no adverse effects on this syndrome. Although some recommend endocarditis prophylaxis for labor and delivery, this is probably not necessary with routine vaginal delivery.

6. What other cardiac lesions are generally well tolerated during pregnancy?

- Aortic and mitral insufficiency if the patient is asymptomatic or only mildly symptomatic.
- Atrial septal defect, ventricular septal defect, and patent ductus arteriosus if corrected or without evidence of large left-to-right shunt or pulmonary hypertension.
- Tricuspid and pulmonary valvular lesions

7. In which cardiac conditions should pregnancy be avoided?
Uncorrected tetralogy of Fallot
Pulmonary hypertension
Eisenmenger's syndrome
Marfan's syndrome with a dilated aortic root
Cardiomyopathy of any cause
Coronary artery disease, especially in women with diabetes

8. What risks are associated with aortic valve disease during pregnancy?
Mild aortic stenosis may not pose significant problems during pregnancy. However, moderate or severe aortic stenosis is associated with significant maternal (17%) and fetal (32%) mortality. Maternal mortality may be as high as 50% after therapeutic abortion.

The transvalvular gradient increases during pregnancy as vascular volume increases and systemic vascular resistance decreases. However, the greatest risk occurs at the time of labor and delivery, when significant decreases in preload can lead to diminished cardiac output and myocardial ischemia, cerebral ischemia, and death. Invasive cardiac monitoring may be required to monitor preload.

9. What are the risks of mitral stenosis during pregnancy?
Mitral stenosis accounts for nearly 90% of rheumatic heart disease during pregnancy. Approximately 25% of women with mitral stenosis have their first symptoms during pregnancy.

As blood volume, heart rate, and cardiac output increase during pregnancy, the increased relative obstruction to flow across the stenosed mitral valve causes increased pulmonary venous congestion which, in turn, may lead to frank **pulmonary edema.** During delivery, the maternal circulation receives an additional 500 ml "autotransfusion" from the placenta, which can cause acute pulmonary edema. Medical management includes bed rest, digoxin if the patient is in atrial fibrillation, and diuresis. Cardioversion may be safely used when necessary. Closed valvulotomy is relatively safe during pregnancy. If this fails, mitral valve replacement has been performed with low fetal mortaltiy.

As indicated, **atrial fibrillation** may complicate mitral stenosis as atrial circumference increases. This leads to congestive heart failure as well as thromboembolic disease. In addition to treatment of the arrhythmia, patients should be chronically anticoagulated, usually with heparin.

During labor, patients with mitral stenosis may require invasive hemodynamic monitoring (remembering that pulmonary capillary wedge pressures do not reflect left ventricular filling pressures, so cardiac output must be monitored). Valsalva maneuver may acutely decrease preload, causing cardiac output to fall precipitously. Tachycardia can also cause diminished cardiac output, so regional anesthesia is generally used to minimize pain.

10. Can cardiac medications be used during pregnancy?
In general, most cardiovascular medications may be used during pregnancy. **Digoxin** crosses the placenta but has not been shown to be teratogenic, although levels must be carefully monitored to avoid toxicity. Serum levels generally fall during pregnancy.

Diuretics cross the placenta but are not teratogenic. Because of their potential effects on uteroplacental perfusion, they are usually not used to treat pregnancy-induced hypertension but may be continued during pregnancy in a woman who is taking them chronically.

Antiarrhythmic agents, such as procainamide and quinidine, have not been shown to be harmful to the fetus. Although concerns about intrauterine growth restriction exist, beta-blockers may also be used if indicated. Experience with newer antiarrhythmics (flecainide, mexiletine, amiodarone) is limited, but so far, no adverse effects have been reported.

Calcium channel blockers are gaining in use during pregnancy and may be used when necessary. These agents cross the placenta and have been used to treat fetal tachycardia in utero.

Angiotensin-converting enzyme inhibitors should be avoided during pregnancy because of reports of fetal loss in animals and because of case reports in humans of anuric renal failure, sometimes fatal, seen in neonates exposed in utero.

11. What risks are associated with cardiac valve prostheses during pregnancy?
Women with prosthetic valves can tolerate the hemodynamic effects of pregnancy without long-term deleterious effects. Maternal risks are increased due to thromboembolic events or hemorrhagic complications from anticoagulation. Prophylaxis against valve thrombosis must be maintained throughout pregnancy, usually with adjusted-dose heparin to keep the activated partial thromboplastin time at 1.5–2.0 times normal at mid-interval between doses. Some data exist to support warfarin use from the second trimester until 36 weeks' gestation, but this is controversial, to say the least.

Some suggest using bioprosthetic valves in young women of child-bearing age, because anticoagulation is often unnecessary with tissue valves. However, these valves are associated with a high failure rate, especially in women who become pregnant, and require replacement significantly more often than mechanical valves. Cryopreserved homografts are an emergency option.

Infective endocarditis is rare during pregnancy and delivery, but the consequences of prosthetic valve endocarditis are often catastrophic, so these women should be candidates for antibiotic prophylaxis during labor and delivery.

12. What other cardiac lesions necessitate endocarditis prophylaxis during delivery?
To be at risk for infective endocarditis, patients must not only have a condition but also undergo a procedure that places them at risk. Cesarean section, uncomplicated vaginal delivery, and therapeutic abortion are procedures not associated with endocarditis risk. There are, therefore, *no* cardiac conditions for which endocarditis prophylaxis is absolutely indicated during delivery.

13. How should a woman with congenital heart disease be counseled during pregnancy?
Most women with congenital heart lesions have no genetic syndrome associated with the lesion. Assuming that teratogenic exposure is not the cause, the overall risk of recurrence in their children appears to be about 5%. Of note, children of affected mothers appear to have a higher risk than those of affected fathers. The explanation for this is not clear.

Many anatomic defects can be diagnosed prenatally, and the use of fetal echocardiography is recommended in all pregnant women with congenital heart disease.

14. Can a woman breast-feed while taking a cardiac medication?
In almost all cases, breast-feeding women should be encouraged to continue. Only an estimated 2% of the maternal dose of a drug is ingested by the baby and is rarely of clinical significance. If necessary, drug levels can be monitored in breastfeeding infants.

Heparin does not get into breast milk, and the amount of warfarin ingested by the baby is too small to affect coagulation. Therefore, women taking warfarin may breast-feed their babies without concern.

BIBLIOGRAPHY

1. Cunningham FG, Pritchard JA, Hankins GDV, et al: Peripartum heart failure: Idiopathic cardiomyopathy or compounding cardiovascular events? Obstet Gynecol 67:157–168, 1986.
2. Easterling TR, Chadwick HS, Otto CM, Benedetti TJ: Aortic stenosis in pregnancy. Obstet Gynecol 72:113–118, 1988.
3. Gianopoulos JG: Cardiac disease in pregnancy. Med Clin North Am 73:639–651, 1989.
4. Lee W, Cotton DB: Peripartum cardiomyopathy: Current concepts and clinical management. Clin Obstet Gynecol 32:54–67, 1989.
5. Pitkin RM, Perloff JK, Koos BJ, Beall MH: Pregnancy and congenital heart disease. Ann Intern Med 112:445–454, 1990.
6. Raymond R, Underwood DA, Moodie DS: Cardiovascular problems in pregnancy. Cleve Clin J 54:95–103, 1987.
7. Sullivan JM, Ramanathan KB: Management of medical problems in pregnancy—Severe cardiac disease. N Engl J Med 313:304–309, 1985.

55. HEART DISEASE AND CANCER CHEMOTHERAPY

Marie E. Wood, M.D.

1. What conditions need to be considered when a cancer patient presents with heart failure?

Potential etiologies of congestive heart failure (CHF) in these individuals include:

- Superior vena caval obstruction or portal hypertension
- Lymphangitic spread of the primary tumor to the lung
- Cardiomyopathy, either intrinsic or drug-induced
- Pericardial disease: effusion or restrictive/constrictive pericarditis
- Infectious disease, such as tuberculosis or coxsackie B-induced pericarditis
- Autoimmune diseases, uremia, or hypothyroidism

2. Which chemotherapy drugs most frequently cause CHF?

The drug most commonly associated with CHF is doxorubicin. Daunorubicin, another anthracycline, also causes CHF but is used less frequently. The newer anthracyclines, mitoxantrone and idarubicin, are less cardiotoxic but, at high total doses, may cause CHF. 5-Fluorouracil and interferon also cause CHF.

3. How do the anthracyclines cause CHF?

The anthracycline (doxorubicin in experimental models) binds to cardiolipin in myocytes. This binding appears to have two consequences: (1) adenosine triphosphate (ATP) synthesis is disrupted, leading to decreased contractility; and (2) free radicals are generated by the anthracycline–cardiolipin complex. Free radical lipid peroxidation occurs and is believed to cause myocyte damage.

4. What increases anthracycline damage?

The most important factor is **dose.** Thirty percent of individuals treated with > 450–550 mg/m^2 develop CHF. Also important is the **route** of administration. When the **dosing schedule** was changed from large doses given once every 3 weeks to weekly dosing or continuous infusion over 24–72 hours, the incidence of toxicity decreased. Thus, fewer people developed CHF when given smaller doses more frequently.

Other factors that contribute to anthracycline-induced CHF include older age, concomitant drugs (mitomycin C may increase risk), prior or subsequent radiation therapy to the heart, and preexisting cardiac conditions (i.e., hypertension or myocardial infarction). The iron status of the individual may be important, with iron-deficient individuals tolerating more anthracycline.

5. How can you monitor for or diagnose anthracycline-induced cardiomyopathy?

The gold standard is endomyocardial biopsy, which can identify myocardial damage prior to the presence of clinical symptoms. This technique is a very expensive as well as invasive way to diagnose cardiomyopathy.

Other studies that may be helpful include echocardiogram and radionuclide cardiac angiography (MUGA). Generally, the anthracycline should be withheld if the left ventricular ejection fraction (LVEF) drops below 50% or decreases 10% during therapy.

6. How is anthracycline-induced cardiomyopathy treated?

Essentially the same as any other type of CHF: inotropic support and afterload reduction. Other than stopping the anthracycline, there are no special methods of treating this type of CHF.

7. Describe the natural history of anthracycline-induced cardiomyopathy.

Anthracycline-induced cardiomyopathy can present acutely (within days), subacutely (up to 30 months after the last dose), or late (6–20 years after the last dose). Most patients show symptomatic improvement with conventional treatment. If diagnosed early, symptoms may completely resolve.

8. How can anthracycline-induced cardiomyopathy be prevented?

Currently, close monitoring of the total dose and LVEF are the primary means of prevention. The drug should be stopped if the LVEF decreases 10% or to < 50% during a course of therapy. Attention to the age of the patient, route of administration, and any concomitant problems help to decrease the incidence of CHF. Cardioprotection against oxidative damage with vitamin E or N-acetylcysteine is being studied but has not shown conclusive benefit. Another cardioprotective agent, the iron-chelator ICRF-187, is being tested and looks promising in clinical trials.

9. Besides CHF, what other cardiac problems does chemotherapy cause?

1. Myocardial ischemia (from ST-T wave changes to infarction)
2. Arrhythmias (atrial and ventricular)
3. Pericardial effusions
4. Myocardial hemorrhage (very rarely)

10. When should chest pain be considered a complication of chemotherapy?

Chest pain and myocardial injury do not commonly occur with chemotherapy, but either can be seen with the vinca alkaloids (vincristine, vinblastine, and navelbine) as well as the new taxane, taxol. However, cancer patients can have myocardial infarctions, just like other individuals with risk factors. Myocardial injury due to the hypercoagulable state of Trousseau's syndrome is an important diagnosis to consider, as the treatment differs from that of other causes of myocardial injury (i.e., chronic heparinization).

11. What chemotherapeutic agents cause pericardial effusions?

Cyclophosphamide can cause a serosanguinous pericardial effusion. This is seen at very high doses when acute cardiac hemorrhage develops. Retinoic acid, interleukin-2 (IL-2), and other biologic agents can cause pericardial effusions as part of a syndrome of fever, dyspnea, edema, and pleural effusions.

12. Does radiation therapy damage the heart?

Yes. The development of shielding techniques has greatly reduced cardiac toxicity associated with mediastinal or lung radiation. Nevertheless, toxicity still occurs, especially when radiation is given along with certain chemotherapeutic agents. Among a host of cardiac abnormalities are pericardial disease, valvular disease, coronary artery disease, conduction abnormalities, and myocardial dysfunction. Prior to the development of shielding techniques, pericarditis and pleural effusions were more common complications. Now, coronary artery disease is the most common problem.

13. How does radiation therapy cause coronary artery disease?

Radiation appears to cause atherosclerotic lesions as well as an increase in coronary spasm. The atherosclerotic plaques develop without the usual cardiac risk factors and histologically have more fibrosis. Individuals with radiation-induced coronary artery disease are more likely to have involvement of the right coronary, left main, or left anterior descending arteries.

CONTROVERSIES

14. Should all patients receiving anthracyclines have LVEF determined before chemotherapy?
For: Any individual is at risk to decrease the LVEF with anthracyclines, and if caught early, severe toxicity may be prevented.
Against: Determination of LVEF may be an unnecessary cost to patients, especially if they are young or are going to receive < 450 mg/m^2 of doxorubicin.

15. Should patients receive endomyocardial biopsy to diagnose anthracycline-induced cardiomyopathy?
For: It is the best test. Endomyocardial biopsy is much more sensitive and specific than echocardiography or MUGA scan.
Against: Endomyocardial biopsy is expensive. It is an invasive procedure with a risk of myocardial perforation, which can be a morbid complication.

BIBLIOGRAPHY

1. Arsenian MA: Heart disease after mediastinal radiotherapy. Post-grad Med 91:211, 1992.
2. Braverman AC, Antin JH, Plappert MT, et al: Cyclophosphamide cardiotoxicity in bone marrow transplantation: A prospective evaluation of new dosing regimens. J Clin Oncol 9:1215–1223, 1991.
3. Casper ES, Gaynor JJ, Hajdu SI, et al: A prospective randomized trial of adjuvant chemotherapy with bolus versus continuous infusion of doxorubicin in patients with high grade extremity soft tissue sarcoma and an analysis of prognostic factors. Cancer 68:1221–1229, 1991.
4. Freeman NJ, Costanza ME: 5-Fluorouracil-associated cardiotoxicity. Cancer 61:36–45, 1988.
5. Hancock SL, Tucker MA, Hoppe RT: Factors affecting late mortality from heart disease after treatment of Hodgkin's disease. JAMA 270:1949–1959, 1993.
6. Naschitz JE, Yeshurun D, Abrahamson J, et al: Ischemic heart disease precipitated by occult cancer. Cancer 69:2712, 1992.
7. Rowinsky EK, McGuire WP, Guarnieri T, et al: Cardiac disturbances during the administration of taxol. J Clin Oncol 9:1704–1712, 1991.
8. Schwartz RG, McKenzie WB, Alexander J, et al: Congestive heart failure and left ventricular dysfunction complicating doxorubicin therapy. Am J Med 82:1109, 1987.
9. Sonnenblick M, Rosin A: Cardiotoxicity of interferon: A review of 44 cases. Chest 99:557, 1991.
10. Speyer JL, Green MD, Kramer E, et al: Protective effect of the bispiperazinedione ICRF-187 against doxorubicin-induced cardiac toxicity in women with advanced breast cancer. N Engl J Med 319:745–752, 1988.
11. Steinherz LJ, Steinherz PG, Tan CT, et al: Cardiac toxicity 4 to 20 years after completing anthracycline therapy. JAMA 266:1672–1677, 1991.

56. RENAL DISEASE AND THE HEART

Harmeet Singh, M.D.

1. What renal complications can occur from cardiac catheterization?

1. **Contrast nephrotoxicity:** acute renal failure occurring within 2–5 days of the procedure, due to nephrotoxic effects of contrast dyes. It is especially common in patients with preexisting chronic renal insufficiency and diabetes mellitus (> 60% incidence when 30 ml of dye was used).

2. **Atheroembolic renal disease:** mechanical disruption of aortic atheroma by the catheter and subsequent microembolization into the kidneys. Clinically, it is characterized by a sudden or slow increase in serum creatinine level, which is usually not completely reversible and occasionally may be associated with eosinophilia, thrombocytopenia, and transient decreases in serum complement levels. Urinary abnormalities may range from benign sediment to hematuria, proteinuria, eosinophiluria, or red cell casts. Embolization to other organs may occur (e.g., livedo reticularis, peripheral cyanosis, bowel ischemia).

2. What precautions can be taken to prevent or minimize contrast nephrotoxocity?

1. Recognize **high-risk individuals** prone to this complication (i.e., those with diabetes mellitus and chronic renal insufficiency).

2. **Volume replete,** because hypovolemic patients are at much higher risk. In patients without congestive heart failure or overt signs of volume excess, diuretics should be stopped at least 1–2 days before the procedure, and intravenous fluids should be started several hours before the test.

3. Intravenous **mannitol,** 25 g given before and after the procedure, may be protective. Monitor intake and output closely, and avoid negative fluid balance with mannitol diuresis. Mannitol is contraindicated in patients with severe renal insufficiency, in whom it can cause pulmonary edema secondary to the osmotic effect of mannitol.

3. Do nonionic, low-osmolality contrast media cause less contrast nephrotoxicity than conventional high-osmolality contrast media?

A lower adverse reaction profile of low-osmolality agents has been suggested, but there is no convincing evidence for decreased nephrotoxicity from controlled randomized human studies. Because these agents are about 20 times more expensive than the conventional high-osmolality agents, their routine use is not justified in the absence of clear evidence of a lower side effect profile.

4. What are the lipid abnormalities associated with renal disease?

- In **nephrotic syndrome,** elevation of total and low-density lipoprotein (LDL) cholesterol is a result of increased hepatic synthesis of lipoprotein B, most likely due to hypoalbuminemia. The hypercholesterolemia is usually severe.
- In **chronic renal failure,** hypertriglyceridemia is seen in 30% of patients. The defect may be due to the reduced lipolysis of triglyceride-rich lipoproteins (mainly very-low-density lipoproteins, VLDL).

5. Should these lipid abnormalities be treated?

The rationale for lowering lipid levels is to reduce the risk for coronary artery disease. The evidence for the independent role of lipids in causing progression of renal disease is largely experimental and *not* a rationale to lower lipid levels in renal disease.

The **hypercholesterolemia of nephrotic syndrome** should be treated, and because of its severity, dietary therapy alone is not sufficient. The drugs of choice are the HMG-CoA reductase inhibitors, which can reduce LDL cholesterol levels by 40–80 mg/dl. If another drug is needed, a bile acid sequestrant (cholestyramine) is the best choice for combination therapy.

For the **hypertriglyceridemia of chronic renal failure,** there is no scientific evidence to support the use of triglyceride-lowering agents in lowering the coronary artery disease risk, but there is ample evidence of a higher incidence of adverse reactions to these agents in this population.

6. What cardiac complications are seen after renal transplantation?
Coronary artery disease is a major cause of morbidity and mortality in the post-renal transplant period. An accelerated atherosclerosis occurs after renal transplant that has a multifactorial basis. These patients already have a high incidence of asymptomatic coronary artery disease (diabetes mellitus and renal insufficiency), and the use of steroids and cyclosporine, both of which cause lipid abnormalities, hastens atherosclerosis. These patients may have hypercholesterolemia, hypertriglyceridemia, or mixed hyperlipidemia. Other factors that contribute to the atherosclerotic risk and independent coronary artery disease risk are post-transplant hypertension, which is very common, and possibly post-transplant erythrocytosis, which may predispose to vascular thrombosis.

7. What should be done to prevent post-transplant coronary artery disease?
Preexisting coronary artery disease is an important predictor of post-transplant ischemic events, and aggressive attempts should be made to identify and treat (medically and surgically) pretransplant patients with coronary artery disease. In diabetic patients there is a high incidence of silent ischemia and pretransplant stress testing should be done. Aggressive pretransplant treatment improves the patient survival in this group.

After transplantion, patients with known coronary artery disease should have regular follow-up, and diagnostic evaluation should be instituted on appearance of the first symptom related to coronary ischemia. Other means of treatment include:
  A. **Lowering lipid levels:**
    1. Achieving ideal body weight.
    2. Eliminate medications that alter lipids (i.e., beta blockers, diuretics).
    3. Decrease prednisone and cyclosporine dose if possible.
    4. Use cholesterol-lowering agents. HMG-CoA inhibitors should be used cautiously because of their high-risk of complications in the post-transplant population.
  B. **Modifying other risk factors:**
    1. Smoking cessation.
    2. Blood pressure control.
    3. Exercise.
    4. Improving glycemic control.

8. Describe the common causes of azotemia seen in congestive heart failure.
There is frequently an elevation of blood urea nitrogen (BUN) and creatinine (Cr) seen in patients with congestive heart failure.

a. Prenal azotemia is the most important cause of acute increases in BUN and Cr in patients with congestive heart failure and is secondary to reduced renal perfusion resulting either from true volume contraction due to diuretic use or from decreased cardiac output. It is manifested by an increased BUN/Cr ratio (normally <10:1), benign urinary sediment, low urine sodium (<20 mEq/L), and a low fractional excretion of sodium (<1%).

b. Acute tubular necrosis results from a prolonged prerenal state resulting in ischemic renal tubular injury with increased BUN and Cr, a normal BUN/Cr ratio, granular casts and renal epithelial cells in urine, high urine sodium (>20 mEq/L), and elevated fractional excretion of sodium (>1%). This is a reversible insult.

c. Ischemic nephropathy is characterized by subacute or chronic deterioration of renal function in patients with congestive heart failure and atherosclerotic disease with or without hypertension. The underlying renal lesion is bilateral renal artery stenosis.

9. Does the use of angiotension-converting enzyme (ACE) inhibitors in heart failure carry any associated risks?

Clearly, the ACE inhibitors are the agents of choice in patients with congestive heart failure because they improve survival. However, ACE inhibitors also can cause renal insufficiency in severe congestive heart failure.

In congestive heart failure, renal hypoperfusion results in elevated renin and angiotensin II levels. Angiotensin II causes efferent more than afferent vasoconstriction and helps maintain the glomerular filtration rate. Because ACE inhibitors block angiotensin II synthesis, the protective effect of angiotensin II to maintain glomerular filtration rate is lost as a result of efferent vasodilatation. This is a reversible phenomenon. In some situations, there is small increase in creatinine with the use of ACE inhibitors which then stabilizes, in these patients, ACE inhibitors may be continued. The survival benefits from the ACE inhibitors outweigh the minor increases in serum creatinine.

10. What are the electrocardiographic (ECG) abnormalities seen in various electrolyte disturbances?

1. **Hypokalemia:** Flattened T waves, U waves, ST depression, arrhythmias (atrial and ventricular arrhythmias), prolonged QT intervals.

2. **Hyperkalemia:** Tall peaked T waves in precordial leads, followed by decreased amplitude of R waves, widened QRS complex, prolonged PR interval, and decreased amplitude and disappearance of P wave; arrhythmias

3. **Hypocalcemia:** Prolonged QT interval, arrhythmias

4. **Hypercalcemia:** Shortened QT interval, arrhythmias

5. **Hypermagnesemia:** Bradycardia, heart block (various degrees)

6. **Hypomagnesemia:** Arrhythmias, prolonged QT interval

11. Are there any risks in using nonsteroidal anti-inflammatory drugs (NSAIDs) in patients with congestive heart failure?

In congestive cardiac failure, decreased renal blood flow results from low cardiac output. There are adaptive attempts to maintain renal blood flow and glomerular filtration rate (GFR) through various mechanisms, both intrinsic and extrinsic to the kidney (such as circulating hormones, e.g., adrenergic system, renin angiotensin system). An important intrinsic adaptation by the kidney is the release of vasodilator prostaglandins (PGE_2, PGI_2), which maintain renal blood flow and GFR by afferent arteriolar vasodilation. Hence, NSAID use in this setting counteracts this physiologic adaptation by inhibiting the production of vasodilator prostaglandins, thereby decreasing GFR.

12. What is uremic pericarditis?

In end-stage renal disease, there are two types of pericarditis: **uremic pericarditis** occurs prior to initiation of dialysis; **dialysis pericarditis** is seen in patients on stable maintenance hemodialysis. The pathogenesis of uremic pericarditis seems to relate to uremic toxins, since it improves with dialysis. The causative factors for dialysis pericarditis are unclear. Fluid overload may contribute to both forms of pericarditis.

13. What are clinical features of uremic pericarditis?

A. Physical findings
1. Chest pain (60–70%)
2. Pericardial rub (> 90%)
3. Fever (60–90%)
4. Hypotension
B. Laboratory abnormalities
1. ECG changes
2. Leukocytosis
3. Abnormal chest x-ray
4. Demonstration of pericardial fluid on echocardiogram

Systemic features and cardiac tamponade are more common in dialysis pericarditis. The pericardial fluid can range from serous, serosanguineous, to hemorrhagic.

14. How is it treated?

The presence of **uremic pericarditis** in patients with end-stage renal disease is an absolute indication to initiate dialysis. Even in **dialysis pericarditis,** increasing intensity of dialysis (frequency and duration) should be the first step, as this results in resolution of disease in many patients. Pericardiocentesis is reserved for patients with hemodynamic compromise secondary to cardiac tamponade. These patients eventually need either pericardiotomy or pericardiectomy. NSAIDs and steroids are generally not beneficial in treating uremic pericarditis.

15. What is uremic cardiomyopathy?

Uremic cardiomyopathy is a broad term and is defined as abnormal left ventricular function seen in patients with end-stage renal disease. The etiology of heart failure in these patients is multifactorial. Hypertension, coronary artery disease, and volume overload seem to be the major causative factors. Others include anemia, arteriovenous fistula, acid-base/electrolyte abnormalities, secondary hyperparathyroidism, nutritional deficiencies, β_2-microglobulin, and uremic toxins.

16. Does hemodialysis result in cardiovascular consequences?

1. **Hypotension:** This is the commonest side effect of hemodialysis, and the etiology is multifactorial.

2. **Electrolyte disturbance:** Rapid changes of serum, potassium, calcium, magnesium, and pH occur which affect cell membrane potential and may lead to cardiac arrhythmias.

3. **Arteriovenous fistula:** A fistula is an area of low resistance that leads to increased cardiac output and workload, which can cause heart failure.

17. List the renal diseases seen in infective endocarditis.

- Renal emboli
- Acute tubular necrosis (secondary to renal ischemia)
- Interstitial nephritis (a complication of antibiotics used)
- Immune-mediated glomerulonephritis (due to immune complex deposition in the kidney)

18. Describe the common electrolyte disorders seen in congestive heart failure.

1. **Hyponatremia:** *Hypervolemic hyponatremia* occurs in the face of excess total body sodium and reflects excessive water retention. *Hypovolemic hyponatremia* occurs in aggressively treated patients on diuretics and is due to true volume depletion from excessive diuresis leading to antidiuretic hormone (ADH) release. Urinary analysis in both the types of hyponatremia shows low urine sodium (< 20 mEq/L), low fractional excretion of sodium (< 1%), and elevated urine osmolality.

2. **Hypokalemia:** Excessive urinary K losses are a result of elevated aldosterone concentrations, due to poor renal perfusion or diuretic use.

3. **Hyperkalemia:** This can occur from low urinary K excretion or use of ACE inhibitors.

4. **Hypomagnesemia:** This results from diuretic use, especially loop diuretics, which cause urinary magnesium losses.

19. What acid-base abnormalities are seen in congestive heart failure?

1. Respiratory alkalosis (due to hyperventilation from hypoxemia)
2. Metabolic acidosis (poor tissue perfusion resulting in anaerobic metabolism
3. Metabolic alkalosis (excessive diuretic use and hypovolemia)
4. Respiratory acidosis (rare except in severe congestive heart failure, when after prolonged hyperventilation, there is respiratory muscle fatigue and elevation of PCO_2

BIBLIOGRAPHY

1. Case records of the Massachusetts General Hospital (case #34-1991). N Engl J Med 325:563, 1991.
2. Comty CM, Wathen RL, Shapiro FL: Uremic pericarditis. Cardiovasc Clin 7:219, 1976.
3. Daugirdas JT: Dialysis hypotension: A hemodynamic analysis. Kidney Int 33:233, 1991.
4. Grundy SM: Management of hyperlipidemia of kidney disease. Kidney Int 37:847, 1990.
5. Hirshfield JW: Low osmolality contrast agents: Who needs them? N Engl J Med 326:482, 1992.
6. Jacobson HR: Ischemic renal disease: An overlooked clinical entity. Kidney Int 34:729, 1988.
7. Kasiske BL, Umen AJ: Persistent hyperlipidemia in renal transplant patients. Medicine 66:309, 1987.
8. Manske CL, Sprafka MJ, Strony JT, Wang Y: Contrast nephrography in azotemic diabetic patients undergoing coronary angiography. Am J Med 89:615, 1990.
9. Neugarten J, Baldwin DS. Glomerulonephritis in bacterial endocarditis. Am J Med 77:297, 1984.
10. Pastan SO, Braunwald E: Renal disorders and heart disease. In Braunwald E: Heart Disease, 4th ed. Philadelphia, W.B. Saunders, 1992.
11. Schrier RW: Pathogenesis of sodium and water retention in high-output and low-output cardiac failure, nephrotic syndrome, cirrhosis and pregnancy. N Engl J Med 319:1065, 1988.
12. Schrier RW, Gottschalk CW. Diseases of the Kidney, 5th ed. Boston, Little, Brown, 1992.

57. ENDOCRINE AND NUTRITIONAL DISORDERS AND HEART DISEASE

Jane Reusch, M.D., and Fred D. Hofeldt, M.D.

1. In acromegaly, what associated cardiac diseases may be seen?
Coexisting cardiovascular diseases are common in acromegaly and are the most common cause of death in untreated acromegalic individuals. Evidence for cardiac enlargement, hypertrophy, diastolic filling abnormalities, congestive heart failure, arrhythmias, myocardiopathy, arterial hypertension, aortic and mitral valve disease, and advanced atherosclerotic diseases (including coronary artery disease) are seen. Diabetes mellitus with associated hyperinsulinism contributes to the increased atherosclerotic occurrence, morbidity, and mortality.

2. What hemodynamic changes are seen in hyperthyroidism?
Patients with hyperthyroidism have a high cardiac output state, characterized by increased stroke volume and increased pulse rate. There is a decreased peripheral vascular resistance, increased blood volume, increased pulse pressure, and a hyperdynamic precordium, resulting from increasing cardiac contractility.

3. What cardiac manifestations may be seen in hyperthroidism?
- Hypertension (particularly isolated systolic hypertension)
- Sinus tachycardia
- Premature atrial contractions
- Paroxysmal atrial tachycardia
- Atrial fibrillation
- Conduction disturbances (varying degrees)
- High output heart failure (with cardiomyopathy)
- Low output failure (with underlying comprised left ventricular function)
- Mitral valve prolapse
- Ischemic heart disease with angina and coronary insufficiency

4. How is atrial fibrillation managed in hyperthyroidism?
Hyperthryoid patients with atrial fibrillation are at an increased risk for peripheral thromboembolism. Anticoagulation is recommended. These patients may be resistant to the usual dosage of digitalis. Beta blockers are frequently helpful.

5. What are the cardiac hemodynamic changes in hypothyroidism?
The hypothyroid patient has decreased cardiac contractility and presents with increased peripheral vascular resistance, decreased blood volume, decreased cardiac output, decreased heart rate, and decreased pulse pressure.

6. What are the cardiovascular presentations of hypothyroidism?
The cardiovascular manifestations of hypothyroidism may include bradycardia, a quiet precordium, diastolic hypertension, and a dilated cardiac silhouette on chest x-ray. Patients may have pericardial effusions accounting for the cardiac enlargement. However, worsening congestive heart failure occurs in the hypothyroid state as thyroid hormone deficiency leads to decreased myocardial contractility. Some patients may present with noncardiac chest pain and elevations in creatinine kinase, with elevation of the MM fraction ruling out myocardial infarction. Electrocardiographic (ECG) abnormalities typically include sinus bradycardia, nonspecific ST-T wave abnormalities, and low voltage. Hypothyroidism has been seen in association with ventricular

arrhythmias, including torsade de pointes. Hypothyroid patients have increased prevalence of atherosclerotic heart disease, which may be related to the dyslipidemia accompanying hypothyroidism.

7. What consideration is needed in hypertensive patients with low potassium?

Excess adrenal mineralocorticoids cause hypertension in < 1% of the population. However, they may be implicated when the hypertension is associated with hypokalemia, particularly in the patient who has a high salt intake or may not be taking diuretics.

8. Which mineralocorticoids cause hypertension?

Aldosterone, 11-desoxycorticosterone (DOC), and corticosterone (B).

9. Which laboratory tests exclude the diagnosis of Cushing's syndrome?

Frequently, a simple overnight **dexamethasone suppression test** will assist in evaluating the patient with suspected Cushing's syndrome. The patient is given 1 mg of dexamethasone at 11 P.M., and the plasma cortisol is measured at 8 A.M. the following morning. Values less than 5 µg/dl indicate normal suppression, values between 5 and 10 µg/dl are borderline, and values >10 µg/dl are abnormal.

An equally helpful test is a 24-hour urine measurement for **free cortisol.** Patients with elevated urinary free cortisol or nonsuppressible cortisol values should be evaluated for Cushing's syndrome.

10. Which laboratory test is used to characterize Cushing's disease?

A failure to suppress to 1-mg overnight dexamethasone (or its equivalent test, 0.5 mg of dexamethasone administered every 6 hours for 2 days) or an elevated 24-hour urine free cortisol is seen in patients with Cushing's syndrome. Cushing's disease (hypothalamic-pituitary Cushing's) is distinguished from the other causes of Cushing's syndrome by a 50% reduction in the plasma cortisol value after an 8-mg overnight dexamethasone suppression or a similar 50% suppression in urinary cortisol metabolites (17-hydroxycorticosteroids or free cortisol) with the long suppression test of 2 mg of dexamethasone every 6 hours for 2 days. Patients with pituitary Cushing's disease have normal to slightly elevated plasma ACTH levels. They show enhanced responsiveness to corticotropin-releasing factor (CRF) testing, which helps distinguish them from patients with adrenal forms of Cushing's syndrome and ectopic Cushing's syndrome, where there is usually no ACTH response to CRF testing. Localization of pituitary Cushing's disease is achieved by inferior petrosal sinus sampling for ACTH during a CRF infusion.

11. What clinical features in a hypertensive patient suggest the presence of pheochromocytoma?

1. Headache, which is characteristically, but not always, pounding and severe
2. Palpitations with or without tachycardia
3. Excessive, inappropriate perspiration

12. How is pheochromocytoma best diagnosed?

For screening purposes, a 24-hour urine collection for vanillylmandelic acid (VMA), total catecholamines (epinephrine, norepinephrine), and metanephrine, normetanephrine, and creatinine will frequently establish the diagnosis in the hypertensive patient. Occasionally, urinary catecholamines and their metabolites collected during a typical "spell" will be helpful in diagnosing the patient with episodic disease. In patients requiring further evaluation, plasma catecholamines can be measured under standardized conditions; patients with pheochromocytoma have plasma catecholamine values > 950 pg/ml (5.62 nmol/L). These values will not suppress on the clonidine suppression test. Provocative stimulation tests for pheochromocytoma such as glucagon, histamine, and tyramine are considered dangerous and should be avoided.

13. What is syndrome X?

This multimetabolic syndrome describes the association of certain clinical features and risk factors predictive of coronary artery disease: abdominal obesity (waist/hip >0.85), hypertension, carbohydrate intolerance or type II diabetes mellitus, and dyslipidemia (hypertriglyceridemia and low high-density lipoprotein [HDL] levels). The unifying associations with these clinical states are hyperinsulinemia and insulin resistance. Other related findings in these patients include hyperuricemia, physical inactivity, and aging. In contrast to this metabolic syndrome X, a cardiac syndrome X exists in which patients have anginal symptoms, normal coronary arteries on catheterization studies, but small, more distal occlusive disease (microvascular angina). Both syndromes may coexist in the same patient.

14. How common is coronary artery disease in patients with diabetes mellitus?

Coronary artery disease is the most common cause of morbidity and mortality in diabetic individuals, being 1.2–6.6 times more prevalent than in the nondiabetic population. Its predominance is even greater in individuals with non-insulin-dependent diabetes and in diabetic females. Seventy-seven percent of all diabetic hospitalizations are related to coronary artery disease.

15. What are the risk factors for coronary artery disease in diabetic patients?

Diabetes alone is an independent cardiovascular risk factor, along with the classic cardiac risk factors of advancing age, male gender, postmenopausal status in females, cigarette smoking, hypertension, family history of coronary artery disease, and dyslipidemia. Diabetes has been noted to amplify the effects of these classic risk factors for coronary artery disease. In patients with insulin-dependent diabetes mellitus, hypertension and proteinuria are the strongest risk factors associated with coronary artery disease. In individuals with non-insulin-dependent diabetes, hypertriglyceridemia and proteinuria are the most potent risk factors.

16. How is proteinuria implicated?

Proteinuria is the strongest predictor of cardiovascular mortality in all individuals with diabetes mellitus. It is frequently associated with hypertension and is a marker of renal disease. It is also associated with increased fibrinogen and increased platelet aggregability, as well as abnormalities in lipid profiles.

17. What is the role of fibrinolysis?

Abnormally slow fibrinolysis is a recently established independent risk factor for coronary artery disease. In individuals with non-insulin-dependent diabetes mellitus, there is an increase in plasma-activating inhibitor-1 activity (PAI-1 activity). This has been associated with insulin resistance, and there is a direct correlation between hyperinsulinemia and an increase in PAI-1 activity.

18. Is it true that in diabetic patients, the atherosclerotic disease is more diffuse and seldom operable?

No. It has long been assumed that diffuse coronary atherosclerosis is associated with diabetes mellitus, implying that these patients have an inoperable disease. Recent data have failed to show any true incidence of more diffuse coronary artery disease in diabetic individuals compared with non-diabetics. This observation is important when considering revascularization by coronary artery bypass graft. The vessels do appear to be similarly operable in both groups.

19. Is there a difference in success rate for coronary artery bypass grafting in diabetic versus nondiabetic patients?

No. Although diabetics have a higher risk of perioperative groin and sternal wound infections, as well as renal insufficiency, the late follow-up after surgery shows a similar survival and symptom-free interval for diabetics compared to nondiabetics. One study suggested a slower flow rate in the grafts of individuals with diabetes, but this has not been confirmed in subsequent studies. Overall, the two groups behave similarly.

20. What is diabetic cardiomyopathy?

Diabetic cardiomyopathy is abnormal cardiac function leading to congestive heart failure symptoms in individuals without coronary artery disease, valvular disease, rheumatic fever, or other known cardiac disease. Hence, individuals with diabetic cardiomyopathy have classic symptoms of congestive heart failure (i.e., paroxysmal nocturnal dyspnea, orthopnea, edema, dyspnea on exertion) in the absence of any obvious cause for their cardiomyopathy besides diabetes mellitus. Pathologically, these individuals have a dilated cardiomegaly and interstitial fibrosis. Some reports have described an interstitial deposition of a periodic acid–Schiff-positive material. Approximately, 15% of the individuals with diabetes and congestive heart failure in the Framingham study were believed to have diabetic cardiomyopathy. As such, this is a common clinical entity.

21. Is angina a reliable marker of ischemic disease in diabetics?

No. Classically, many individuals with diabetes have been thought to have silent ischemia. Individuals with diabetic autonomic neuropathy clearly have an increased incidence of silent myocardial infarction secondary to abnormal enervation of the heart. However, despite a plethora of studies, it has not been shown conclusively whether silent ischemia is more common in diabetics without autonomic neuropathy.

Because there is a significant incidence of autonomic neuropathy that could impair angina or anginal equivalents in individuals with diabetes, it is important to do an aggressive workup of nonspecific symptoms or those of early congestive heart failure, especially in individuals with long-standing diabetes.

22. In acute myocardial infarction, what are the implications of concurrent diabetes?

Overall, individuals with diabetes do significantly worse than nondiabetics in the setting of acute myocardial infarction. They suffer from an increased frequency of events during their initial hospitalization as well as long-term.

In the acute setting, individuals with diabetes are more prone to develop shock, congestive heart failure, myocardial rupture, and reinfarction, all of which are associated with increased mortality. Because of the increased catecholamine surge associated with acute myocardial infarction a transient increase in glucose concentration frequently develops.

Delayed complications of acute myocardial infarction are also more common among diabetics. The survival following myocardial infarction at 1, 2, and 5 years is 82%, 78%, and 58% in diabetics compared with 94%, 92%, and 82% in nondiabetics. Although β-blockers are relatively contraindicated in diabetes, they are of benefit after myocardial infarction and should be given. An associated asymptomatic hypoglycemia may be present and requires frequent monitoring in patients on insulin and oral agents.

23. What is beriberi? Who gets it?

Beriberi is a thiamine deficiency which is relatively uncommon in the United States. In the Middle East and Asia, it is seen among people who wash their rice before they eat it. They develop a thiamine deficiency while replete in other vitamin status (wet beriberi). It is characterized by malaise and fatigue, an increased cardiac output secondary to decreased systemic vascular resistance and increased venous return, and edema with enlarged cardiac silhouettes and pulmonary effusions. They respond very well to thiamine replacement.

Dry beriberi is thiamine deficiency in generalized protein calorie malnutrition and is more commonly seen in the United States. Individuals with poor caloric intake which is relatively high in carbohydrates, e.g., alcoholics, are at risk. The usual clinical picture is an elevated heart rate with warm hands (representing the decreased systemic vascular resistance), and a generalized neuropathy (including motor deficits and decreased reflexes). This can be associated with a nutritional cirrhosis or paresthesias of the extremities. Treatment is with thiamine replacement but may include early digitalis and diuretics.

BIBLIOGRAPHY

1. Becker C: Hypothyroidism and atherosclerotic heart disease. Endocr Rev 6:432–440, 1985.
2. Bravo EL, Gifford RW: Pheochromocytoma: Diagnosis, localization and management. N Engl J Med 311:1298–1303, 1984.
3. Donahue RP, Orchard TJ: Diabetes mellitus and macrovascular complications: an epidemiological perspective. Diabetes Care 15:1141–1155, 1992.
4. Fein FS, Scheuer J: Heart disease in diabetes. In Rifkin H, Porte D (eds): Ellenberg and Rifkin's Diabetes Mellitus: Theory and Practice, 4th ed. New York, Elsevier, 1990, pp 812–823.
5. Fuh MM, Jeng C, Young M, et al: Insulin resistance, glucose intolerance and hyperinsulinemia in a patient with microvascular angina. Metabolism 42:1090–1092, 1993.
6. Ganda OP, Arkin CF: Hyperfibrinogenemia: An important risk factor for vascular complications in diabetes. Diabetes Care 15:1245–1250, 1992.
7. Gwynne JT, McMillan DE: Summary and highlights of the XIV International Diabetes Federation Satellite Sympoisum on Macrovascular Complications of Diabetes. Diabetes 41(suppl 2):116–119, 1992.
8. Jarrett RJ: Risk factors for coronary heart disease in diabetes mellitus. Diabetes 41:1–3, 1992.
9. Koskinen P, Mänttäri M, Manninen V, et al: Coronary heart disease incidence in NIDDM patients in the Helsinki Heart Study. Diabetes Care 15:820–825, 1992.
10. LeMar HJ, West SG, Hofeldt FD, et al: Covert hypothyroidism presenting as a cardiovascular event. Am J Med 91:549–552, 1991.
11. Liao Y, Cooper RS, Ghali JK, Lansky D, Cao G, Lee J: Sex differences in the impact of coexistent diabetes on survival in patients with coronary heart disease. Diabetes Care 16:708–713, 1993.
12. Schneider DJ, Nordt TK, Sobel BE: Attenuated fibrinolysis and accelerated atherogenesis in Type II diabetic patients. Diabetes 42:1–7, 1993.
13. Sheps SG, Jiang N, Klee GG: Diagnostic evaluation of pheochromocytoma. Endocr Metab Clin North Am 17:397–414, 1988.
14. Sniderman A, Michel C, Racine N: Heart disease in patients with diabetes mellitus. In Draznin B, Eckel R (eds): Diabetes and Atherosclerosis: Molecular Basis and Clinical Aspects. New York, Elsevier, 1993, pp 255–274.
15. Stamler J, Vaccaro O, Neaton JD, Wentworth D: Diabetes, other risk factors, and 12-yr cardiovascular mortality for men screened in the Multiple Risk Factor Intervention Trial. Diabetes Care 16:434–444, 1993.
16. Williams GH, Braunwald E: Endocrine and nutritional disorders and heart disease. In Braunwald E (ed): Heart Disease: A Textbook of Cardiovascular Medicine, 4th ed. Philadelphia, W.B. Saunders, 1992, pp 1827–1855.

58. CARDIAC MANIFESTATIONS OF RHEUMATOLOGIC DISORDERS

Richard W. Erickson, M.D., and Mark Malyak, M.D.

1. What are the cardiovascular manifestations of Marfan syndrome?

Marfan syndrome is an example of an heritable disorder of connective tissue that may have cardiovascular manifestations. It is an autosomal dominant disease that in many cases appears to be due to a mutation in the gene encoding for fibrillin, a component of the connective tissue microfibril. The characteristic skeletal abnormalities of the classic form of Marfan syndrome include increased limb length, pectus excavatum or carinatum, spinal deformities, and arachnodactyly. Excessive height is due to long lower extremities; therefore, the ratio of upper segment (top of head to pubis) to lower segment (pubis to heel) is abnormally low. Ocular abnormalities include subluxation of the lens and myopia.

Cardiovascular abnormalities, particularly sequelae of dilatation of the ascending aorta, are responsible for the majority of excessive deaths in Marfan syndrome. Aortic insufficiency results primarily from dilatation of the annulus and the ascending aorta. Compared with the mitral valve, myxomatous degeneration of the aortic valve leaflets probably plays only a minor role. The most feared complication of Marfan syndrome is acute dissection or rupture of the aorta, which often results in the patient's death. The degree of dilatation of the ascending aorta appears to correlate with the risk of aortic regurgitation, aortic dissection, and aortic rupture. Mitral valve prolapse potentially leading to severe mitral regurgitation is also commonly seen in patients with Marfan syndrome. As opposed to aortic insufficiency, the primary pathologic process occurs within the mitral valve leaflets themselves, termed myxomatous degeneration.

Simple bedside examination, chest radiography, and electrocardiography are insufficiently sensitive to diagnose and assess the degree of aortic dilatation, the best predictor of impending acute aortic dissection or rupture. Therefore, annual echocardiography is recommended in all patients with Marfan syndrome. Once the diameter of the aortic root reaches 45–50 mm, it is reasonable to assess the patient every 3 months; once the diameter reaches 55–60 mm, prophylactic surgery should be considered. Pharmacologic beta-adrenergic antagonism may be beneficial in patients with dilated aortic roots who are not yet candidates for surgery. Isometric exercise should be avoided. In addition to assessment of the aorta and aortic valve, echocardiography also allows evaluation of the mitral valve. Finally, antibiotic prophylaxis for infective endocarditis is necessary in patients with mitral or aortic regurgitation.

2. What other heritable disorders of connective tissue may result in cardiovascular abnormalities?

Ehlers-Danlos syndrome
Osteogenesis imperfecta
Homocystinuria

3. Polyarteritis nodosa causes what cardiac abnormalities?

Polyarteritis nodosa (PAN) is a primary vasculitis syndrome that results in necrotizing vasculitis of medium and small-sized muscular arteries. Though by no means definite, immune complex deposition within vessel walls is likely responsible. In certain patients the antigen has been identified, and in such cases is most commonly hepatitis B surface antigen (HBsAg). The manifestations of the disease result from systemic inflammation (constitutional symptoms such as fatigue, malaise, anorexia, and weight loss that are likely manifestations of circulating cytokines) and focal tissue ischemia and infarction as a consequence of vascular compromise resulting from the vasculitic process. Focal aneurysms of vessels may occur and occasionally rupture.

Involvement of the renal vasculature commonly results in hyperreninemic hypertension, which may lead to secondary cardiovascular disease. Primary involvement of the heart is also common in PAN, usually due to vasculitis of the medium and small-sized muscular arteries. The vessels involved are usually smaller and more distal than those involved in atherosclerotic heart disease. Occlusion of these vessels due to vasculitis may result in recurrent and usually small myocardial infarctions, leading to patchy myocardial fibrosis on pathologic examination. It may manifest clinically as angina pectoris, acute myocardial infarction, sudden death, dysrhythmias, or congestive heart failure. Fibrinous pericarditis due to the underlying inflammatory disease may occur, but is more commonly due to uremia. Finally, conduction defects may occur as a result of ischemia/infarction or inflammation extending beyond vessels into the SA and AV nodes.

The treatment for PAN includes high-dose glucocorticoids and often cytotoxic therapy, particular the administration of daily, oral cyclophosphamide.

4. What other primary vasculitic syndrome may affect the cardiovascular system?

Allergic angiitis and granulomatosis (Churg-Strauss syndrome)
Hypersensitivity vasculitis syndromes
Wegener's granulomatosis
Giant cell arteritis (temporal arteritis)
Takayasu's arteritis
Behçet's disease
Kawasaki disease

5. Can subacute bacterial endocarditis mimic a primary arthritic condition?

Yes. Extracardiac manifestations of subacute bacterial endocarditis (SBE) may be due to circulating cytokines, deposition of immune complexes, or embolic phenomena. Since SBE is an inflammatory process, cytokines may be elaborated into the circulation and result in symptoms such as fever, fatigue, malaise, anorexia, and weight loss, findings common in primary rheumatologic disorders. Circulating immune complexes due to the chronic antigenemia are common; these may deposit in a variety of end organs such as the kidney where they may lead to acute glomerulonephritis, also a common finding in a variety of rheumatologic disorders. This mechanism likely also contributes to the arthritis which may be present in SBE. Additionally, direct infection of joints (septic arthritis) may occur secondary to the chronic bacteremia. Embolic disease may result in infarction of a variety of end organs, including the brain and heart. To make the situation even more confusing, 24-50% of patients with SBE are rheumatoid factor positive due to the chronic antigenemia. Therefore, blood cultures should be obtained in every patient with fever and arthritis to exclude the possibility of SBE.

6. Rheumatoid arthritis rarely affects the heart. True or false?

Rheumatoid arthritis (RA) is a systemic autoimmune disease of unknown etiology that manifests predominantly as a chronic, symmetric, inflammatory synovitis of the peripheral joints. Extraarticular manifestations are quite variable and usually mild but occasionally severe and life-threatening. Extraarticular manifestations are usually due to vasculitis of small blood vessels or to granulomatous infiltration in end organs.

Although only 2% of patients with RA manifest symptoms of pericarditis, evaluation of patients by echocardiography or during postmortem examination reveals evidence of pericardial inflammation in approximately 30% of patients. Most patients with symptomatic pericarditis respond to treatment with nonsteroidal anti-inflammatory drugs (NSAIDs). Pericardial tamponade and constrictive pericarditis are unusual but well-described complications.

Like pericarditis, focal or diffuse granulomatous infiltration of the myocardium, endocardium, and valves is a fairly common pathologic finding that rarely manifests clinically. Microscopically, this finding resembles the rheumatoid nodule, with which it likely shares a common pathologic origin. Clinical manifestations, when they occur, include congestive heart failure, valvular dysfunction, and dysrhythmias.

Inflammation of the coronary arteries is demonstrable in approximately 20% of patients on postmortem examination but, like the other cardiac manifestations of RA, rarely manifests clinically as myocardial ischemia.

7. How may systemic lupus erythematosus affect the heart?

Systemic lupus erythematosus (SLE) is a systemic autoimmune disease of unknown etiology characterized by the production of various autoantibodies, including antibodies directed against nucleic acids and (deoxy)ribonucleoproteins, cell membrane epitopes (blood cells, neurons), and phospholipids. Clinical manifestations result from deposition of immune complexes or through the interaction of antibodies that directly interfere with cellular or coagulation function.

The most common cardiac manifestation of SLE is **pericarditis,** which is found in up to 80% of postmortem examinations. Clinical manifestations of pericarditis, either characteristic pain or an auditory rub on auscultation, may be present at some time in up to 50% of patients. SLE tends to be an episodic disorder characterized by remissions and exacerbations; pericarditis associated with SLE tends to follow this general rule. Cardiac compression due to large effusions or to constrictive pericarditis has been reported but is unusual.

Congestive heart failure in the patient with SLE may be secondary to various extracardiac causes, including renal failure and hypertension. Occasionally, myocarditis due to infiltration of the myocardium by inflammatory cells may manifest clinically as congestive heart failure or dysrhythmias.

Endocarditis caused by Libman-Sacks vegetations is present in up to 75% of patients with SLE on postmortem examination. These small 1–4 mm lesions are found on the edge of the mitral and aortic valves most commonly but occasionally involve the right-sided valves, valve rings, papillary muscles, and endocardium. They are usually clinically silent but occasionally may lead to valvular compromise, embolic phenomenon, and bacterial endocarditis.

Premature coronary artery disease due to atherosclerosis is becoming a common problem as patients with SLE survive longer. Potential causes of this premature atherosclerosis include hypertension, glucocorticoid therapy, and chronic immune complex deposition within coronary artery walls.

Finally, patients with SLE and **antiphospholipid antibodies** may have the same manifestations as patients with primary antiphospholipid antibody disease (see question 11).

8. What is the neonatal lupus syndrome?

The neonatal lupus syndrome is a disease of the fetus and neonate that likely results from maternal transfer of the autoantibodies anti-Ro (SS-A) and/or anti-La (SS-B) to the fetal circulation. Clinical manifestations are variable and include dermatitis, hepatitis, hemolytic anemia, and thrombocytopenia. The most common cardiac manifestation of the neonatal lupus syndrome is complete congenital heart block; this lesion is responsible for the major morbidity and mortality of this disorder. Many patients require permanent pacemaker therapy.

9. Polymyositis and dermatomyositis result in inflammation of skeletal muscle. Is cardiac muscle ever involved?

Both polymyositis and dermatomyositis are autoimmune disorders of unknown etiology; their primary clinical manifestation is weakness due to inflammation and necrosis of skeletal muscle. Helpful clinical findings include proximal muscle weakness, elevated serum enzymes (such as creatine phosphokinase), and characteristic electromyographic and biopsy abnormalities. Dermatomyositis is characterized by dermatologic findings in addition to myositis.

Up to 40% of patients with polymyositis and dermatomyositis may have cardiac abnormalities. Supraventricular tachyarrhythmias are most common. Various degrees of conduction defects and ventricular tachyarrhythmias also have been noted. An inflammatory myopathy of cardiac muscle resulting in congestive heart failure has occasionally been observed. Finally, pericarditis with varying degrees of effusion may occur. Coronary arteritis and valvular lesions are unusual.

10. What are the cardiac manifestations of scleroderma (systemic sclerosis)?

Systemic sclerosis is an autoimmune disorder of unknown etiology that results in a diffuse bland vasculopathy and variable fibrosis of skin and various end organs, particularly the heart, lungs, kidneys, and gastrointestinal tract. The diffuse vasculopathy may lead to varying degrees of ischemia and infarction in the skin and various end organs; the consequence of these diffuse ischemic events may be the characteristic fibrosis of the disease. Two major subcategories are often recognized. The first is systemic sclerosis with limited cutaneous scleroderma or CREST syndrome (calcinosis, Raynaud's phenomenon, esophageal dysmotility, sclerodactyly, and telangiectasia). The other is systemic sclerosis with diffuse cutaneous scleroderma.

The heart in systemic sclerosis may be involved directly, in the form of myocardial fibrosis, or indirectly, as a result of pulmonary or renal involvement. Clinical features include congestive heart failure, supraventricular and ventricular tachyarrhythmias, conduction disturbances, and syndromes of myocardial ischemia, including angina, acute myocardial infarction, and sudden death. Pericarditis also may be present, either as a primary manifestation or secondary to uremia.

11. What is the antiphospholipid antibody syndrome?

The antiphospholipid antibody syndrome (APS) is a disorder characterized by circulating antiphospholipid antibodies and manifesting clinically as variable degrees of recurrent arterial and venous thromboses, recurrent spontaneous abortions, and thrombocytopenia. The disease may be primary or associated with another disorder such as SLE. It remains unclear how the antiphospholipid antibodies result in clinical expression. Antiphospholipid antibodies may be recognized by the presence of the lupus anticoagulant (elevated partial thromboplastin time not corrected by addition of normal sera and not due to antibodies directed against specific clotting factors), a false-positive serologic test for syphilis, or the presence of anticardiolipin antibodies as determined by enzyme-linked immunosorbent assay.

Cardiac manifestations of APS include thromboses of the coronary arteries that lead to myocardial ischemia and/or infarction. Cardiac valvular abnormalities also may be present, including sterile vegetations and aortic and mitral regurgitation. Such lesions may occur in patients with primary APS as well as APS associated with SLE.

BIBLIOGRAPHY

1. Braunwald E (ed): Heart Disease: A Textbook of Cardiovascular Medicine, 4th ed. Philadelphia, W.B. Saunders, 1992.
2. Kelly WN, Harris ED Jr, Ruddy S, Sledge CB (eds): Textbook of Rheumatology, 4th ed. Philadelphia, W.B. Saunders, 1993.
3. Klippel JH, Dieppe PA (eds): Rheumatology. St. Louis, Mosby, 1994.
4. McCarty DJ, Koopman WJ (eds): Arthritis and Allied Conditions, 12th ed. Philadelphia, Lea & Febiger, 1993.
5. Schlant RC, Alexander RW (eds): Hurst's The Heart: Arteries and Veins, 8th ed. New York, McGraw-Hill, 1994.

59. SUBSTANCE ABUSE AND THE HEART

Olivia V. Adair, M.D.

1. When should alcohol cardiomyopathy be suspected?

All patients with dilated cardiomyopathy should be asked about alcohol consumption. In addition, macrocytosis is a good indicator of chronic alcohol abuse, even when liver function tests are normal. Susceptibility to the adverse effects of alcohol on the heart is apparently individual. Susceptibility is demonstrated by the presence of immunoglobin A on the sarcolemma and muscle of small blood vessels at biopsy of patients with alcoholic cardiomyopathy.

2. Does the type of alcoholic drink influence the effect on the heart?

No. Studies show no difference in the abnormalities observed in patients using predominantly wine, beer, or whiskey. Moreover, no consistent pattern of drinking is associated with heart failure. Possible additives in home brew and/or moonshine alcoholic substances may cause additional toxic damage.

3. Describe the presentation of patients who develop myocardial damage secondary to chronic alcoholism.

Alcohol abuse causes the diffuse myocardial damage seen in other primary myocardial diseases. However, fewer than one-half of patients present with symptoms of congestive heart failure (CHF), whereas in other primary myocardial diseases CHF is the predominant feature. A significant number of patients with alcoholic cardiomyopathy present with arrhythmias and chest pain.

4. Are specific electrocardiographic (ECG) changes associated with alcoholic cardiomyopathy?

The ECG of patients with alcohol cardiomyopathy may be normal or display nonspecific changes. As disease of the ventricle progresses, poor R wave progression is common, reflecting conduction delay. In addition, enlargement of the left ventricle and left and/or right atrium is common, whereas left or right bundle branch block is seen in 10% of patients.

5. What common arrhythmias are associated with alcohol ingestion?

Supraventricular arrhythmias predominate in patients without overt cardiomyopathy and in patients with acute intoxication; atrial fibrillation is the most prominent. The etiology appears to be moderate delays in conduction, which cause acute arrhythmias or "holiday heart." Acute arrhythmias are seen in heavy, binge drinking, in chronic abuse, or in special circumstances (e.g., prolonged sleeplessness) without chronic abuse. The risk of supraventricular arrhythmias with 6 or more drinks/day is increased by 2.6.

6. Are the arrhythmias seen during withdrawal the same as acute intoxication arrhythmias?

During withdrawal concentrations of plasma catecholamines are high, and patients may have frequent ventricular ectopy. Ventricular ectopy may help to explain the sudden deaths in young and middle-aged alcoholics without coronary artery disease. The threshold for ventricular fibrillation is reduced, and moderate alcohol levels suggest a declining blood level at the time of cardiac arrest.

7. What is the prognosis in alcoholic cardiomyopathy?

The prognosis is variable, depending on the extent of cardiac involvement. If the patient continues to drink, the prognosis is particularly grave. In one study, patients who remained abstinent over a

4-year period experienced a 9% mortality rate, whereas of those who continued to drink, > 50% died during the same 4 years. Unfortunately, the recovery rate with abstinence is not as great as previously reported; earlier studies probably observed and reported cases of milder cardiac involvement. Only a minority of patients with moderate-to-severe alcoholic cardiomyopathy show clinical improvement with abstinence; after a certain stage of disease, the prognosis most likely continues to be poor, regardless of abstinence or therapy.

8. How common is cocaine use in the United States? Why is it important in cardiac problems?
An estimated 8 million people regularly use cocaine in the United States by inhalation, smoking, or intravenous injection. Recent surveys show that the number of hard-core cocaine users has increased. The mean age of hard-core cocaine users is rising as addicts age. Older or aging cocaine users experience a higher incidence of cardiac abnormalities.

9. How is cocaine use diagnosed as the cause of a specific cardiac problem?
All patients presenting with coronary artery disease syndrome, cardiac arrhythmias, myocardial dysfunction, myocarditis, or endocarditis should be questioned about use of cocaine and other drugs. The age, gender, and social status of the patient are not determining factors; grandmothers, stockbrokers, and all sorts of people use illicit drugs. Patients should be examined for marks from intravenous use, nasal redness, nasal septum irritation, or other physical signs of use. Urine should be analyzed for metabolites of cocaine if there is a concern, as it remains positive for 1–2 or sometimes several days, whereas plasma half-life is approximately 50–90 minutes.

10. How does cocaine affect the heart?
The cardiovascular effects of cocaine are multifactoral and complex. Cocaine has been shown to cause or to be associated with cardiomyopathy, myocarditis, endocarditis, ventricular arrhythmias, myocardial infarction, coronary artery spasm and angina, and sudden death. Cocaine inhibits the neuronal or presynaptic reuptake of norepinephrine and the neuronal uptake of catecholamine hormones. This pharmacologic action increases the synaptic cleft concentration of norepinephrine and the circulating levels of both norepinephrine and epinephrine.

Cardiovascular Complications of Cocaine

Sudden death
Acute myocardial infarction
Chest pain without myocardial infarction
Acute, reversible myocarditis
Irreversible heart muscle disease
Acute, severe hypertension
Acute aortic dissection, rupture
Electrocardiographic changes: sinus tachycardia, premature ventricular complexes, Wolff-Parkinson-White arrhythmias, ventricular tachycardia, torsade de pointes, ventricular fibrillation, prolongation of QTc, and early repolarization (ST segment) changes
Pneumopericardium
Stroke
Subarachnoid hemorrhage
Accelerated coronary atherosclerosis
Intimal hyperplasia of coronary vessels

From Crawley IS, Schlant RC: Effect of noncardiac drugs, electricity, poisons, and radiation on the heart. In Schlant RC, Alexander RW (eds): Hurst's The Heart, 8th ed. New York, McGraw Hill, 1994, with permission.

11. What is the most common clinical presentation in cocaine abuse?
Chest pain is the most common symptom, whereas acute myocardial infarction (MI) is the most common clinical presentation.

12. How does cocaine abuse cause an acute MI?

Cocaine affects the heart in multiple ways, both directly and indirectly. Cocaine abuse may result in myocardial infarction in patients with normal coronary arteries, coronary artery spasm, or previous coronary artery disease. The mechanisms include (1) increased oxygen demand (secondary to increases in heart rate and blood pressure), (2) decreased coronary artery blood flow (secondary to vasospasm or thrombosis with increased platelet aggregation), and (3) myocarditis (secondary to toxic effect or hypersensitivity). Cocaine use also promotes intimal proliferation in coronary arteries.

13. How significant is the cardiomyopathy associated with cocaine use?

The link between cocaine and the development of cardiomyopathy has been supported by animal studies that show the drug's depressant effect on cardiac function. Acute as well as chronic left ventricular dilatation and dysfunction may lead to significantly depressed cardiac function. Other causes of cardiomyopathy should be ruled out, (e.g., ischemia, cardiomyopathy associated with acquired immunodeficiency syndrome [AIDS]). Patients may present with significant cardiomyopathy and heart failure, in a large study at the University of Colorado, 13% of a young population (mean age: 36 years) of cocaine users had left ventricular dysfunction or ejection fraction < 50%.

With symptoms of shortness of breath and fatigue, the diagnosis may be missed. All cocaine users with symptoms suggestive of congestive heart failure should be elevated by echocardiogram for cocaine-induced cardiomyopathy. In a significant number of patients (7%, according to one study) asymptomatic cardiomyopathy may promote arrhythmias.

14. What electrophysiologic abnormalities are seen in cocaine users?

Cocaine blocks the fast sodium channels in the myocardium, thus producing a depression of depolarization and a slowing of conduction velocity. The refractoriness of the atrial and ventricular muscle is also prolonged. Cocaine is similar in its electrophysiologic properties to class 1 antiarrhythmic agents, and QT prolongation and ventricular arrhythmias, including torsade de pointes, occur. Transient heart block of the second and third degrees also has been reported. Heart block as well as arrhythmias may respond to correction of acidosis, hypokalemia, and hypomagnesemia.

15. What ECG changes are seen in cocaine users?

A study of cocaine users presenting to the emergency department (ED) found significant ECG abnormalities in 50% of patients. The major abnormalities included prolonged PR, QRS, and QT intervals (with an increase in atrial and ventricular refractoriness), tachycardias or bradycardias, increased QRS voltage, poor R wave progression, nonspecific ST-T wave changes, early repolarization, and ST elevation (with possible ischemia), and ventricular and atrial arrhythmias. Another study of asymptomatic cocaine users found abnormal ECGs in up to 29%. During the first weeks of withdrawal cocaine abusers frequently develop silent myocardial ischemia, manifested as ST elevation, during ambulatory ECG monitoring. These changes were believed to be associated with coronary vasospasm.

16. How should patients with cocaine-induced chest pain be evaluated? Should they be admitted to the hospital?

The etiology of chest pain after cocaine use is most likely multifactoral, myocardial ischemia, infarction, and aortic dissection must not be overlooked. Chest radiographs should be considered to rule out cocaine-induced pneumomediastinum, pneumothorax, and widened mediastinum. Prompt EKG is important to evaluate patients with ischemia because of the common occurrence of early repolarization. The creatinine kinase level may be elevated as a result of rhabdomyolysis; although the pattern is different from that in acute MI, the distinction is not helpful in the ED. In one study, angina was ruled out in 101 consecutive cocaine users presenting to the ED with suggestive chest pain, but there was no work-up for cardiac risk. Another study looked at risk stratification in cocaine users (mean age: 37 years) presenting with chest pain and found a significant amount of coronary artery disease (40% with > 70% stenosis and 21% with ≤ 70%

stenosis). Young cocaine users, therefore, seem to be predisposed to myocardial ischemia, coronary artery disease, or infarction. As a result, many authors recommend admission of cocaine users who present with typical or atypical chest pain to a coronary care unit or monitored bed if infarction is suspected. Even hours after cocaine use, coronary spasm and arrhythmias may occur.

17. Is endocarditis frequently seen in cocaine users?
Yes. Intravenous cocaine abuse has strong association with endocarditis; *Staphylococcus aureus* is the most commonly isolated organism. Unfortunately, because the staphylococci may be resistant, drug sensitivity must be established. Moreover, rare organisms may be the culprit. In intravenous users, the tricuspid valve is more commonly involved in the endocarditis, patients are prone to develop paravalvular abscess, which may require transesophageal echocardiography.

18. Which arrhythmias are most commonly seen with cocaine abuse?
The most common arrhythmias are tachycardia and premature ventricular beats, which are usually transient and do not require treatment. Cocaine-induced supraventricular tachycardia, ventricular tachycardia, and ventricular fibrillation are also seen; management depends on etiology and hemodynamic status of the patient. The underlying problems may be myocardial infarction or ischemia, QT interval prolongation, reperfusion after coronary spasm, or electrolyte imbalance. Bradycardia also has been reported in the absence of infarction, but it is transient.

BIBLIOGRAPHY

 1. Adair OV, Rainguet S, Pearson T, et al: Echocardiography abnormalities in chronic cocaine users [abstract]. Circulation 23 (Suppl):150A, 1994.
 2. Bertolet BD, Freund G, Martin CA, et al: Unrecognized left ventricular dysfunction in an apparent healthy cocaine abuse population. Clin Cardiol 13:323–328, 1990.
 3. Chakko S, Fernandez A, Mellman TA, et al: Cardiac manifestations of cocaine abuse: A cross-sectional study of asymptomatic men with history of long-term abuse of "crack" cocaine. J Am Coll Cardiol 20:1168–1174, 1992.
 4. Chokshi SK, Moore R, Pandian NG, Isner JM: Reversible cardiomyopathy associated with cocaine intoxication. Ann Intern Med 111:1039–1040, 1989.
 5. Cohen EJ, Klatsky AL, Armstrong MA: Alcohol use and supraventricular arrhythmia. Am J Cardiol 62:971–973, 1988.
 6. Cregler LL: Cocaine: The newest risk factor for cardiovascular disease. Clin Cardiol 14:449–456, 1991.
 7. Diamond I: Alcoholic myopathy and cardiomyopathy (editorial). N Engl J Med. 320:458, 1989.
 8. Karch SB, Billingham ME: The pathology and etiology of cocaine-induced heart disease. Arch Pathol Lab Med 112:225, 1988.
 9. Kupari M, Koskinen P, Suokas A, Ventila M: Left ventricular filling impairment in asymptomatic chronic alcoholics. Am J Cardiol 661:1473–1477, 1990.
10. Lange RA, Cigarroa RG, Yancy CW, et al: Cocaine-induced coronary artery vasoconstriction. N Engl J Med 321:1577, 1989.
11. McCall D: Alcohol and the cardiovascular system. Curr Probl Cardiol 12:351, 1987.
12. Nademanee K, Adair O, Havranek E, et al: A prospective study of cocaine related cardiovascular morbidity and mortality: Chronic cocaine users vs post-angioplasty patients. Circulation (abstract) 1994.
13. Nademanee K, Gorelick DA, Josephson MA, et al: Myocardial ischemia during cocaine withdrawal. Ann Intern Med 111:878–880, 1989.
14. Nademanee K: The cardiovascular toxicity of cocaine. Primary Cardiol 17(3):40–49, 1991.
15. Om A: Cardiovascular compliations of cocaine. Am J Med Sci 303:333–339, 1992.
16. Om A, Ellaham S, DiSciascio G: Management of cocaine-induced cardiovascular complications. Am Heart J. 125:471, 1993.
17. Patel R, McArdle JJ, Regan TJ. Increased ventricular vulnerability in a chronic ethanol model despite reduced electrophysiologic responses to catecholamines. Alcohol Clin Exp Res. 15:785–789, 1991.
18. Urbano-Marquez A, Estruch R, Navarro-Lopez F, et al: The effects of alcoholism on skeletal and cardiac muscle. N Engl J Med 320:409–415, 1989.
19. Vikhert AM, Tsiplenkova VG, Cherpachenka NM: Alcoholic cardiomyopathy and sudden cardiac death. J Am Coll Cardiol 8:3A–11A, 1986.

60. CARDIAC MANIFESTATIONS OF AIDS

Olivia V. Adair, M.D.

1. How commonly is the heart affected in patients with AIDS?
Cardiac involvement has been reported in from one-quarter to one-half of the patients with AIDS, as defined by echocardiographic, endomyocardial biopsy, or autopsy findings. This involvement may cause clinically apparent manifestations in only 10–25% of patients, depending on the stage of disease and whether the patients are hospitalized.

2. List the common lesions in cardiac involvement in AIDS.
    1. Metastatic or primary involvement of Kaposi's sarcoma or other malignant lymphomas involving the myocardium, epicardium, or pericardium
    2. Myocarditis (infectious, viral, lymphocytic, noninfectious), endocarditis, or pericarditis
    3. Pericardial effusions
    4. Cardiomyopathy (right, left, or biventricular)
    5. Vasculitis
    6. Toxic effects of drugs used against the infectious or anti-HIV drugs

3. What are the most common clinical manifestations of AIDS when there is heart involvement?
- Myocarditis (40–52%)
- Pericarditis (in up to 15% of cases, with an effusion in 18%–40%)
- Congestive heart failure due to left ventricular dilatation and dysfunction (10–42%)

These lesions may present as angina, dyspnea, fatigue, and dyspnea on exertion. Also ventricular arrhythmias, endocarditis, and right-heart failure may be presenting abnormalities. Anderson and Virman proposed the use of four clinical categories of AIDS heart disease: (1) endocardial disease, (2) myocardial disease, (3) pericardial disease, and (4) neoplasms.

4. When a patient with HIV infection presents with dyspnea, should we have concerns about a cardiac etiology?
Yes. AIDS patients have multiple symptoms for which the system involved may be unclear. For example, chest pain, dyspnea, fatigue, edema, and palpitations are general symptoms which may have multisystem etiologies. Because these patients may not have overt clinical evidence for cardiac disease, only through a heightened awareness of the frequent involvement of the heart will correct diagnosis and management be initiated.

5. Describe the diagnostic workup for the AIDS patient with dyspnea.
The physical examination may help implicate a pulmonary or cardiac etiology. However, usually this is not sufficient, and a chest x-ray may be inconclusive since old and/or new pulmonary infiltrates do not rule out a cardiac problem. An echo-Doppler study, however, may be very helpful in evaluating a patient for pericardial effusion, tamponade, cardiomyopathy, valve disease, (especially tricuspid regurgitation secondary to pulmonary hypertension), or segmental wall motion abnormalities. Many of these patients also may have risk factors for coronary artery disease (i.e., male smokers) and ischemia or infarction should be considered; therefore, an electrocardiogram should be routinely obtained.

6. Why is it important to perform an echocardiogram on an AIDS patient with chest pain or shortness of breath?
Because there may be specific findings on the echocardiogram that will change the management, improve the quality of life, and provide symptomatic improvement for the patient. For example, if the patient has a cardiomyopathy, diuretics and angiotensin-converting enzyme (ACE)-

inhibitors may markedly alleviate the shortness of breath not otherwise treated if the patient is diagnosed as having a chronic pulmonary infection. Also, specific antibiotics are indicated for infectious myocarditis and pericarditis, as well as antineoplastic therapy for specific neoplasms. When a pericardial effusion is present, arrangements need to be made for pericardiocentesis and possibly biopsy for specific diagnosis. Tuberculous pericarditis often presents with tamponade and requires urgent drainage.

7. How common is pericarditis in AIDS, and what are the common etiologies?
Pericarditis occurs in 5–15% of patients with AIDS and usually presents as chest pain. The causes may be viral disease, bacterial infection, tuberculosis, neoplasm, or fungal infection.

8. Does the patient's clinical status affect the likelihood of cardiac abnormalities?
Only a few studies have looked at this issue. It was shown that patients with more advanced disease, i.e., AIDS, had more cardiac abnormalities on echo-Doppler than patients who were HIV-positive but pre-AIDS. Also, patients with CD4+ lymphocyte counts $\leq 100/mm^3$ had a higher prevalence of abnormalities on echo-Doppler compared to patients with higher CD4+ counts. The presence of an active opportunistic infection, however, did not correlate with the presence of abnormalities. One study showed an association of opportunistic infection with more cardiac abnormalities but no association with left ventricular dysfunction. They also showed that the highest relationship with a low CD4+ count was pericardial effusion.

9. How common is endocarditis in AIDS patients?
Endocarditis is not a common finding in AIDS patients. Because most of the larger studies have been done in centers where the major HIV-positive population is not intravenous drug abusers though, this may be an unidentified area of concern. We have reported in a study of a large group of patients who were HIV-positive intravenous drug abusers frequent valve abnormalities (67%). However, only 7% of the patients had active endocarditis at the time of evaluation.

10. Which patients develop cardiomyopathy and poor left ventricular function?
This is controversial. One study showed a correlation between the CD4+ counts of $\leq 100/mm^3$ and the presence of left ventricular (LV) dysfunction. Levy et al. showed that patients with CD4+ counts $\leq 100/mm^3$ and AIDS had the most cases (55%) of LV dysfunction, whereas those with a CD4+ count $> 100/mm^3$ and active AIDS or pre-AIDS had approximately the same percentage of cases of LV dysfunction (17% and 16%, respectively). However, in a young population, even these numbers are unexpectedly high. These findings suggest that HIV itself, directly or indirectly, influences the cardiac pathology.

11. What are the suggested therapies for dilated cardiomyopathy and heart failure in HIV-positive patients, and what is their prognosis?
Unfortunately, congestive heart failure in HIV-positive patients has been reported to have a rapidly progressive downward course. Despite the poor outcome, however, the heart failure initially responds to conventional therapy with ACE inhibitors and diuretics. Zidovudine therapy does not appear to change the poor outcome or prevent the development of dilated cardiomyopathy.

12. What are the major cardiac malignancies in AIDS?
Two types of malignancies affecting the heart have been described in AIDS—Kaposi's sarcoma and malignant lymphoma, with Kaposi's sarcoma being the more common. Kaposi's sarcoma is found mostly in HIV-positive male homosexuals, with primary Kaposi's sarcoma being rare and having declined in incidence since the early 1980s. Kaposi's sarcoma may involve the epicardium (a common location), myocardium, and/or pericardium.

   Malignant cardiac lymphoma may be primary or secondary and is usually high-grade, with Burkitt-like cells (small and noncleaved) or large-cell immunoblastic plasmacytoid types. In most cases, they appear to originate from B cells.

13. Do cardiac abnormalities improve in AIDS patients?

There have been few specific follow-up studies of AIDS-related cardiac findings. In one study, Blanchard et al. reported approximately 1 year's follow-data on AIDS and asymptomatic HIV-positive patients. Over the follow-up, 44% of the AIDS patients and only 5% of the asymptomatic HIV-positive patients died. Echocardiographic abnormalities were common in both groups, but persistent LV dysfunction was more prevalent in the AIDS group and had the grim prognosis of 100% mortality in 1 year. Resolution of cardiac abnormalities was seen with LV dysfunction in 43%, right ventricular enlargement in 44%, and without specific intervention, pericardial effusion resolution in 42%.

14. Why are the cardiac lesions occasionally transient?

This issue needs further study, but it is possible that infectious myocarditis may be the major cause of LV dysfunction and pericarditis and that there is transient occurrence of these cardiopathic agents. The right ventricular transient changes are most likely due to changes in pulmonary hypertension associated with opportunistic pulmonary infections. Therefore, it is important to have patients re-evaluated, especially if symptoms change, as medications may need frequent adjustments. We perform echo-Doppler studies on our AIDS patients as symptoms dictate or electively every year if they have significant cardiac involvement or advanced disease.

15. What are the clinical manifestations of AIDS myocarditis?

The clinical manifestations of AIDS myocarditis depend on the severity of the inflammatory process, i.e., focal or diffuse, and/or the location of the lesion. For example, if the focus is in the His bundle, the patient presents with conduction abnormalities; diffuse disease presents with full-blown congestive heart failure or with chest pain, shortness of breath, or significant arrhythmias. Most patients have no clinical manifestations or only subtle clinical findings.

BIBLIOGRAPHY

1. Acierno LJ: Cardiac complications in acquired immunodeficiency syndrome (AIDS): A review. Am Coll Cardiol 1989; 13:1144–1154, 1989.
2. Adair OV, Mendoza RE, Chebaclo M, Vacarrino R: A prospective study of sixty-seven acquired immunodeficiency syndrome patients for evaluation of cardiac abnormalities. Clin Res 38(2):361A, 1990.
3. Anderson DW, Yirmani R, Reilly JM, et al: Prevalent myocarditis at necropsy in the acquired immunodeficiency syndrome. J Am Coll Cardiol 11:792–799, 1988.
4. Baroldi G, Coralo S, Morini M, et al: Focal lymphocytic myocarditis in acquired immunodeficiency syndrome (AIDS): A correlative morphologic and clinical study in 26 consecutive fatal cases. Am Coll Cardiol 12:463–469, 1988.
5. Blanchard DG, Hagenhoff C, Chow LC, et al: Reversibility of cardiac abnormalities in human immunodeficiency virus (HIV)-infected individuals: A serial echocardiography study. J Am Coll Cardiol 17:1270–1276, 1991.
6. Cammarosano C, Lewis W: Cardiac lesions in acquired immunodeficiency syndrome (AIDS). J Am Coll Cardiol 5:703–706, 1985.
7. Cotton P: AIDS giving rise to cardiac problems. JAMA 263(16):2149, 1990.
8. Himelman RB, Chung WS, Chernoff DN, et al: Cardiac manifestations in human immunodeficiency virus: A two-dimensional echocardiography study. J Am Coll Cardiol 13:1030–1036, 1989.
9. Klima M, Esudier SM: Pathologic findings in the hearts of patients with acquired immunodeficiency syndrome. Texas Heart Inst J 18:116–121, 1991.
10. Levy WS, Simon GL, Rios JC, Ross AM: Prevalence of cardiac abnormalities in human immunodeficiency virus infection. Am J Cardiol 63:86–89, 1989.
11. Lewis W, Grody WW: AIDS and the heart: Review and consideration of pathogenetic mechanisms. 1:53–64, 1992.

61. EXERCISE AND THE HEART

Bruce E. Andrea, M.D.

1. Describe the central mechanisms underlying the cardiovascular responses to exercise.
With anticipation of, and in early exercise, there is an immediate and progressive withdrawal of vagal tone, causing an increase in heart rate. Venous return is augmented by the action of muscular contraction, resulting in increased preload and thus stroke volume via the Frank-Starling mechanism. Concurrently, there is an increase in catecholamine release, further increasing heart rate as well as contractility.

2. What adaptive cardiovascular features are noted in conditioned endurance athletes?
1. Increased blood volume and red blood cell mass
2. Increased skeletal muscle capillary density, mitochondrial mass, and oxidative capacity
3. Increased left ventricular mass, end-diastolic dimension, and stroke volume
4. Increased diameter of coronary arteries
5. Decrease in resting heart rate
6. Likely increase in ventricular fibrillation threshold

3. Explain the different cardiovascular responses to volume overload and pressure overload.
Exercise is commonly characterized as being either endurance or strength-promoting. Most activities have some component of each. At the two extremes are pure endurance training as exemplified by long-distance running, and strength training as exemplified by weight-lifting. These two forms of exercise exert different loads on the cardiovascular system.

The **endurance athlete** experiences long periods of elevated cardiac output and heart rate, resulting in **increased preload.** Blood pressure is elevated modestly.

In contrast, the **power athlete** performs short bursts of intense exercise, with extreme elevations in blood pressure and only small increases in cardiac output. Intra-arterial pressures of 500/200 mmHg have been measured during maximal lifting in elite power athletes. The result is **increased afterload.**

In afterload stress, septal and free wall thickness increase to normalize myocardial wall stress. Left ventricular cavity dimension does not change. In preload stress, the increase is primarily in ventricular end-diastolic cavity dimension, with a proportional increase in septal and free wall thickness to normalize myocardial wall stress.

4. What is VO$_2$max?
VO$_2$max is the abbreviation for maximal oxygen consumption per minutes. Maximal oxygen consumption is measured by collecting expired air during progressive exercise. When the difference between inspired and expired O$_2$ content and the volume of air ventilated are known, oxygen consumption can be calculated. Such testing is used to measure maximal endurance capacity in athletes, evaluate patients with heart disease, and distinguish pulmonary from cardiovascular limitation in exercise.

Average VO$_2$max for Various Groups

80 mL/kg/min —	World-class male endurance athlete
65–70 —	World class female endurance athlete
60 —	Long-term endurance training
45 —	Normal young males
16–20 —	New York Heart Association Class II heart failures
<13 —	Indication for heart transplantation in appropriate candidate

5. What is the lactate threshold?

As the workload is progressively increased during exercise, an equilibrium point is reached between the production and clearance of lactic acid. This is termed the lactate threshold (or anaerobic threshold). At higher workloads, lactic acid accumulates.

Practically speaking, this point can be measured noninvasively using gas exchange. As lactic acid is buffered, CO_2 is released and ventilation must be increased. The lactate threshold is identified as the point where the ratio of minute ventilation to O_2 consumption increases while the ratio of minute ventilation to CO_2 production is constant.

This transition, referred to as the ventilatory threshold, has also been labeled the anaerobic threshold. Yet the inference that the body suddenly shifts to anaerobic metabolism as the workload increases or that there is inadequate oxygen delivery at the tissue level is hotly debated. In fact, radioisotope studies reveal that lactate is a by-product and a fuel at lower work rates, and can serve as a substrate shuttle between less active muscle groups and active groups, allowing for some degree of local glycogen sparing during prolonged exercise.

A better explanation for the progressive net appearance of lactate in the blood beyond some exercise threshold relates to increased reliance on muscle fibers with less oxidative capacity and decreased lactate clearance. As work rate increases, there is increased recruitment of motor units that have less oxidative capacity and greater glycolytic capacity (fast-twitch muscle fibers). In essence, these fibers are biased toward glycolysis, and thus their recruitment results in increased lactic acid release. Concurrently, as the work rate increases, there is proportionate decrease in splanchnic—namely, hepatic—blood flow and thus less lactate clearance. Other factors likely contribute but are beyond the scope of this discussion.

6. Is peak endurance performance limited by the cardiovascular system or by respiration?

Maximal cardiac output is the limiting factor in otherwise normal subjects exercising at sea level. It has been shown consistently that with progressive exercise to maximal performance, oxygen consumption plateaus along with cardiac output while minute ventilation continues to increase. At high altitude, lung disease, or in respiratory musculoskeletal disorders, respiratory gas exchange can limit maximal exercise performance.

7. What is the risk of sudden death or myocardial infarction during or soon after exercise?

In young and middle-aged joggers in Rhode Island between 1976 and 1980, there was 1 death/400,000 exercise hours. In a cohort of U.S. Air Force recruits, there was 1 death/3,000,000 exercise hours. Although the likelihood for sudden death is 5–10 times increased during or shortly after vigorous exercise, regular exercise over time probably decreases the risk of sudden death. The Framingham Study documented a lower incidence of sudden death and all cardiovascular events in individuals with good exercise habits.

The relative risk of having an infarction during or within 1 hour of heavy exertion is 1.3 to 20, though only 5% of myocardial infarctions are triggered by heavy exertion. This risk for triggered infarction is lowest in those who exercise regularly (4 times/wk). Sedentary individuals run the highest risk for a myocardial infarction being triggered by strenuous activity.

8. List the most common causes of exercise-induced sudden death in people younger than 35.

In this group, hypertrophic cardiomyopathy is the most common cause of sudden cardiac death, accounting for over 50% in most series. Other causes in decreasing order are anomalous coronary artery origin and course, coronary artery disease, cystic medial necrosis (Marfan's syndrome) with aortic rupture, and idiopathic concentric left ventricular hypertrophy. Other rare causes include myocarditis, aortic stenosis, mitral valve prolapse with significant myxomatous changes, right ventricular dysplasia, conduction system abnormalities (including long QT syndrome), amyloidosis, sarcoidosis, and cardiac tumors.

Two potential etiologies which need further study relate to the illicit use of anabolic steroids and cocaine by athletes. Anabolic steroid use may result in an excessive hypertrophic response to exercise conditioning and, as such, predispose to decreased left ventricular compliance and possibly sudden death. Anabolic steroids also affect lipid metabolism and platelet function in an adverse way, thus increasing the risk for atherosclerotic disease. Cocaine promotes atherosclerosis, impairs normal coronary vasodilation, promotes coronary spasm, and can trigger myocardial infarction and arrhythmias. Cocaine may also be a cause of focal cardiomyopathy or focal myocarditis and thus trigger exercise-related sudden cardiac death long after its discontinuation.

9. What is hypertrophic cardiomyopathy?

Hypertrophic cardiomyopathy (HCM) is the encompassing term used to describe the pathologic state of malignant myocardial hypertrophy which is out of proportion to expected hemodynamic load. Macroscopically, there is significant increased wall thickness which appears out of proportion to left ventricular cavity size. Idiopathic concentric left ventricular hypertrophy is a less common cause of exercise-induced sudden death. Whereas morphologically it appears similar to HCM, with concentric hypertrophy out of proportion to eccentric left ventricular cavity enlargement, there is no evident histologic abnormality and no genetic link has been identified. Whether this is purely an excessive hypertrophic response to physiologic hemodynamic loads, a variation of HCM, or a pathologic state induced by anabolic steroid use is not known.

10. Describe the clinical features of HCM.

Although most patients with HCM are asymptomatic, the initial presentation in some may be sudden death, and others may have complaints of new exertional dyspnea, chest pains, palpitations, dizziness, or syncope. The pathophysiologic processes underlying these symptoms include an interrelation between systolic and diastolic dysfunction, with or without dynamic left ventricular outflow obstruction, with or without ischemia, and with or without brady- or tachyarrhythmias. It is easy to see how extreme exercise can exacerbate symptoms in HCM, including triggering sudden death.

11. Numerous electrocardiographic "abnormalities" have been noted among athletes, attributable to physiologic hypertrophy and increased vagal tone. Name several.

1. Sinus bradycardia
2. Sinus pauses
3. Wandering atrial pacemaker
4. First-degree atrioventricular block
5. Second-degree atrioventricular block (most commonly Wenckebach)
6. Incomplete right bundle branch block
7. Left ventricular hypertrophy
8. Right ventricular hypertrophy
9. Right atrial enlargement
10. Vertical axis
11. Early repolarization (J-point elevation)
12. T-wave inversion

12. What echocardiographic features differentiate physiologic left ventricular (LV) hypertrophy in the athlete from HCM?

Characteristics of the Physiologic Athletic Heart

Upper limit of LV thickness rarely ≥ 13 mm, except in world-class athletes
Uniform hypertrophy, with adjacent wall segments never differing by > 2 mm
Septal-to-free wall thickness ratio ≤ 1.3 (except in highly trained weight-lifters)
Proportionality of LV thickness to LV internal dimension (LVID)
    Endurance athlete—Septum:LVID < 0.22
    Power athlete—Septum:LVID < 0.28
Proportionate papillary muscle hypertrophy
Normal LV outflow tract dimensions
Normal left atrial size (< 45 mm)
Normal systolic function
Absence of clinically relevant mitral regurgitation
Normal Doppler transmitral LV filling pattern

Systolic anterior motion of the mitral valve suggests HCM. Transmitral Doppler evidence of impaired LV filling, including diminished early filling phase, augmented late filling of atrial contraction, and prolongation of deceleration between early and late filling phases, also suggest HCM if there is significant left ventricular hypertrophy without hypertension. Left atrial enlargement and mitral valve thickening are abnormal findings in a normotensive athlete and suggest HCM.

13. Are there gender and racial differences in the expression of physiologic left ventricular hypertrophy seen in athletes?

There are limited data on women, but of the elite female endurance athletes studied, LV septal thickness did not exceed 12 mm and the ratio of LV septum to LV free wall remained ≤ 1.3. In a study of male athletes, 11% of 265 black collegiate athletes had septal thickness ≥ 13 mm, compared with only 1.7% of elite white athletes with septal thickness ≥ 13 mm. This more pronounced hypertrophy seen among black athletes may represent a racial difference. However, black and white athletes were not matched for type of activity.

14. Outline a cost-effective approach to athletic preparticipation screening.

1. History
    Family history of possible premature sudden cardiac death?
    Family history of congenital heart disease?
    Use of anabolic steroids or cocaine?
    Excessive dyspnea or decreasing exercise tolerance?
    Significant palpitations?
    Exertional dizziness or syncope?
    Exertional chest pain?
2. Physical examination (seeks to rule out hypertension, Marfan habitus, aortic stenosis or coarctation, and hypertrophic obstructive cardiomyopathy)
    Brief musculoskeletal survey
    Bilateral brachial blood pressures
    Cardiac auscultation in seated or standing position
        Reduces or eliminates innocent flow murmurs.
        Enhances the murmur of hypertrophic obstructive cardiomyopathy
        Increases physiologic splitting of S_2 (possible atrial septal defect if fixed splitting)
        Include Valsalva maneuver
Based on abnormal screening findings, it is possible that as many as 10–20% of athletes could be referred for more costly evaluations, including ECG, echocardiogram, or evaluation by a cardiologist. An alternative approach would be to perform a limited echocardiogram at the time of mass screening of a group of athletes. Data on this approach are incomplete.

15. When should an athlete's participation in competitive-level or high-intensity sports be restricted?

The American College of Cardiology recommendations are:
    Restricted activity
        Uncontrolled hypertension
        Hypertrophic cardiomyopathy
        Marfan's syndrome
        Aortic stenosis (more than mild)
        If question of congenital or acquired coronary artery disease, restrict participation, until athlete is further evaluated.
    Partially restricted activity
        Moderate aortic insufficiency (discourage isometric/power training)
        Other congenital heart lesions (appropriate medical follow-up necessary)

BIBLIOGRAPHY

1. American College of Sports Medicine: Clinical exercise physiology. In ACSM: Guidelines for Exercise Testing and Prescription, 4th ed. Philadelphia, Lea & Febiger, 1991, pp 11–34.
2. Curfman GD: Is exercise beneficial—or hazardous—to your health? N Engl J Med 329:1730–1731, 1993.
3. Dilsizian V, Bonow RO, Epstein SE, et al: Myocardial ischemia detected by thallium scintigraphy is frequently related to cardiac arrest and syncope in young patients with hypertrophic cardiomyopathy. J Am Coll Cardiol 22:796–804, 1993.
4. Lewis JF, Maron BJ, Diggs JA, et al: Pre-participation echocardiographic screening for cardiovascular disease in a large, predominantly black population of collegiate athletes. Am J Cardiol 64:1029–1033, 1989.
5. Maron BJ (ed): The athlete's heart. Cardiol Clin 10:197–339, 1992.
6. Maron BJ, Epstein SE, Roberts WC: Causes of sudden death in competitive athletes. J Am Coll Cardiol 7:204–214, 1986.
7. Mittleman MA, Maclure M, Tofler GH, et al: Triggering of acute myocardial infarction by heavy physical exertion: Protection against triggering by regular exercise. N Engl J Med 329:1677–1683, 1993.
8. Oakley GDG: The athletic heart. Cardiol Clin 5:319–329, 1987.
9. Pelliccia A, Maron BJ, Spataro A, et al: The upper limit of physiologic cardiac hypertrophy in highly trained elite athletes. N Engl J Med 324:295–301, 1991.
10. Thompson PD: Athletes, athletics, and sudden cardiac death. Med Sci Sports Exerc 25:981–984, 1993.
11. Thompson PD, Funk EJ, Carleton RA, et al: Incidence of death during jogging in Rhode Island from 1976 through 1980. JAMA 247:2535, 1982.
12. Zehender M, Meinertz T, Keul J, et al: ECG variants and cardiac arrhythmias in athletes: Clinical relevance and prognostic importance. Am Heart J 119:1378–1391, 1990.

INDEX

Page numbers in **boldface** type indicate complete chapter.